Development, Characterization, and Application of Bioactive Peptides, Diagnostic Biomarkers, and Pharmaceutical Proteins

Development, Characterization, and Application of Bioactive Peptides, Diagnostic Biomarkers, and Pharmaceutical Proteins

Guest Editors

Hyung-Sik Won
Ji-Hun Kim

MDPI

Basel • Beijing • Wuhan • Barcelona • Belgrade • Novi Sad • Cluj • Manchester

Guest Editors
Hyung-Sik Won
Department of Biotechnology
Konkuk University
Chungju-si
Korea, South

Ji-Hun Kim
College of Pharmacy
Chungbuk National
University
Cheongju
Korea, South

Editorial Office
MDPI AG
Grosspeteranlage 5
4052 Basel, Switzerland

This is a reprint of the Special Issue, published open access by the journal *Biomolecules* (ISSN 2218-273X), freely accessible at: www.mdpi.com/journal/biomolecules/special_issues/9Q206MEP3T.

For citation purposes, cite each article independently as indicated on the article page online and using the guide below:

Lastname, A.A.; Lastname, B.B. Article Title. *Journal Name* **Year**, *Volume Number*, Page Range.

ISBN 978-3-7258-3564-5 (Hbk)
ISBN 978-3-7258-3563-8 (PDF)
https://doi.org/10.3390/books978-3-7258-3563-8

Contents

Sang-Woo Han and Hyung-Sik Won
Advancements in the Application of Ribosomally Synthesized and Post-Translationally Modified Peptides (RiPPs)
Reprinted from: *Biomolecules* **2024**, *14*, 479, https://doi.org/10.3390/biom14040479 . . . . **1**

Surajit Bhattacharjya, Zhizhuo Zhang and Ayyalusamy Ramamoorthy
LL-37: Structures, Antimicrobial Activity, and Influence on Amyloid-Related Diseases
Reprinted from: *Biomolecules* **2024**, *14*, 320, https://doi.org/10.3390/biom14030320 . . . . **22**

Gwansik Park, Hyosuk Yun, Hye Jung Min and Chul Won Lee
A Novel Dimeric Short Peptide Derived from -Defensin-Related Rattusin with Improved Antimicrobial and DNA-Binding Activities
Reprinted from: *Biomolecules* **2024**, *14*, 659, https://doi.org/10.3390/biom14060659 . . . . **51**

Yoshifumi Kimira, Konosuke Osawa, Yoshihiro Osawa and Hiroshi Mano
Preventive Effects of Collagen-Derived Dipeptide Prolyl-Hydroxyproline against Dexamethasone-Induced Muscle Atrophy in Mouse C2C12 Skeletal Myotubes
Reprinted from: *Biomolecules* **2023**, *13*, 1617, https://doi.org/10.3390/biom13111617 . . . . **63**

Tatevik Sargsyan, Lala Stepanyan, Henrik Panosyan, Heghine Hakobyan, Monika Israyelyan and Avetis Tsaturyan et al.
Synthesis and Antifungal Activity of Fmoc-Protected 1,2,4-Triazolyl--Amino Acids and Their Dipeptides Against *Aspergillus* Species
Reprinted from: *Biomolecules* **2025**, *15*, 61, https://doi.org/10.3390/biom15010061 . . . . **75**

Naveenkumar Radhakrishnan, Sukumar Dinesh Kumar, Song-Yub Shin and Sungtae Yang
Enhancing Selective Antimicrobial and Antibiofilm Activities of Melittin through 6-Aminohexanoic Acid Substitution
Reprinted from: *Biomolecules* **2024**, *14*, 699, https://doi.org/10.3390/biom14060699 . . . . **96**

Júlia García-Gros, Yolanda Cajal, Ana Maria Marqués and Francesc Rabanal
Synthesis of the Antimicrobial Peptide Murepavadin Using Novel Coupling Agents
Reprinted from: *Biomolecules* **2024**, *14*, 526, https://doi.org/10.3390/biom14050526 . . . . **109**

Minho Seo, Kyeong-Ju Lee, Bison Seo, Jun-Hyuck Lee, Jae-Hyeon Lee and Dong-Wook Shin et al.
Analysis of Self-Assembled Low- and High-Molecular-Weight Poly-L-Lysine–Ce6 Conjugate-Based Nanoparticles
Reprinted from: *Biomolecules* **2024**, *14*, 431, https://doi.org/10.3390/biom14040431 . . . . **120**

Yulia Ilina, Paul Kaufmann, Michaela Press, Theo Ikenna Uba and Andreas Bergmann
Enhancing Stability and Bioavailability of Peptidylglycine Alpha-Amidating Monooxygenase in Circulation for Clinical Use
Reprinted from: *Biomolecules* **2025**, *15*, 224, https://doi.org/10.3390/biom15020224 . . . . **132**

Kong-Nan Zhao, Goce Dimeski, Paul Masci, Lambro Johnson, Jingjing Wang and John de Jersey et al.
Generation of Rapid and High-Quality Serum by Recombinant Prothrombin Activator Ecarin (RAPClot™)
Reprinted from: *Biomolecules* **2024**, *14*, 645, https://doi.org/10.3390/biom14060645 . . . . **144**

Graham E. Jackson, Marc-Antoine Sani, Heather G. Marco, Frances Separovic and Gerd Gäde
The Adipokinetic Hormone (AKH) and the Adipokinetic Hormone/Corazonin-Related Peptide (ACP) Signalling Systems of the Yellow Fever Mosquito *Aedes aegypti*: Chemical Models of Binding
Reprinted from: *Biomolecules* **2024**, *14*, 313, https://doi.org/10.3390/biom14030313 . . . . **165**

Andra V. Krauze, Yingdong Zhao, Ming-Chung Li, Joanna Shih, Will Jiang and Erdal Tasci et al.
Revisiting Concurrent Radiation Therapy, Temozolomide, and the Histone Deacetylase Inhibitor Valproic Acid for Patients with Glioblastoma— Proteomic Alteration and Comparison Analysis with the Standard-of-Care Chemoirradiation
Reprinted from: *Biomolecules* **2023**, *13*, 1499, https://doi.org/10.3390/biom13101499 . . . . **188**

biomolecules

MDPI

Review

Advancements in the Application of Ribosomally Synthesized and Post-Translationally Modified Peptides (RiPPs)

Sang-Woo Han [1] and Hyung-Sik Won [1,2,*]

1 Department of Biotechnology, Research Institute (RIBHS) and College of Biomedical & Health Science, Konkuk University, Chungju 27478, Chungbuk, Republic of Korea; swhan524@kku.ac.kr
2 BK21 Project Team, Department of Applied Life Science, Graduate School, Konkuk University, Chungju 27478, Chungbuk, Republic of Korea
* Correspondence: wonhs@kku.ac.kr

Abstract: Ribosomally synthesized and post-translationally modified peptides (RiPPs) represent a significant potential for novel therapeutic applications because of their bioactive properties, stability, and specificity. RiPPs are synthesized on ribosomes, followed by intricate post-translational modifications (PTMs), crucial for their diverse structures and functions. PTMs, such as cyclization, methylation, and proteolysis, play crucial roles in enhancing RiPP stability and bioactivity. Advances in synthetic biology and bioinformatics have significantly advanced the field, introducing new methods for RiPP production and engineering. These methods encompass strategies for heterologous expression, genetic refactoring, and exploiting the substrate tolerance of tailoring enzymes to create novel RiPP analogs with improved or entirely new functions. Furthermore, the introduction and implementation of cutting-edge screening methods, including mRNA display, surface display, and two-hybrid systems, have expedited the identification of RiPPs with significant pharmaceutical potential. This comprehensive review not only discusses the current advancements in RiPP research but also the promising opportunities that leveraging these bioactive peptides for therapeutic applications presents, illustrating the synergy between traditional biochemistry and contemporary synthetic biology and genetic engineering approaches.

Keywords: bioactive peptides; genetic engineering; heterologous expression; high-throughput screening; RiPPs; synthetic biology

Citation: Han, S.-W.; Won, H.-S. Advancements in the Application of Ribosomally Synthesized and Post-Translationally Modified Peptides (RiPPs). *Biomolecules* **2024**, *14*, 479. https://doi.org/10.3390/biom14040479

Academic Editor: Leonard B. Maggi Jr.

Received: 19 March 2024
Revised: 12 April 2024
Accepted: 13 April 2024
Published: 15 April 2024

1. Introduction

Bioactive peptides are a fascinating group of natural products with significant potential in pharmaceuticals and biotechnology. The potent biological activities of bioactive peptides, including antimicrobial, antiviral, and antitumor properties, make them prime candidates for drug development. Bioactive peptides are classified into the following two major groups based on biosynthetic pathways: (1) ribosomally synthesized and post-translationally modified peptides (RiPPs) and (2) non-ribosomal peptides (NRPs). RiPPs (e.g., lanthipeptides and lasso peptides) have unique biosynthetic pathways that combine ribosomal synthesis with highly diverse and complex post-translational modifications [1], while NRPs (e.g., penicillin and vancomycin) are assembled by non-ribosomal peptide synthetases independently of the ribosome [2].

RiPPs constitute a significant class of natural products found across all domains of life, from bacteria to humans. Because of their bioactive properties, stability, and specificity, RiPPs have gained attention from various industries. In the pharmaceutical sector, RiPPs are investigated for their potential as novel therapeutics including antibiotics [3], antivirals [4], and anticancer agents [5], many of which are undergoing clinical trials or are FDA-approved (Figure 1) [6]. In agriculture, they are considered for use as eco-friendly biopesticides [7], contributing to sustainable farming practices. The food industry employs RiPPs, such as nisin, as natural preservatives to combat spoilage and pathogenic bacteria, thereby extending product shelf life while ensuring safety [8]. The wide-ranging utility of RiPPs highlights their significant value across various industries.

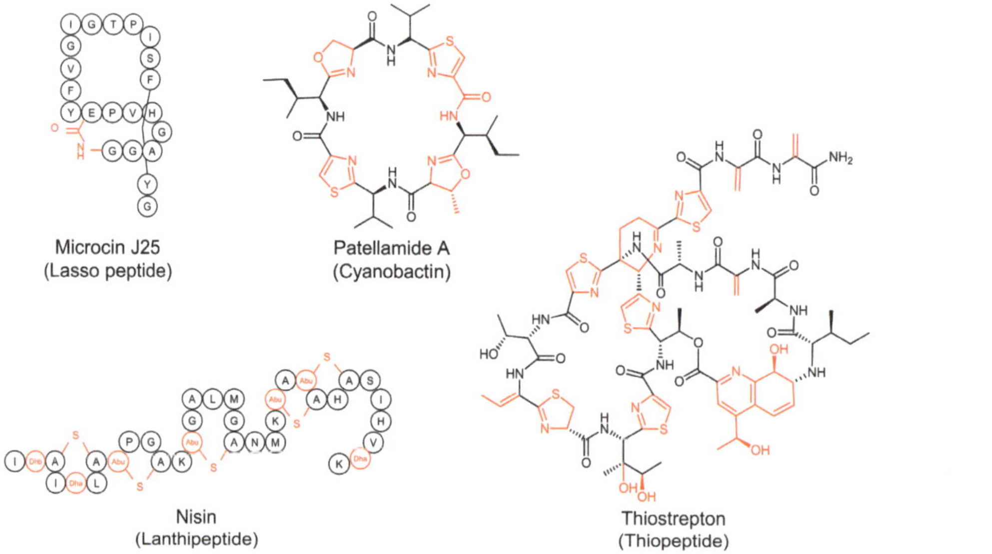

Figure 1. Representative therapeutic RiPPs and their classes. Letters in circles represent amino acids, and moieties undergoing modification are highlighted in red.

RiPPs originate from precursor peptides that are synthesized on ribosomes from the corresponding mRNA. These precursors typically consist of a leader peptide (or in some cases, a follower peptide) guiding post-translational modifications (PTMs) and a core peptide undergoing PTMs. After ribosomal synthesis, the precursor peptides undergo a series of PTMs that are responsible for the remarkable diversity in the structure and function of RiPPs. The PTMs can include processes like cyclization, dehydration, methylation, and cleavage of leader peptides [9–11]. Leader peptides are particularly important for PTMs owing to their effects on the specificity and activity of tailoring enzymes, sometimes keeping RiPPs inactive until the modifications are completed [12]. PTMs play a pivotal role in optimizing the therapeutic efficacy of RiPPs through a variety of mechanisms. By introducing modifications that increase lipophilicity or facilitate membrane interactions, PTMs can significantly enhance cell permeability, thereby enabling RiPPs to effectively target intracellular pathways [13]. These modifications not only improve the stability of RiPPs in biological environments by conferring resistance to proteolytic degradation and stabilizing their structures but also induce significant changes in their three-dimensional conformation, which is crucial for their biological activities [14]. Moreover, PTMs can adjust the binding characteristics and affinity of RiPPs towards specific targets, enabling more effective interactions at lower concentrations and introducing new functional groups or biochemical properties [15]. This selective post-translational tailoring enhances the physicochemical and biological attributes of RiPPs, positioning them as versatile and potent candidates for various therapeutic applications by fine-tuning their pharmacological properties to address specific clinical needs effectively.

RiPPs can be easily predicted and engineered because of their direct genetic encoding. Notably, advancements in genome sequencing have played a crucial role in the identification and characterization of RiPPs. The ribosomal origin of these peptides allows for the prediction of their chemical structures from genomic data, facilitating genome-driven RiPP discovery. This characteristic renders RiPPs an attractive target for bioengineering and synthetic biology efforts aimed at producing novel bioactive compounds. Heterologous expression of RiPP gene clusters in hosts like *Escherichia coli* [12,16–21] and *Streptomyces* sp. [22,23] is essential for elucidating these peptides and generating novel derivatives. Recent advances in synthetic biology and bioinformatics have significantly impacted research on RiPPs, particularly in the discovery of novel RiPPs and their engineering. The integration of high-throughput genome sequencing with sophisticated bioinformatic algorithms has enabled the prediction of RiPP biosynthetic pathways directly from genetic material. For example, specialized tools such as AntiSMASH [24], PRISM [25], and RODEO [26] have been developed for mining and annotating RiPP biosynthetic gene clusters, leading to an accelerated identification of new RiPPs [27,28]. On the other hand, synthetic biology facilitates in vivo and in vitro synthesis and screening of RiPPs by heterologous expression under diverse generic circuits [29]. Furthermore, these advances have exploited the inherent promiscuity within RiPP biosynthetic systems to generate a diverse array of engineered compounds with enhanced bioactivities and stability [29]. However, translating these gene clusters into known chemical entities remains challenging because of the complex nature of the PTMs and enzyme–substrate interactions within the cell. The lack of understanding of RiPPs restricts our ability to predict the complexity of RiPP biosynthetic gene clusters (BGCs), comprising multiple genes encoding peptides and proteins necessary for the biosynthetic process, and the diversity of PTMs. Therefore, the structural analysis of RiPP requires a multifaceted approach employing tandem mass spectrometry (MS) to identify PTMs and Nuclear Magnetic Resonance (NMR) to elucidate structural details and dynamics upon binding [30,31]. However, structural characterization is often hindered by low isolation yields from natural sources. To address these challenges, recent strategies have included the activation of silent biosynthetic gene clusters [23,32–35], the refactoring of biosynthetic gene clusters [22,36–38], and in vitro reconstruction of biosynthetic pathways [39–41].

In this work, we provide a comprehensive analysis of RiPPs, highlighting recent developments of synthetic biological systems and their applications in the production and engineering of RiPPs (Table 1).

Table 1. A summary of the recently discovered or engineered RiPPs described in this review.

RiPP Product	Class	Biological Activity	Ref.
Thiovarsolin	Thioamitides	Unidentified	[23]
Daptide	Daptide	Hemolytic activity	[22]
Imiditide	Imiditide	Unidentified	[38]
Mycetolassin	Lasso peptide	Unidentified	[42]
7 RiPPs	Lanthipeptide, lasso peptide, LAP	Unidentified	[32]
30 RiPPs	Lanthipeptide, lasso peptide, graspetide, glycocin, LAP, thioamitide	Antimicrobial activity against ESKAPE pathogens	[37]
24 RiPPs	Lanthipeptide, lasso peptide	Antimicrobial activity against human pathogens	[36]
Octreotide analogs	Ranthipeptide	Unidentified	[43]
Hybrid RiPPs	Lanthipeptide	Antimicrobial activity against antibiotic-resistant MRSA strain	[44]
Hybrid RiPPs	Lanthipeptide	Antimicrobial activity against antibiotic-resistant MRSA strain	[45]
Hybrid RiPPs	Cyanobactin, microviridin	Unidentified	[46]
Prenylated lanthipeptides	Lanthipeptide	Unidentified	[47]
Cycle peptides	Cyanobactin	Unidentified	[48]
Cycle peptides	Cyanobactin	Unidentified	[40]
Pantocin A analogs	Pantocin	Unidentified	[49]
Lactazole analogs	Thiopeptide	Unidentified	[50]
Freyrasin analogs	Ranthipeptide	Binding to the SARS-CoV-2 Spike receptor	[51]
Ubonodin analogs	Lasso peptide	Antimicrobial activity against opportunistic human pathogens	[52]
Cycle peptides	Lasso peptide	Anticancer activity	[39]
XY3-3	Lanthipeptide	Inhibition to HIV infection	[53]
Hybrid RiPPs	Lanthipeptide	Antimicrobial activity against pathogenic bacteria	[54]
Halα analogs	Lanthipeptide	Antimicrobial activity	[21]

Our discussion begins with the synthesis of precursor peptides on cellular ribosomes, detailing the specific and highly controlled PTMs such as cyclization, methylation, hydroxylation, acylation, and proteolysis, which are critical for maturing these precursors into bioactive compounds. We further explore the role of these modifications in enhancing RiPP stability and bioactivity, illustrating the cellular machinery's precision in generating these molecules. The advances in synthetic biology for RiPP production are also examined, including strategies for heterologous expression and genetic refactoring to produce novel RiPP analogs. We highlight the substrate tolerance of tailoring enzymes as a key factor in generating diverse RiPP analogs and discuss the importance of leader peptides in directing

PTMs. Finally, we introduce the latest screening methods for identifying functional RiPPs, preparing readers to appreciate the depth of research and technological innovation in the field of RiPP biosynthesis and function.

2. Biosynthetic Pathways of RiPPs

The biosynthesis of RiPPs commences in the cellular ribosomes, where precursor peptides are synthesized based on genetic information. These precursors typically consist of the following two distinct regions: the leader peptide and the core peptide (Figure 2). The leader peptide, positioned at the N-terminus (or occasionally at the C-terminus as a follower peptide), plays a critical role within the cell by guiding the subsequent PTMs of the core peptide. This leader peptide–core peptide architecture is essential for the controlled and specific modifications that the core peptide undergoes. The cellular machinery recognizes these leader peptides as targets for a series of enzymatic transformations that eventually result in the mature RiPP.

Within the cell, the core peptide undergoes various PTMs, a critical process for the functional diversity of RiPPs. Common modifications include the addition or alteration of functional groups, cyclization, and the formation of unique bond structures, such as thioether linkages. These modifications are not only diverse but also highly specific, often occurring at precise locations within the core peptide. The cellular environment thus plays a critical role in ensuring the correct folding and processing of these peptides, which is essential for the biological activity of the final RiPP product.

Major PTMs of RiPPs include cyclization, methylation, hydroxylation, acylation, and proteolysis. During cyclization, amino acid side chains can bridge across the chain, creating rings within the peptide backbone and forming circular structures, as exemplified by lanthipeptides [55]. Radical *S*-adenosylmethionine (SAM) enzymes, for instance, establish covalent bonds between side chains within the backbone (e.g., lanthipeptides) or head-to-tail connections (e.g., lasso peptides), generating complex cyclic scaffolds. These rings not only enhance stability but also influence interactions with target molecules, affecting biological activity. On the other hand, methyltransferases append methyl groups ($–CH_3$) to specific nitrogen or oxygen atoms, subtly altering the RiPP's structure. Methylation affects properties such as pK_a, membrane interactions, and stability, thereby tuning the RiPP's interaction with its biological targets. *N*-methylation, for example, increases stability against protease [56], while *O*-methylation in lanthipeptides and lasso peptides can adjust binding affinity [57,58]. Also, P450 enzymes incorporate hydroxyl groups (–OH) onto specific carbon atoms within the RiPP scaffold. This precise modification can activate RiPPs by modifying solubility and stability, with hydroxylation playing a vital role in antimicrobial activity in families like lassomycin [59]. Lastly, acyltransferases attach various acyl groups, such as acetyl or propionyl, to specific side chains. In surfactin A, acetylation affects surface properties, enhancing interactions with membranes and contributing to potent surfactant activity [60].

The precursor peptide contains the sequences for proteases beside the core peptides. Proteases cleave at specific peptide bonds, releasing the core peptide region from the precursor peptide that acts as a protective form of the RiPP. This proteolysis event not only activates the RiPP but also influences its final structure, such as revealing the active site. For more detailed information about proteolytic events, we refer to a comprehensive review published recently [11]. On the other hand, research efforts focusing on the tailoring enzymes for PTMs have provided a biochemical understanding of RiPP biosynthesis and strategies for engineering RiPPs. For example, previous studies have demonstrated the flexibility of tailoring enzymes for substrates (i.e., core peptides) [38,61,62]. The significant substrate tolerance of tailoring enzymes has not only highlighted the natural diversification of RiPPs but also facilitated the engineering of novel RiPP analogs. By exploiting this substrate tolerance and using synthetic biology techniques to manipulate genes encoding RiPP precursors, RiPP analogs have been synthesized with desired biological functions, such as enhanced antibiotic potency [44] and increased stability [45,63].

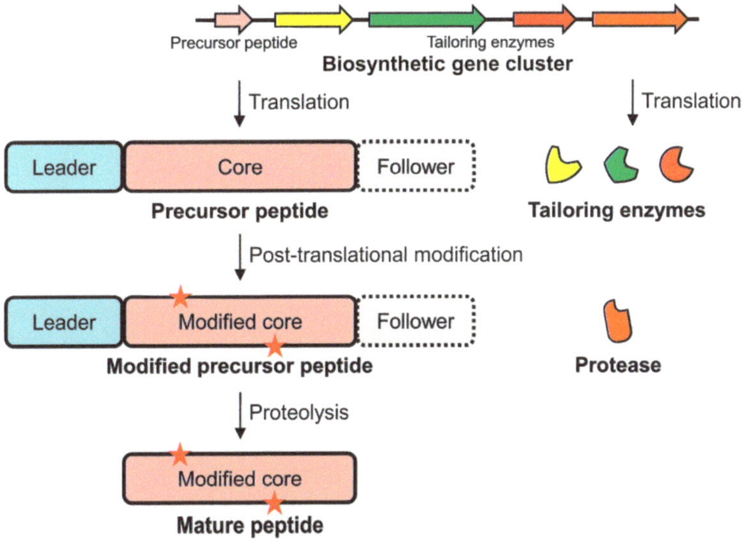

Figure 2. Schematic representation of the RiPP biosynthetic pathway. The biosynthetic gene cluster, which includes various genes responsible for RiPP synthesis, is translated into a precursor peptide and tailoring enzymes. After translation, tailoring enzymes, recruited by the leader (and/or follower) peptide, modify the core peptide. Subsequently, a protease cleaves the leader (and/or follower) peptide, resulting in the production of the mature peptide. Red stars represent the occurrence of PTM.

3. Advances in Synthetic Biology for RiPP Expression and Production

Synthetic biology provides innovative solutions to overcome the challenges associated with expression, engineering, and screening. A key advancement is the development of strategies targeting multiple synthetic biology levels, including individual proteins, pathways, metabolic flux, and host optimization. This approach significantly enhances the feasibility and effectiveness of RiPP preparation by tailoring the host's metabolic machinery to support RiPP biosynthesis. Moreover, synthetic biology enables the engineering of RiPPs by reconstituting precursor peptides, wherein different functional groups are added to the core peptides. This interchangeability of substrate elements is crucial to tailoring RiPPs both in vivo and in vitro, thereby expanding the chemical and functional space of RiPPs.

RiPPs are produced via two distinct approaches including (1) natural biosynthesis and (2) heterologous expression. Natural biosynthesis utilizes the organism's inherent metabolic pathways to produce RiPPs. Producing RiPPs in their native environment ensures correct folding and PTMs essential for their biological activity, as well as the natural diversity of RiPP structures and bioactivities. However, natural biosynthesis is limited by scalability, variability in yield, purity, and gene silencing [64]. To address these issues, considerable research efforts have focused on heterologous expression in surrogate hosts like *E. coli* or *Streptomyces* sp. Heterologous expression allows researchers to circumvent the complexity and the limitations of native genetic systems, typically using model organisms whose genetic manipulation and scale-up are easier than source organisms. This approach, however, presents challenges such as the complexity of reconstituting native biosynthetic machinery in a heterologous host and stability issues with precursor peptides [18–20]. Additionally, PTMs may occur differently between the host and the native producer, potentially affecting the final RiPP structure and activity. Despite these challenges, heterologous expression (Figure 3) has offered opportunities for discovery and innovation beyond the capabilities of natural biosynthesis.

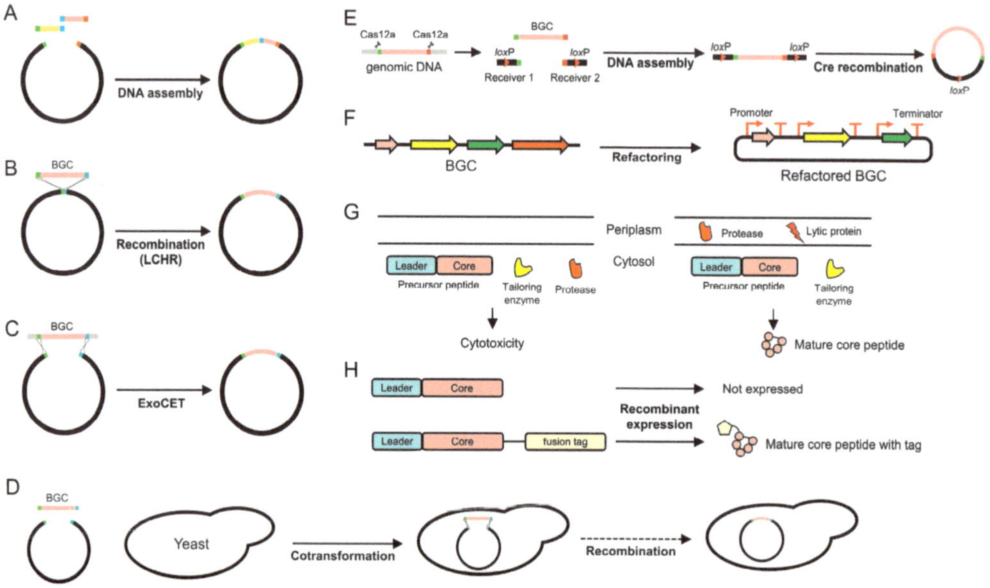

Figure 3. Genetic engineering for heterologous RiPP expression. (**A**) In DNA assembly methods such as Gibson assembly, multiple PCR products are ligated into an expression vector through a single isothermal reaction. (**B**) RecET facilitates homologous recombination between a lengthy linear fragment of a BGC and a vector (circular or linear) containing homologous regions. (**C**) ExoCET employs an exonuclease in addition to promoting recombination with longer fragments of BGC that carry non-homologous overhangs. (**D**) Upon transformation into yeast with fragments of BGC and a vector with homologous regions, the DNA fragments are assembled via the yeast's native recombination system. (**E**) In the CAPTURE technique, the BGC fragment, isolated from genomic DNA by Cas12a, is ligated into synthetic receivers with *lox*P sites using DNA assembly methods, followed by circularization with the Cre enzyme. (**F**) Replacing native regulatory elements with uncharacterized mechanisms into well-understood systems facilitates the heterologous expression of selected BGC components, crucial for the biosynthesis of mature RiPP. (**G**) The expression of RiPP with bioactive properties triggers cell death in the host strain. However, by transporting a protease and a lytic protein to the periplasmic region and delaying the expression of the lytic protein, maturation of RiPP occurs, allowing the host cell to survive. (**H**) The addition of a fusion tag to a precursor peptide increases its stability and expression level, leading to an accumulation of mature RiPP in a heterologous cell.

3.1. Genetic Manipulation for Heterologous Expression

To address the complexities inherent in the genetic systems of RiPPs, two innovative strategies stand out including heterologous expression and genetic refactoring. Heterologous expression is a promising approach for activating silent BGCs identified by bioinformatic tools but not expressed under laboratory conditions. This method involves transferring BGCs to more manageable host organisms, such as *E. coli*, enabling the activation of these silent BGCs often under a foreign promoter. However, the cloning method based on PCR amplification is impractical for large BGCs, especially because of the introduction of mutations during PCR amplification [65].

To minimize PCR errors, methods that join multiple DNA fragments, occasionally coupled with de novo DNA synthesis, have emerged as reliable alternatives (Figure 3A). For instance, Gibson assembly facilitates the simultaneous assembly of multiple overlapping DNA fragments in a single reaction by combining exonuclease, polymerase, and ligase activities [66]. Using assembly-based methods, Wuisan et al. cloned darobactin A BGCs from various *Photorhabdus khanii* substrains [35]. However, assembly methods face severe limitations due to length [67] and GC content [68]. Direct cloning can simplify the cloning process and reduce the effort required to obtain desired BGCs. This approach bypasses the construction of genomic libraries and captures BGCs directly from genomic DNA without PCR amplification, proceeding through homologous recombination.

RecET recombination, originally identified in the Rac prophage of *E. coli*, comprises two proteins including RecE exonuclease and RecT annealing protein [69]. These proteins facilitate homologous recombination, integrating linear DNA fragments into the chromosome or plasmids of *E. coli* (Figure 3B). Fu et al. developed cloning tools mediated by RecET, termed linear plus linear homologous recombination (LLHR) and linear plus circular homologous recombination (LCHR), which are mechanistically distinct from conventional recombineering mediated by λ Redαβ [70]. Exonuclease can enhance the performance of RecET recombination especially in cloning large genomic regions (>50 kb) [34]. Wang et al. described the exonuclease combined with RecET recombination (ExoCET), which entails associating two DNA molecules outside the cell through a combination of in vitro exonuclease treatment and annealing facilitated by RecET homologous recombination (Figure 3C). However, the direct application of RecET-based recombination is primarily in *E. coli*, as the system relies on specific interactions with its cellular machinery [69]. For application in other organisms, analogous systems or engineered versions of RecET adapted to the cellular environment of the host organism are necessary. For example, *Saccharomyces cerevisiae* possesses a natural homologous recombination system, leading to the development of transformation-associated recombination (TAR) [71]. In TAR, a vector containing two homology arms is linearized and co-transformed with genomic DNA harboring the BGCs of interest into *S. cerevisiae* (Figure 3D). The yeast's recombination machinery facilitates the integration of DNA fragments into the vector. For instance, Santos-Aberturas et al. successfully captured 31.7 kb of the thiovarsolin BGC, comprising 25 genes from *Streptomyces varsoviensis*, utilizing TAR [23].

In contrast, the Cre-*lox* recombination system, originating from bacteriophage P1, offers a genetic engineering platform applicable across a broad spectrum of organisms beyond its origins [72]. This system consists of the Cre recombinase enzyme and *lox*P recognition sites, enabling the seamless integration of DNA based on the orientation and placement of *lox*P sites. Unlike organism-specific methods such as TAR [71] and RecET [69], which are tailored to yeast and *E. coli*, respectively, the simplicity and universality of the Cre/*lox*P mechanism allow for its application in a diverse range of microbial systems [33]. Recently, Enghiad et al. described CAPTURE (Cas12a-assisted precise targeted cloning using in vivo Cre-*lox* recombination), which combines the precision of CRISPR-Cas12a genome editing with the flexibility of the Cre-*lox* recombination system (Figure 3E) [32]. CAPTURE employs the Cas12a enzyme for DNA digestion, T4 DNA polymerase for DNA assembly, and Cre-*lox* recombination for in vivo circularization of DNA, addressing the challenges of conventional cloning such as high GC content and sequence repeats. The researchers successfully cloned 43 uncharacterized BGCs, including probable lanthipeptide and lasso peptide BGCs, within 3–4 days, with sizes up to 113 kb. In another study, CAPTURE was applied to clone BGCs for daptide, a novel class of RiPPs characterized by an unusual (*S*)-N_2,N_2-dimethyl-1,2-propanediamine-modified C-terminus. Ren et al. [22] cloned daptide BGCs from *Microbacterium paraoxydans* DSM 15019 and expressed them in *Streptomyces albus* J1074, a versatile host for natural product pathway expression. This approach enabled the production, isolation, and detailed characterization of these unique peptides. Through heterologous expression, the team identified and analyzed daptides, revealing their distinctive bioactivities, including hemolytic activity.

3.2. Refactoring

Approaches to cloning entire BGCs may face challenges because of complex regulatory mechanisms inherent within BGCs and compatibility issues with heterologous hosts. Refactoring BGCs could overcome this challenge by circumventing the natural regulatory network [29]. This process simplifies and optimizes BGCs by selecting and reorganizing essential genes into operons and introducing synthetic regulatory elements, thereby fostering modularity and simplification (Figure 3F). Codon randomization is often employed to eliminate unidentified regulatory elements and promote efficient translation [29]. Cao et al. utilized refactoring to enhance the heterologous production of a novel RiPP, imiditides, whose BGC comprises a precursor peptide of NmaA and a tailoring enzyme of NmaM [38]. The refactoring involved the co-expression of genes by placing His_6-SUMO-*NmaA* and untagged NmaM on separate expression plasmids. This approach enabled the successful heterologous expression and the PTM of imiditides. For more complex BGCs, researchers have implemented a plug-and-play refactoring strategy, where each gene module is constructed, assembled into a single plasmid, and interchangeably used within clusters. Ren et al. applied plug-and-play refactoring to identify essential genes for daptide biosynthesis using the mpa BGC [22]. Each codon-optimized mpa gene (mpaABCDM) was subcloned onto helper plasmids and combined via Golden Gate assembly to construct different versions of biosynthetic pathways, demonstrating the essential function of mpaABCDM in dipeptide production. Although refactoring offers numerous advantages, it requires significant time to prepare modular fragments. Leveraging robotics can provide one promising solution. Ayikpoe et al. developed a high-throughput pathway refactoring platform based on DNA synthesis and robotic assembly using Type IIS restriction enzymes [37]. With the refactoring of 96 bacterial RiPP BGCs identified by the RODEO tool [26], they successfully isolated 30 peptides spanning six RiPP classes [lanthipeptide, lasso peptide, graspetide, glycocin, linear azol(in)e-containing peptide (LAP), and thioamitide], with three peptides exhibiting antibiotic activity against multidrug-resistant bacterial pathogens known as ESKAPE. This platform facilitated the rapid evaluation of uncharacterized BGCs through automated pathway refactoring and heterologous expression. BGCs can be reconstituted by substituting existing genes and elements with synthetic counterparts. In 2023, King et al. demonstrated the systematic mining of lanthipeptide and lasso peptide BGCs from 2229 human microbiome genomes to identify antimicrobial peptides [36]. To address the challenges presented by the diverse origins of BGCs, they engineered synthetic gene clusters by incorporating codon optimization, synthetic regulatory elements including ribosome binding sites and terminators, a SUMO tag for precursor peptide stabilization, and a His tag for peptide purification. The synthetic gene clusters also featured a TEV protease site, replacing natural leader cleavage sites for simplified cleavage. Among seventy BGCs identified by the antiSMASH tool [24], twenty-three peptides (19 lanthipeptides and four lasso peptides) were functionally characterized, leading to the discovery of several RiPPs exhibiting activity against multidrug-resistant pathogens, including three RiPPs effective against vancomycin-resistant *Enterococci*. These findings underscore the potential of refactoring and heterologous expression as a potent strategy for the discovery of novel bioactive compounds, making a significant contribution to antimicrobial research.

3.3. Compartmentation

One major challenge in the production of RiPPs is the potential cytotoxicity of mature RiPPs to heterologous hosts, which hinders the discovery of novel RiPPs and the development of high-yield production systems. To mitigate this cytotoxicity, research efforts have focused on exploiting natural resistance mechanisms, such as efflux systems including peptide translocation [73,74] and transporters [75–77]. A notable study employed a compartmentation strategy for the expression of RiPPs, particularly focusing on lanthipeptides, through a synthetic biology approach in *E. coli* (Figure 3G) [12]. This strategy is crucial for overcoming the challenge of leader peptide removal—a bottleneck in heterologous RiPP production—by temporally programming leader peptide cleavage through protease compartmentalization and inducible cell autolysis. Specifically, it involves expressing the precursor peptide and biosynthetic enzymes in the cytosol, while compartmentalizing the protease to the periplasmic space to avoid premature interaction and potential cytotoxicity. Autolysis is induced using a temperature-controlled lysis gene cassette from bacteriophage λ, enabling the release of bioactive peptides after PTMs have been completed in the cytosol. Remarkably, this method simplifies the RiPP production process by facilitating in vivo leader peptide removal, significantly improving the throughput for discovering, characterizing, and engineering RiPPs. It also demonstrates the system's effectiveness in producing bioactive lanthipeptides, such as haloduracin and lacticin 481, highlighting the method's potential scalability and applicability to other RiPP classes, thereby revolutionizing RiPP engineering and discovery efforts.

3.4. Fusion Tags

The diversity of maturation mechanisms across different RiPPs presents a challenge in developing a universally applicable production system. For instance, transporters are indispensable for the maturation of certain RiPPs [78], but not essential for lasso peptide maturation [79]. A strategy that is applicable to a wide range of RiPPs involves the stabilization of RiPPs through the attachment of an additional tag to the N- or C-terminus of the precursor peptide (Figure 3H). One widely utilized tag is a small ubiquitin-like modifier (SUMO), which, when fused to proteins, beneficially influences their expression, folding, and solubility [16,17]. In 2022, Glassey et al. described the broad applicability of the SUMO fusion to 11 RiPP classes originating from diverse species [18]. They aimed to overcome the inherent challenges of peptide instability and functional expression in heterologous hosts such as *E. coli*. By fusing a SUMO tag to either the N- or C-terminus of the precursor peptides, this strategy stabilizes the expression of a broad spectrum of RiPPs, with the SUMO tag being proteolytically removed after PTMs. Remarkably, they successfully expressed 24 functional peptides out of 50 tested in *E. coli*, facilitating high-throughput screening and discovery of diverse RiPPs predicted by bioinformatic tools. Indeed, recent studies have exploited the SUMO fusion strategy for genome mining of RiPPs [36,38].

Fusion with fluorescent proteins, which are attractive partners for enhancing the solubility of recombinant proteins [80], is also applicable to RiPP expression. In a study by Vermeulen et al., plantaricin 423 and mundticin ST4SA, when fused with GFP at their N-terminus, were expressed in soluble forms in the host *E. coli* [19]. Additionally, Van Zyl et al. utilized mCherry for the heterologous expression of lanthipeptides such as nisin and clausin with N-terminal fusion [20]. Compared with other strategies, fluorescent tags enable the evaluation of RiPP expression levels through real-time fluorescence monitoring. For instance, the fluorescent intensity of GFP-MunX was compared under various conditions (e.g., IPTG concentration, expression time, and temperature) to optimize expression conditions, resulting in a yield of 12.4 mg of mundticin per liter of culture in *E. coli* [19].

3.5. Plasmid Copy Number

Very recently, Fernandez et al. highlighted the importance of selecting the appropriate plasmid vector and replicon, which can influence host cell viability and plasmid stability, for achieving high RiPP production yields [81]. Using capistruin—a lasso peptide—as a model system, the BGC was incorporated into different plasmids with varying replicons and then heterologously expressed in *Burkholderia* sp. FERM BP-3421. By increasing the plasmid copy number, they achieved a production yield of 240 mg/L, representing a 1.6-fold improvement over the previously optimized overproducer clone [42]. Interestingly, an increased plasmid copy number was associated with a prolonged lag phase during cell culture, indicating potential growth defects likely due to the antibiotic effect of the produced capistruin. This strategy was applied to the production of mycetolassin-15 and mycetolassin-18, novel lasso peptides originating from *Mycetohabitans* sp. B13. Contrary to capistruin, a higher plasmid copy number resulted in approximately a 2-fold reduction in production yield and a shorter lag phase, indicating that the effectiveness of the production system depends on the type of RiPP. This approach provided insights into the role of plasmid copy number in balancing peptide production with host cell viability and growth.

4. Strategies and Innovations in RiPP Engineering

Protein engineering for RiPPs (Figure 4) holds significant promise for both fundamental research and practical applications, ranging from discovering new bioactive compounds with therapeutic potentials to understanding biological mechanisms. This process aids in elucidating cellular processes and disease mechanisms through the modification of RiPPs and plays a crucial role in combating antibiotic resistance by providing new antimicrobial agents. Engineering RiPPs enhances their specificity, activity, stability, and bioavailability, making them more effective as therapeutic agents with fewer side effects.

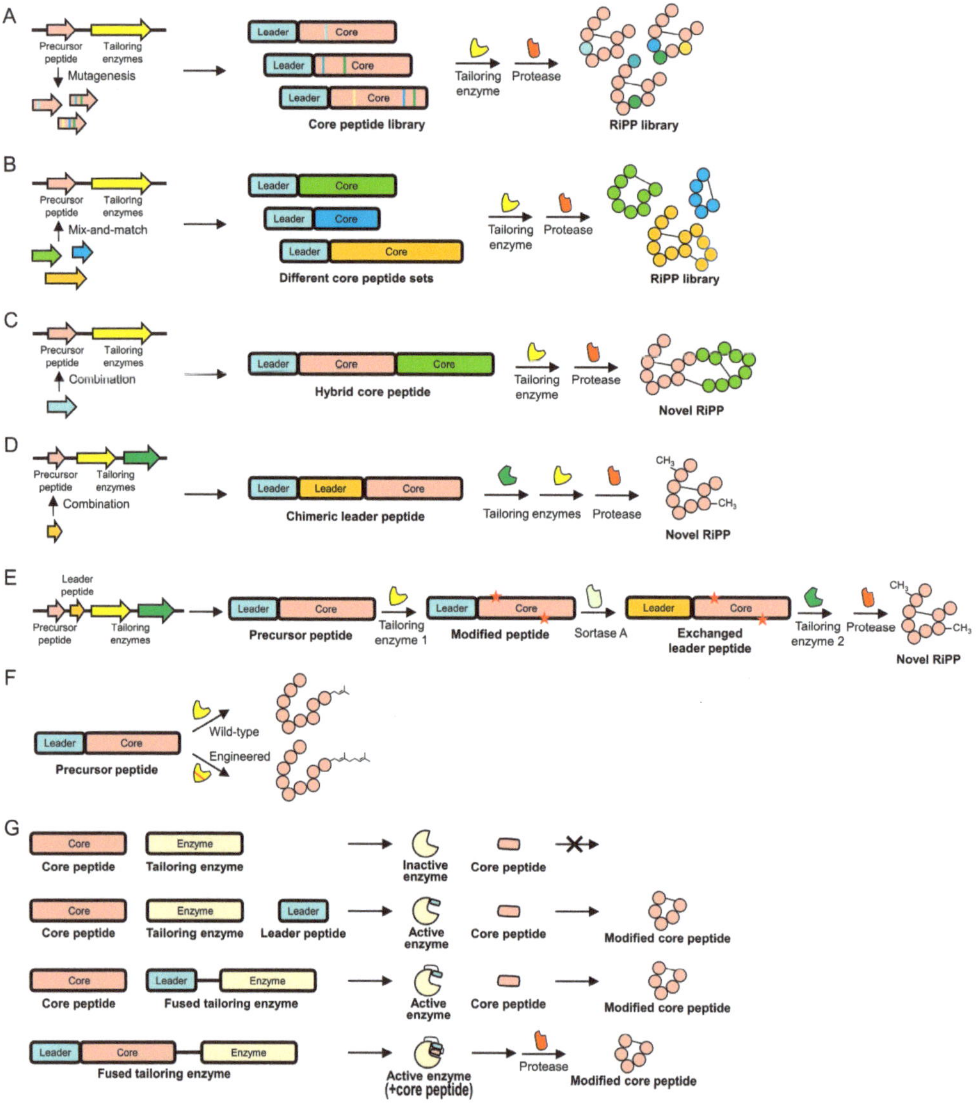

Figure 4. Strategies of RiPP engineering with respect to core peptides (**A–C**), leader peptides (**D**,**E**), and tailoring enzymes (**F**,**G**). (**A–C**) Addressing core peptides, substrate flexibilities of tailoring enzymes enable site-directed mutations (**A**), incorporation of foreign core peptides (**B**), and creation of hybrid core peptides with multiple domains (**C**), leading to a variety of RiPPs. (**D**,**E**) Utilizing leader peptides' properties in guiding PTMs, diverse combinations of PTMs can be introduced on a single core peptide through chimeric leader peptides with multiple domains to guide PTMs (**D**) and leader peptide exchange using sortase A (**E**). (**F**) Protein engineering can enhance the substrate range

of tailoring enzymes, broadening their application in generating RiPP variants. (**G**) The regulatory mechanism in tailoring enzyme activation can be simplified by introducing a free leader peptide and by fusing a tailoring enzyme with both a leader and a precursor peptide, simplifying the RiPP biosynthesis process.

4.1. Core Peptides

One interesting feature of the RiPP biosynthetic system is the substrate tolerance of tailoring enzymes, which implies the versatility of these enzymes with various core peptides. Previous studies have reported that only several residues of core peptides are critical for tailoring enzymes to catalyze PTMs, independent of the types and numbers of other residues [40,43,82]. This feature suggests an engineering strategy of introducing mutations into tolerant sites to generate myriad RiPP analogs (Figure 4A) [21,43]. For instance, a radical SAM enzyme encoded by *PapB* from *Paenibacillus polymyxa*, which catalyzes thioether cross-links between Cys and acidic residues (i.e., Asp and Glu) across diverse sequences, can accept various core peptides containing a Cys-X_n-Asp motif (n = 0~6), even with D-amino acids at cross-linking sites [43,83]. Such capability extends the enzyme's utility beyond conventional substrate specificities, enabling peptide engineering by introducing diverse amino acids at tolerant sites and incorporating D-amino acids at either of the intolerant sites to alter their biological activities. The enzyme's flexibility facilitates the incorporation of unconventional amino acids and the crafting of complex peptide architectures, which are typically challenging via standard synthetic routes. Leveraging this unique substrate tolerance, researchers prepared an analog of the FDA-approved therapeutic agent octreotide, whose disulfide bond is replaced with a Cys-Glu thioether linkage. Although the analog's biological function has not yet been profiled, this strategy presents a prospect for developing new peptide-based therapeutics, potentially improving biological effectiveness, stability, or pharmacological attributes.

The substrate tolerance of tailoring enzymes facilitates extensive engineering through the mix-and-match of diverse tailoring enzymes and core peptides, which is unprecedented in nature (Figure 4B). A recent study by Nguyen et al. exemplified this combinatorial strategy for macrocyclization using diverse core peptide backbones [82]. The researchers combined the tailoring enzymes MprC (cyclodehydratase), MprD (flavin-dependent oxidase), and PatG (subtilisin-like protease) with the core peptides MprE2, MprE5, MprE10, and PatE from *Methylovulum psychrotolerans*, aiming to create novel macrocyclized proteusin analogs with unique structural features. MprC facilitates the cyclodehydration of serine and threonine residues, MprD oxidizes azoline-containing peptides to azole-containing peptides, and PatG guides head-to-tail macrocyclization by recognizing an AYD sequence at the C-terminus of peptides. This approach leveraged the enzymes' substrate tolerance to engineer RiPPs, demonstrating their potential as versatile biotechnological tools for generating diverse natural product libraries.

Zhao and Kuipers produced novel macrocyclic lanthipeptides, named thanacin and ripcin, by substituting the core peptide region in nisin BGCs with those of the antimicrobial peptides thanatin and rip-thanatin, respectively [44]. The capability of tailoring enzymes to catalyze foreign core peptides raised questions about whether PTMs occur simultaneously when core peptides are concatenated. They prepared a hybrid precursor peptide including the core peptide regions for both nisin and ripcin, generating a series of novel peptides named ripcin B–G depending on the length of the ripcin core peptide (13–18 residues) (Figure 4C). These hybrid lanthipeptides exhibited enhanced antimicrobial activity against *Staphylococcus aureus* and tested Gram-negative pathogens compared with either nisin or ripcin alone. Ripcin B–G were notable for their resistance to the nisin resistance protein, making them particularly attractive for selective antimicrobial applications in complex microbial environments.

Guo et al. combined two strategies—mutagenesis and hybrid construction—to enhance antimicrobial efficacy and stability [45]. They first created hybrid peptides by fusing domains from various nisin variants—nisin A, cesin, and rombocin—to produce novel entities like nirocin A and cerocin A. These hybrids exhibited improved action against methicillin-resistant *Staphylococcus aureus*. Subsequently, mutagenesis was employed to increase the peptides' proteolytic stability, resulting in the discovery of cerocin V, which showed minimal degradation by trypsin. Their study highlighted the potential of combining domain modifications and targeted mutations to manipulate biological and physicochemical properties, generating novel bioactive molecules with promising therapeutic potential.

4.2. Leader Peptides

The leader peptide plays a crucial role in directing PTMs, guiding tailoring enzymes, and controlling the maturation of RiPPs, suggesting another strategy to modify RiPP properties. By altering leader peptides, researchers can influence the efficiency and type of PTMs, thereby creating RiPP variants with unique structures and activities. Burkhart et al. hypothesized that by fusing two leader peptides to construct a single chimeric leader peptide, two tailoring enzymes would bind to their respective regions on the chimeric leader peptide, facilitating the combination of PTMs originating from different RiPPs (Figure 4D) [84]. Specifically, the researchers combined an azoline-forming cyclodehydratase (HcaD/F) with a lanthipeptide synthetase (NisB/C) as a feasibility test. This approach demonstrated the potential to create hybrid RiPP products with diverse structural features, laying the groundwork for a broadly applicable platform for combinatorial RiPP biosynthesis. One potential issue with the chimeric leader peptide strategy is the maximum combination of leader peptides. The fusion of leader peptides could reduce the PTM efficiency, even with the repetition of identical leader peptides [85]. Additionally, some tailoring enzymes could work with a leader peptide comprising only one amino acid [86], indicating the possible production of a mixture of RiPPs, including molecules undergoing undesired PTMs. Thus, the sophisticated preparation of RiPP analogs through the fusion of multiple leader peptides requires an extensive understanding of enzyme–substrate recognition.

The leader peptide exchange strategy described by Franz and Koehnke offers a "plug-and-play" solution that can circumvent the complexity of the biosynthetic system (Figure 4E) [46]. They leveraged sortase A, which catalyzes transpeptidation, to exchange a pre-existing leader peptide with another, allowing a precursor peptide to carry only one leader peptide at a time. Specifically, sortase A cleaves a peptide bond within a specific recognition sequence (LPXTG) in the leader peptide and then forms a new peptide bond between the core peptide and the N-terminus of another leader peptide carrying the sortase recognition sequence. They modified the MdnA core peptide sequentially with cyclodehydration and macrocyclization by LynD and MdnC, leading to the preparation of a heterocycle-containing graspetide. This proof-of-concept demonstrates the leader peptide exchange as a potent tool that can facilitate the synthesis of innovative compounds with broad biological activities.

4.3. Tailoring Enzymes

Engineering tailoring enzymes, which directly contribute to the structural and functional diversity of RiPPs through PTMs, is pivotal for advancing RiPP engineering and providing synthetic biology tools (Figure 4F). For instance, prenyltransferases, which catalyze the attachment of prenyl groups to acceptor molecules, could enhance the biological activities of RiPPs by altering molecule lipophilicity and facilitating interaction with cellular targets. However, the broader application of prenyltransferases in producing diverse compounds has been limited by their strict specificity for prenyl donors. To overcome these limitations, Estrada et al. focused on PirF, a Tyr prenyltransferase with C10 isoprene donor (geranyl pyrophosphate, GPP) specificity [47]. Intriguingly, PirF shares over 70% sequence identity with prenyltransferases (e.g., PagF) that are only active toward dimethylallyl pyrophosphate (C5 isoprene donor, DMAPP) and not GPP. Through structure determination, the researchers identified that Gly221 in PirF corresponds to Phe222 in PagF in three-dimensional structures, likely influencing the size and hydrophobicity of the active site. Indeed, substituting Phe222 with alanine or glycine in PagF shifted the substrate preference from a C5 to a C10 isoprene donor, allowing for the use of alternative prenyl donors and expanding the applications of the tailoring enzyme.

The regulatory mechanism of tailoring enzymes, often requiring cognate leader peptides to exhibit activity, could obstruct the applications of engineered enzymes. Interestingly, a previous study by Levengood et al. revealed that supplying a leader peptide apart from a cognate core peptide (in *trans*) activated the tailoring enzyme for PTMs (Figure 4G) [87], suggesting a feasible strategy to mitigate the regulatory system. However, the requirement for large amounts of synthetic peptide made in *trans* activation economically unattractive. An alternative strategy is the fusion of a tailoring enzyme with a leader peptide, where they are covalently bound by additional linker sequences, to constitutively activate the enzyme. Following Oman et al.'s demonstration of the feasibility of this in *cis* activation with lantibiotic synthetase (Figure 4G) [88], subsequent studies demonstrated the generality of in *cis* activation for various enzymes, such as ATP-grasp ligases [89,90] and ATP-dependent cyclodehydratases [91]. Very recently, Lacerna et al. proposed an approach where both the leader and the core peptide were covalently attached to the tailoring enzyme (Figure 4G) [48]. By integrating the leader and core peptides into the enzyme, this method increases reaction efficiency because of the substrate's proximity to the catalytic site, thereby enhancing the specificity and fidelity of complex cyclization reactions. Moreover, this method simplifies the production and purification processes of cyclic peptides, offering a streamlined approach to their isolation.

4.4. Combinatorial Approach

The engineering strategies involving leader peptides, core peptides, and tailoring enzymes can be synergistically combined. A recent study by Sarkar et al. employed multifaceted approaches to produce a broad range of *N*-methylated peptides [40]. Initially, they designed an in vivo expression system wherein OphMA (omphalotin methyltransferase) was fused to the N-terminal of an artificial peptide comprising various core peptides and two recognition sequences for PatA (protease) and PCY1/PsnB (macrocyclase). During heterologous expression, *N*-methylation occurred on the core peptide autocatalytically by in *cis*-activated OphMA. Subsequently, further PTMs involving peptide cleavage and macrocyclization were introduced in vitro by sequentially adding purified PatA and PCY1 (or PsnB), resulting in diverse *N*-methylated peptides. One challenge identified in their study is the limited substrate tolerance of OphMA, in contrast to PatA and PCY1, which have broad substrate specificity. This underscores the importance of promiscuous tailoring enzymes in RiPP engineering.

5. High-Throughput Screening Methods

Recent research efforts have focused on genome mining and peptide engineering to discover novel functional RiPPs as pharmaceutical candidates, through various screening assays as follows: (1) protein binding assays for affinity and binding inhibition tests, (2) growth inhibition assays for antimicrobial activity tests, and (3) cellular assays for cytotoxicity tests. To expedite the process, researchers rely on primary screening conducted in a high-throughput manner. High-throughput screening methods not only enable the identification of RiPPs with desired properties from a vast pool of candidates but also facilitate the characterization of their maturation mechanisms. Key strategies in these efforts include surface display [92–95], two-hybrid systems [53], and mRNA display [39,49,50,96], allowing researchers to rapidly screen peptide libraries. These screening methods rely on protein–RiPP interactions as well as the zone of inhibition assay [21,54] to assess physiological functions (Figure 5).

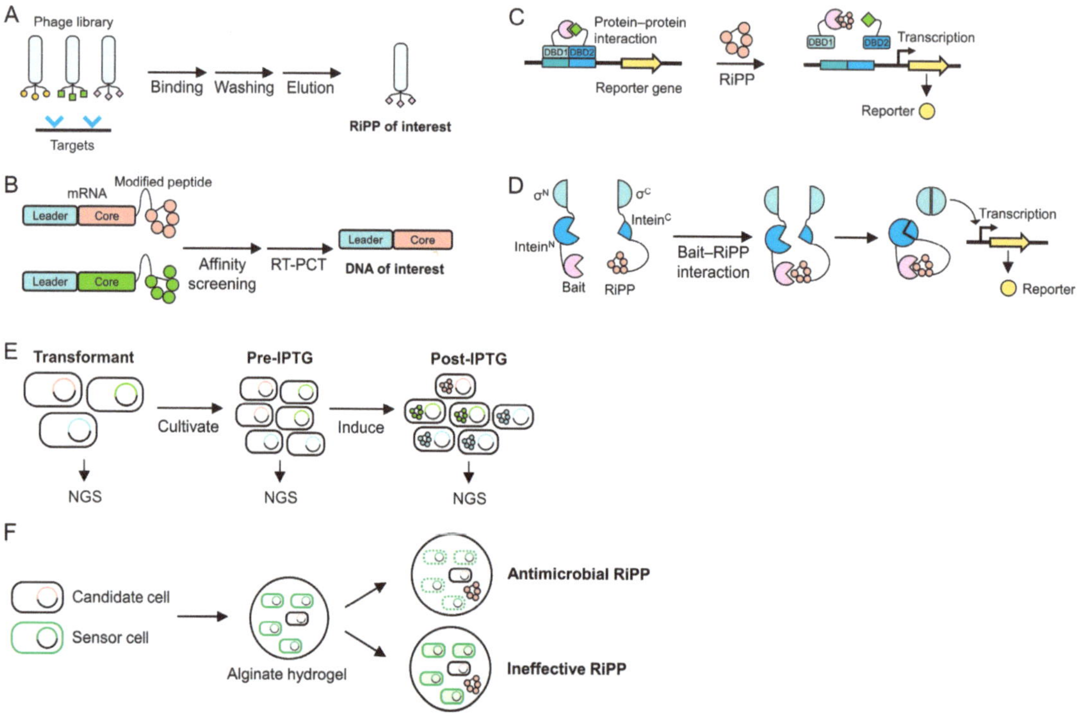

Figure 5. High-throughput screening methods utilized in RiPP research. (**A**) Phage display and (**B**) mRNA display techniques facilitate the straightforward detection of interactions between RiPPs and proteins or molecules. (**C**) The two-hybrid system can identify RiPPs that inhibit protein–protein interactions associated with diseases and infections. (**D**) Another in vivo screening method employs a genetic circuit based on intein, wherein the interaction between a RiPP and a target protein triggers the transcription of a reporter gene, allowing for the detection of RiPP–protein interactions. The antimicrobial activity of RiPPs can be assessed by their ability to inhibit the growth of (**E**) host cells and (**F**) neighboring cells. (**E**) Inhibition of host cell growth correlates with the concentration of RiPPs, as determined by NGS; a lower RiPP concentration signifies higher antimicrobial activity. (**F**) Inhibition of neighboring cell growth is evaluated using sensor cells that express a fluorescent protein; decreased fluorescence intensity indicates higher antimicrobial activity.

5.1. Surface Display

Surface display presents peptides or proteins on the surface of host cells, such as bacteria, yeast, or phages, directly linking the phenotype with its genotype. By genetically fusing the protein of interest to a cell wall or an anchor protein, this technique facilitates easy screening and selection of RiPPs with high affinity and specificity toward particular targets. This is crucial in drug development and enables the detailed study of RiPP–target interactions to understand their mechanisms of action. Despite challenges such as the need for proper peptide folding, display, and host-specific PTMs, surface display remains a powerful method for the high-throughput screening and engineering of RiPPs. It offers versatile platforms like bacterial [92], yeast [95], and phage display [93–95] for RiPP screening. For instance, phage display fuses the peptide of interest to either the N-terminus or C-terminus of a coat protein, such as pIII or pVIII of the M13 bacteriophage, enabling the rapid screening of libraries for targets by exposing the peptide on the surface of bacteriophages (Figure 5A) [97]. Urban et al. implemented the Sec pathway-based phage display to select lanthipeptide libraries specific to urokinase plasminogen activator and streptavidin [94]. Interestingly, PTMs only occurred with fusion to the C-terminus of coat protein pIII, not with N-terminal fusion. This is likely because N-terminal fusion directed the lanthipeptides toward the periplasm on the inner membrane during phage display, making them inaccessible to tailoring enzymes because the Sec pathway translocated the peptide in an unfolded state [94]. Conversely, the lanthipeptide with C-terminal fusion to pIII faced toward the cytoplasm during the assembly of coat proteins, ensuring sufficient time for PTMs. However, peptide fusion to the C-terminus of coat proteins may display inactive RiPPs because maturation typically accompanies the cleavage of a leader peptide by proteases [11]. Hetrick et al. addressed this issue by exploiting the Tat pathway, where translocation is accomplished in the folded state, by fusing NisA, the nisin-encoding gene, to the N-terminus of pIII [95]. They succeeded in displaying mature nisin on bacteriophages with the treatment of NisP protease to detach the leader peptide from the displayed nisin.

5.2. *mRNA Display*

Surface display technologies, while powerful, are subject to several limitations as follows: restricted library sizes (~10^9) [96], the avidity effect arising from displaying multiple copies of peptides [98], and in vivo biases during processes such as transformation and translocation [99]. In contrast, mRNA display, wherein the phenotype (i.e., peptide) is covalently connected to the genotype (i.e., mRNA) via a puromycin link, offers significant advantages by accommodating larger library sizes (~10^{13}), facilitating display in a monomeric context, and employing a simple display scaffold (Figure 5B) [96]. For instance, Bowler et al. utilized mRNA display to screen peptide libraries (~5×10^{11}) against two cancer targets including the calcium and integrin-binding protein CIB1 and the immune checkpoint protein B7-H3 [39]. In constructing the library, they utilized microbial transglutaminase, a versatile enzyme for lysine–glutamine cyclization, to generate diverse macrocyclic peptides, followed by trypsin treatment to distinguish between cyclized and non-cyclized substrates. Subsequently, they selected potent peptides through affinity selection against CIB1 and B7-H3, leading to the high-throughput discovery of specific inhibitors.

mRNA display is also instrumental in the field of post-translational enzymology. Fleming et al. applied mRNA display to study the interaction between the tailoring enzyme PaaA and approximately 34 million PaaP variants, wherein six specific sites from T6 to I11 were randomly mutated, during the biosynthesis of the antibiotic Pantocin A [49]. This technique enabled them to explore the tailoring enzyme's substrate tolerance and the impact of various mutations on enzyme activity, enhancing their understanding of peptide–protein interactions and the synthesis of novel RiPPs. Recent advances in computer science have opened a new era to predict biological interaction. Recently, Vinogradov et al. combined mRNA display with deep learning to investigate the substrate fitness landscapes of Ser dehydratase and YcaO cyclodehydratase involved in lactazole A biosynthesis [50]. This innovative approach generates extensive datasets from mRNA display, which are then analyzed using deep learning algorithms to predict enzymatic substrate preferences. By integrating deep learning, this platform offers a more precise mapping of catalytic preferences of tailoring enzymes, elucidating the molecular basis of cellular processes.

5.3. *Two-Hybrid System*

The ribosomal synthesis of RiPPs makes the two-hybrid system amenable to high-throughput screening for target proteins. This system is instrumental in detecting peptide–protein interactions in vivo by fusing the peptide/protein of interest to separate domains of a transcription factor (Figure 5C) [100]. The interaction between the peptide and the protein reconstitutes a functional transcription factor that activates a reporter gene, leading to color development or growth on selective media. Applied to RiPPs, the two-hybrid system facilitates the identification of novel tailoring enzymes essential for PTMs and RiPP candidates for drug development. Yang et al. employed a lanthipeptide library screening in an *E. coli* host cell through a bacterial reverse two-hybrid system based on the chimeric operator and the repressor of a bacteriophage regulatory system [53]. To identify a lanthipeptide inhibiting the critical protein–protein interaction necessary for HIV budding, they designed two fusion proteins including 434-human TSG101 UEV and P22-HIV p6. The bacteriophage proteins 434 and P22 create a functional repressor complex that inhibits the expression of reporter genes HIS3 and Kan^R, which is essential for cell survival on specific media. The repression depends on the p6 and UEV protein–protein interaction, where the binding of a lanthipeptide disrupts the p6-UEV interaction, conferring a growth advantage. Screening approximately 10^6 libraries led to the identification of a potent inhibitor, XY3-3, heralding a new era in the discovery and development of novel therapeutic agents.

5.4. Intein-Based Genetic Circuit

On the other hand, King et al. leveraged a split intein system for in vivo detection of protein–protein interactions, addressing the challenge of identifying peptides that bind to "undruggable" targets without predefined binding sites [51]. Inteins are protein segments capable of excising themselves and ligating the remaining proteins into a new protein through protein splicing. By constructing two chimeric proteins comprising the σ factorN (N-terminal domain)-NpuN-bait and RiPP-NpuC (C-terminal domain)-σ factorC, they converted peptide–protein binding events into the transcription of reporter genes such as GFP and luciferase through a genetic circuit (Figure 5D). Utilizing *E. coli* as the host, this system tested 10^8 RiPP variants simultaneously, significantly surpassing traditional methods in throughput and specificity. By using the SARS-CoV Spike receptor-binding domain as bait, this approach identified AMK-1057, a probable therapeutic against the SARS-CoV-2 virus, underscoring its potential as a powerful tool for drug discovery based on synthetic biology and offering a promising outlook for targeting proteins previously considered undruggable.

5.5. Next-Generation Sequencing

For the high-throughput screening of novel antibiotics to inhibit RNA polymerase, Thokkadam et al. utilized next-generation sequencing (NGS) to analyze lasso peptide ubonodin variants (Figure 5E) [52]. The screening process involved a library of cells, each producing a distinct ubonodin variant. Upon induction, cells harboring ubonodin variants that inhibited RNA polymerase (RNAP) would perish, while those with either inactive or immature variants would survive. The variants retaining RNAP inhibition activity were identified by sequencing the plasmids from the surviving cell library. To ensure accuracy, five stages of sequencing were performed as follows: the naive library, cloning transformation, screen transformation, pre-IPTG, and post-IPTG. PCR amplification with barcoded primers was used to achieve an over-representation of library samples, ensuring adequate coverage during sequencing on an Illumina MiSeq platform. The analysis focused on the relative frequencies of amino acid substitutions, with increases indicating a loss in RNAP inhibition activity. This method not only facilitated the discovery of potential antibiotics for treating infections caused by *Burkholderia cepacia* complex pathogens but also enabled a comprehensive structure–activity analysis of ubonodin variants.

5.6. Zone of Inhibition Assay

The antimicrobial feature of RiPPs can be screened using the zone of inhibition assay, where microbes grow only in regions devoid of antibiotics. A limitation of this method is its labor-intensive nature and low throughput. Schmitt et al. developed an innovative strategy called nanoFleming to screen antibiotic candidates through the growth inhibition of target bacteria (Figure 5F) [54]. This method miniaturizes and parallelizes Fleming's inhibition zone assay into a high-throughput format to screen large libraries of lanthipeptide variants that inhibit the growth of pathogenic bacteria. For the assay, two types of cells were prepared including mCherry-producing candidate cells that also secreted pre-lanthipeptide variants and GFP-producing sensor cells. These were immobilized in a 500 μm/65 nL alginate hydrogel compartment with a soluble protease. When a secreted lanthipeptide variant exhibited antimicrobial activity, the growth of the sensor cell was inhibited, leading to a decrease in green fluorescence intensity. Using this assay, they identified 11 peptides effective against bacteria showing immunity or resistance to nisin. Focusing on growth inhibition as a measure of antimicrobial activity, the nanoFleming platform emerges as particularly valuable in the development of new therapies to combat antibiotic-resistant bacteria.

The zone of growth inhibition is also an attractive method for robotic screening. In 2022, Guo et al. developed a semi-automated workflow in which lanthipeptide variant libraries were robotically constructed, expressed, and screened [21]. This workflow included an antimicrobial screening step by the zone of growth inhibition using microtiter plates to ensure compatibility with robotic automation. Using this workflow, they constructed a library of 380 single-site and 1373 triple-site mutants of HalA1, resulting in one variant with enhanced antimicrobial activity. Despite a few limitations, such as the poor correlation between the zone of growth inhibition assay using cell lysates and the specific activity using purified peptides, this automated workflow exemplifies the integration of synthetic biology and automation for the rapid and high-throughput characterization of natural products.

6. Conclusions

In this comprehensive analysis, we explore the vibrant and multifaceted landscape of biotechnological innovation and potential therapeutic discovery presented by RiPPs. The intricate biosynthetic pathways highlight the biological significance and complexity of RiPPs. The various PTMs that RiPPs undergo not only exemplify the diversity and specificity inherent in biological systems but also underscore the delicate balance between structure and function, crucial for the peptides' bioactivity.

Advancements in synthetic biology and genetic engineering techniques have significantly broadened the scope of RiPP production and modification, overcoming previous limitations and opening new avenues for exploration. By engineering precursor peptides, tailoring enzymes, and host organisms, scientists can produce RiPPs with enhanced properties or entirely novel functions.

The evolution of screening methods, from traditional assays to cutting-edge technologies like mRNA display and next-generation sequencing, enables researchers to efficiently screen through vast libraries of variants. These techniques expedite the discovery of promising candidates and facilitate a deeper understanding of the intricate relationships between peptide structure, function, and biosynthetic machinery. Leveraging high-throughput and precise methodologies, the field is poised to uncover RiPPs with unique and potent biological activities, marking a significant stride toward addressing the need for new antimicrobial agents and therapeutic peptides.

In conclusion, the study of RiPP biosynthesis, engineering, and screening exemplifies the power of synthetic biology in unlocking nature's mysteries and highlights the potential of RiPPs as a rich source of innovative therapeutic agents. As research progresses, the integration of advanced genetic engineering strategies and high-throughput screening methods will undoubtedly continue to push the boundaries of what is possible, leading to the development of novel RiPP-based applications in medicine, agriculture, and biotechnology.

Author Contributions: S.-W.H. conceived the outline. S.-W.H. and H.-S.W. drafted and revised this manuscript. All authors have read and agreed to the published version of the manuscript.

Funding: This paper was supported by Konkuk University in 2021.

Conflicts of Interest: The authors declare no conflicts of interest.

References

1. Arnison, P.G.; Bibb, M.J.; Bierbaum, G.; Bowers, A.A.; Bugni, T.S.; Bulaj, G.; Camarero, J.A.; Campopiano, D.J.; Challis, G.L.; Clardy, J.; et al. Ribosomally Synthesized and Post-Translationally Modified Peptide Natural Products: Overview and Recommendations for a Universal Nomenclature. *Nat. Prod. Rep.* **2012**, *30*, 108–160. [CrossRef] [PubMed]

2. Fischbach, M.A.; Walsh, C.T. Assembly-Line Enzymology for Polyketide and Nonribosomal Peptide Antibiotics: Logic, Machinery, and Mechanisms. *Chem. Rev.* **2006**, *106*, 3468–3496. [CrossRef] [PubMed]
3. Hudson, G.A.; Mitchell, D.A. RiPP Antibiotics: Biosynthesis and Engineering Potential. *Curr. Opin. Microbiol.* **2018**, *45*, 61–69. [CrossRef] [PubMed]
4. Fu, Y.; Jaarsma, A.H.; Kuipers, O.P. Antiviral Activities and Applications of Ribosomally Synthesized and Post-Translationally Modified Peptides (RiPPs). *Cell. Mol. Life Sci.* **2021**, *78*, 3921–3940. [CrossRef] [PubMed]
5. Frattaruolo, L.; Lacret, R.; Cappello, A.R.; Truman, A.W. A Genomics-Based Approach Identifies a Thioviridamide-Like Compound with Selective Anticancer Activity. *ACS Chem. Biol.* **2017**, *12*, 2815–2822. [CrossRef]
6. Pfeiffer, I.P.-M.; Schröder, M.-P.; Mordhorst, S. Opportunities and Challenges of RiPP-Based Therapeutics. *Nat. Prod. Rep.* 2024, *Online ahead of print.* [CrossRef]
7. Zhou, D.; Wang, X.; Anjago, W.M.; Li, J.; Li, W.; Li, M.; Jiu, M.; Zhang, Q.; Zhang, J.; Deng, S.; et al. Borrelidin-Producing and Root-Colonizing *Streptomyces Rochei* is a Potent Biopesticide for Two Soil-Borne Oomycete-Caused Plant Diseases. *Biol. Control* **2024**, *188*, 105411. [CrossRef]
8. Gharsallaoui, A.; Oulahal, N.; Joly, C.; Degraeve, P. Nisin as a Food Preservative: Part 1: Physicochemical Properties, Antimicrobial Activity, and Main Uses. *Crit. Rev. Food Sci. Nutr.* **2016**, *56*, 1262–1274. [CrossRef] [PubMed]
9. Rodríguez, V. Insights into Post-Translational Modification Enzymes from RiPPs: A Toolkit for Applications in Peptide Synthesis. *Biotechnol. Adv.* **2022**, *56*, 107908. [CrossRef]
10. Fu, Y.; Xu, Y.; Ruijne, F.; Kuipers, O.P. Engineering Lanthipeptides by Introducing a Large Variety of RiPP Modifications to Obtain New-to-Nature Bioactive Peptides. *FEMS Microbiol. Rev.* **2023**, *47*, fuad017. [CrossRef]
11. Eslami, S.M.; van der Donk, W.A. Proteases Involved in Leader Peptide Removal during RiPP Biosynthesis. *ACS Bio Med Chem Au* **2024**, *4*, 20–36. [CrossRef]
12. Si, T.; Tian, Q.; Min, Y.; Zhang, L.; Sweedler, J.V.; van der Donk, W.A.; Zhao, H. Rapid Screening of Lanthipeptide Analogs via In-Colony Removal of Leader Peptides in *Escherichia coli*. *J. Am. Chem. Soc.* **2018**, *140*, 11884–11888. [CrossRef]
13. Duan, H.; Zhang, X.; Figeys, D. An Emerging Field: Post-Translational Modification in Microbiome. *Proteomics* **2023**, *23*, 2100389. [CrossRef]
14. Wang, G. Post-Translational Modifications of Natural Antimicrobial Peptides and Strategies for Peptide Engineering. *Curr. Biotechnol.* **2012**, *1*, 72–79. [CrossRef]
15. Gualillo, O.; Lago, F.; Casanueva, F.F.; Dieguez, C. One Ancestor, Several Peptides: Post-Translational Modifications of Preproghrelin Generate Several Peptides with Antithetical Effects. *Mol. Cell. Endocrinol.* **2006**, *256*, 1–8. [CrossRef]
16. Sun, Z.; Xia, Z.; Bi, F.; Liu, J.-N. Expression and Purification of Human Urodilatin by Small Ubiquitin-Related Modifier Fusion in *Escherichia coli*. *Appl. Microbiol. Biotechnol.* **2008**, *78*, 495–502. [CrossRef]
17. Li, J.F.; Zhang, J.; Zhang, Z.; Ma, H.W.; Zhang, J.X.; Zhang, S.Q. Production of Bioactive Human Beta-Defensin-4 in *Escherichia coli* Using SUMO Fusion Partner. *Protein J.* **2010**, *29*, 314–319. [CrossRef]
18. Glassey, E.; King, A.M.; Anderson, D.A.; Zhang, Z.; Voigt, C.A. Functional Expression of Diverse Post-Translational Peptide-Modifying Enzymes in *Escherichia coli* under Uniform Expression and Purification Conditions. *PLoS ONE* **2022**, *17*, e0266488. [CrossRef]
19. Vermeulen, R.R.; Van Staden, A.D.P.; Dicks, L. Heterologous Expression of the Class IIa Bacteriocins, Plantaricin 423 and Mundticin ST4SA, in *Escherichia coli* Using Green Fluorescent Protein as a Fusion Partner. *Front. Microbiol.* **2020**, *11*, 535667. [CrossRef]
20. Van Zyl, W.F.; Van Staden, A.D.; Dicks, L.M.T.; Trindade, M. Use of the mCherry Fluorescent Protein to Optimize the Expression of Class I Lanthipeptides in *Escherichia coli*. *Microb. Cell Factories* **2023**, *22*, 149. [CrossRef]
21. Guo, E.; Fu, L.; Fang, X.; Xie, W.; Li, K.; Zhang, Z.; Hong, Z.; Si, T. Robotic Construction and Screening of Lanthipeptide Variant Libraries in *Escherichia coli*. *ACS Synth. Biol.* **2022**, *11*, 3900–3911. [CrossRef] [PubMed]
22. Ren, H.; Dommaraju, S.R.; Huang, C.; Cui, H.; Pan, Y.; Nesic, M.; Zhu, L.; Sarlah, D.; Mitchell, D.A.; Zhao, H. Genome Mining Unveils a Class of Ribosomal Peptides with Two Amino Termini. *Nat. Commun.* **2023**, *14*, 1624. [CrossRef] [PubMed]
23. Santos-Aberturas, J.; Chandra, G.; Frattaruolo, L.; Lacret, R.; Pham, T.H.; Vior, N.M.; Eyles, T.H.; Truman, A.W. Uncovering the Unexplored Diversity of Thioamidated Ribosomal Peptides in Actinobacteria Using the RiPPER Genome Mining Tool. *Nucleic Acids Res.* **2019**, *47*, 4624–4637. [CrossRef] [PubMed]
24. Blin, K.; Shaw, S.; Augustijn, H.E.; Reitz, Z.L.; Biermann, F.; Alanjary, M.; Fetter, A.; Terlouw, B.R.; Metcalf, W.W.; Helfrich, E.J.N.; et al. antiSMASH 7.0: New and Improved Predictions for Detection, Regulation, Chemical Structures and Visualisation. *Nucleic Acids Res.* **2023**, *51*, W46–W50. [CrossRef] [PubMed]
25. Skinnider, M.A.; Johnston, C.W.; Gunabalasingam, M.; Merwin, N.J.; Kieliszek, A.M.; MacLellan, R.J.; Li, H.; Ranieri, M.R.M.; Webster, A.L.H.; Cao, M.P.T.; et al. Comprehensive Prediction of Secondary Metabolite Structure and Biological Activity from Microbial Genome Sequences. *Nat. Commun.* **2020**, *11*, 6058. [CrossRef] [PubMed]
26. Tietz, J.I.; Schwalen, C.J.; Patel, P.S.; Maxson, T.; Blair, P.M.; Tai, H.-C.; Zakai, U.I.; Mitchell, D.A. A New Genome-Mining Tool Redefines the Lasso Peptide Biosynthetic Landscape. *Nat. Chem. Biol.* **2017**, *13*, 470–478. [CrossRef] [PubMed]
27. Kloosterman, A.M.; Medema, M.H.; van Wezel, G.P. Omics-Based Strategies to Discover Novel Classes of RiPP Natural Products. *Curr. Opin. Biotechnol.* **2021**, *69*, 60–67. [CrossRef] [PubMed]

28. Russell, A.H.; Truman, A.W. Genome Mining Strategies for Ribosomally Synthesised and Post-Translationally Modified Peptides. *Comput. Struct. Biotechnol. J.* **2020**, *18*, 1838–1851. [CrossRef] [PubMed]
29. Smanski, M.J.; Zhou, H.; Claesen, J.; Shen, B.; Fischbach, M.A.; Voigt, C.A. Synthetic Biology to Access and Expand Nature's Chemical Diversity. *Nat. Rev. Microbiol.* **2016**, *14*, 135–149. [CrossRef]
30. Thibodeaux, C.J. The Conformationally Dynamic Structural Biology of Lanthipeptide Biosynthesis. *Curr. Opin. Struct. Biol.* **2023**, *81*, 102644. [CrossRef]
31. Lohans, C.T.; Vederas, J.C. Structural Characterization of Thioether-Bridged Bacteriocins. *J. Antibiot.* **2014**, *67*, 23–30. [CrossRef]
32. Enghiad, B.; Huang, C.; Guo, F.; Jiang, G.; Wang, B.; Tabatabaei, S.K.; Martin, T.A.; Zhao, H. Cas12a-Assisted Precise Targeted Cloning Using in Vivo Cre-Lox Recombination. *Nat. Commun.* **2021**, *12*, 1171. [CrossRef] [PubMed]
33. Wang, G.; Zhao, Z.; Ke, J.; Engel, Y.; Shi, Y.-M.; Robinson, D.; Bingol, K.; Zhang, Z.; Bowen, B.; Louie, K.; et al. CRAGE Enables Rapid Activation of Biosynthetic Gene Clusters in Undomesticated Bacteria. *Nat. Microbiol.* **2019**, *4*, 2498–2510. [CrossRef] [PubMed]
34. Wang, H.; Li, Z.; Jia, R.; Yin, J.; Li, A.; Xia, L.; Yin, Y.; Müller, R.; Fu, J.; Stewart, A.F.; et al. ExoCET: Exonuclease in Vitro Assembly Combined with RecET Recombination for Highly Efficient Direct DNA Cloning from Complex Genomes. *Nucleic Acids Res.* **2018**, *46*, e28. [CrossRef] [PubMed]
35. Wuisan, Z.G.; Kresna, I.D.M.; Böhringer, N.; Lewis, K.; Schäberle, T.F. Optimization of Heterologous Darobactin A Expression and Identification of the Minimal Biosynthetic Gene Cluster. *Metab. Eng.* **2021**, *66*, 123–136. [CrossRef]
36. King, A.M.; Zhang, Z.; Glassey, E.; Siuti, P.; Clardy, J.; Voigt, C.A. Systematic Mining of the Human Microbiome Identifies Antimicrobial Peptides with Diverse Activity Spectra. *Nat. Microbiol.* **2023**, *8*, 2420–2434. [CrossRef] [PubMed]
37. Ayikpoe, R.S.; Shi, C.; Battiste, A.J.; Eslami, S.M.; Ramesh, S.; Simon, M.A.; Bothwell, I.R.; Lee, H.; Rice, A.J.; Ren, H.; et al. A Scalable Platform to Discover Antimicrobials of Ribosomal Origin. *Nat. Commun.* **2022**, *13*, 6135. [CrossRef]
38. Cao, L.; Do, T.; Zhu, A.; Duan, J.; Alam, N.; Link, A.J. Genome Mining and Discovery of Imiditides, a Family of RiPPs with a Class-Defining Aspartimide Modification. *J. Am. Chem. Soc.* **2023**, *145*, 18834–18845. [CrossRef] [PubMed]
39. Bowler, M.M.; Glavatskikh, M.; Pecot, C.V.; Kireev, D.; Bowers, A.A. Enzymatic Macrolactamization of mRNA Display Libraries for Inhibitor Selection. *ACS Chem. Biol.* **2023**, *18*, 166–175. [CrossRef]
40. Sarkar, S.; Gu, W.; Schmidt, E.W. Applying Promiscuous RiPP Enzymes to Peptide Backbone N-Methylation Chemistry. *ACS Chem. Biol.* **2022**, *17*, 2165–2178. [CrossRef]
41. Liu, R.; Zhang, Y.; Zhai, G.; Fu, S.; Xia, Y.; Hu, B.; Cai, X.; Zhang, Y.; Li, Y.; Deng, Z.; et al. A Cell-Free Platform Based on Nisin Biosynthesis for Discovering Novel Lanthipeptides and Guiding Their Overproduction In Vivo. *Adv. Sci.* **2020**, *7*, 2001616. [CrossRef]
42. Kunakom, S.; Eustáquio, A.S. Heterologous Production of Lasso Peptide Capistruin in a Burkholderia Host. *ACS Synth. Biol.* **2020**, *9*, 241–248. [CrossRef] [PubMed]
43. Eastman, K.A.S.; Kincannon, W.M.; Bandarian, V. Leveraging Substrate Promiscuity of a Radical S-Adenosyl-L-Methionine RiPP Maturase toward Intramolecular Peptide Cross-Linking Applications. *ACS Cent. Sci.* **2022**, *8*, 1209–1217. [CrossRef] [PubMed]
44. Zhao, X.; Kuipers, O.P. Nisin- and Ripcin-Derived Hybrid Lanthipeptides Display Selective Antimicrobial Activity against Staphylococcus Aureus. *ACS Synth. Biol.* **2021**, *10*, 1703–1714. [CrossRef] [PubMed]
45. Guo, L.; Stoffels, K.; Broos, J.; Kuipers, O.P. Engineering Hybrid Lantibiotics Yields the Highly Stable and Bacteriocidal Peptide Cerocin V. *Microbiol. Res.* **2024**, *282*, 127640. [CrossRef]
46. Franz, L.; Koehnke, J. Leader Peptide Exchange to Produce Hybrid, New-to-Nature Ribosomal Natural Products. *Chem. Commun.* **2021**, *57*, 6372–6375. [CrossRef]
47. Estrada, P.; Morita, M.; Hao, Y.; Schmidt, E.W.; Nair, S.K. A Single Amino Acid Switch Alters the Isoprene Donor Specificity in Ribosomally Synthesized and Post-Translationally Modified Peptide Prenyltransferases. *J. Am. Chem. Soc.* **2018**, *140*, 8124–8127. [CrossRef] [PubMed]
48. Lacerna, N.I.; Cong, Y.; Schmidt, E.W. An Autocatalytic Peptide Cyclase Improves Fidelity and Yield of Circular Peptides In Vivo and In Vitro. *ACS Synth. Biol.* **2024**, *13*, 394–401. [CrossRef]
49. Fleming, S.R.; Himes, P.M.; Ghodge, S.V.; Goto, Y.; Suga, H.; Bowers, A.A. Exploring the Post-Translational Enzymology of PaaA by mRNA Display. *J. Am. Chem. Soc.* **2020**, *142*, 5024–5028. [CrossRef] [PubMed]
50. Vinogradov, A.A.; Chang, J.S.; Onaka, H.; Goto, Y.; Suga, H. Accurate Models of Substrate Preferences of Post-Translational Modification Enzymes from a Combination of mRNA Display and Deep Learning. *ACS Cent. Sci.* **2022**, *8*, 814–824. [CrossRef]
51. King, A.M.; Anderson, D.A.; Glassey, E.; Segall-Shapiro, T.H.; Zhang, Z.; Niquille, D.L.; Embree, A.C.; Pratt, K.; Williams, T.L.; Gordon, D.B.; et al. Selection for Constrained Peptides That Bind to a Single Target Protein. *Nat. Commun.* **2021**, *12*, 6343. [CrossRef]
52. Thokkadam, A.; Do, T.; Ran, X.; Brynildsen, M.P.; Yang, Z.J.; Link, A.J. High-Throughput Screen Reveals the Structure–Activity Relationship of the Antimicrobial Lasso Peptide Ubonodin. *ACS Cent. Sci.* **2023**, *9*, 540–550. [CrossRef]
53. Yang, X.; Lennard, K.R.; He, C.; Walker, M.C.; Ball, A.T.; Doigneaux, C.; Tavassoli, A.; van der Donk, W.A. A Lanthipeptide Library Used to Identify a Protein–Protein Interaction Inhibitor. *Nat. Chem. Biol.* **2018**, *14*, 375–380. [CrossRef]
54. Schmitt, S.; Montalbán-López, M.; Peterhoff, D.; Deng, J.; Wagner, R.; Held, M.; Kuipers, O.P.; Panke, S. Analysis of Modular Bioengineered Antimicrobial Lanthipeptides at Nanoliter Scale. *Nat. Chem. Biol.* **2019**, *15*, 437–443. [CrossRef]

55. Zhang, Q.; Yu, Y.; Vélasquez, J.E.; van der Donk, W.A. Evolution of Lanthipeptide Synthetases. *Proc. Natl. Acad. Sci. USA* **2012**, *109*, 18361–18366. [CrossRef]
56. McBrayer, D.N.; Gantman, B.K.; Tal-Gan, Y. N-Methylation of Amino Acids in Gelatinase Biosynthesis-Activating Pheromone Identifies Key Site for Stability Enhancement with Retention of the Enterococcus Faecalis Fsr Quorum Sensing Circuit Response. *ACS Infect. Dis.* **2019**, *5*, 1035–1041. [CrossRef]
57. Su, Y.; Han, M.; Meng, X.; Feng, Y.; Luo, S.; Yu, C.; Zheng, G.; Zhu, S. Discovery and Characterization of a Novel C-Terminal Peptide Carboxyl Methyltransferase in a Lassomycin-like Lasso Peptide Biosynthetic Pathway. *Appl. Microbiol. Biotechnol.* **2019**, *103*, 2649–2664. [CrossRef]
58. Acedo, J.Z.; Bothwell, I.R.; An, L.; Trouth, A.; Frazier, C.; van der Donk, W.A. O-Methyltransferase-Mediated Incorporation of a β-Amino Acid in Lanthipeptides. *J. Am. Chem. Soc.* **2019**, *141*, 16790–16801. [CrossRef]
59. Gavrish, E.; Sit, C.S.; Cao, S.; Kandror, O.; Spoering, A.; Peoples, A.; Ling, L.; Fetterman, A.; Hughes, D.; Bissell, A.; et al. Lassomycin, a Ribosomally Synthesized Cyclic Peptide, Kills *Mycobacterium Tuberculosis* by Targeting the ATP-Dependent Protease ClpC1P1P2. *Chem. Biol.* **2014**, *21*, 509–518. [CrossRef]
60. Maget-Dana, R.; Ptak, M. Interactions of Surfactin with Membrane Models. *Biophys. J.* **1995**, *68*, 1937–1943. [CrossRef] [PubMed]
61. He, B.-B.; Cheng, Z.; Zhong, Z.; Gao, Y.; Liu, H.; Li, Y.-X. Expanded Sequence Space of Radical S-Adenosylmethionine-Dependent Enzymes Involved in Post-Translational Macrocyclization**. *Angew. Chem. Int. Ed.* **2022**, *61*, e202212447. [CrossRef] [PubMed]
62. Yu, Y.; van der Donk, W.A. Biosynthesis of 3-Thia-α-Amino Acids on a Carrier Peptide. *Proc. Natl. Acad. Sci. USA* **2022**, *119*, e2205285119. [CrossRef]
63. Guo, L.; Stoffels, K.; Broos, J.; Kuipers, O.P. Altering Specificity and Enhancing Stability of the Antimicrobial Peptides Nisin and Rombocin through Dehydrated Amino Acid Residue Engineering. *Peptides* **2024**, *174*, 171152. [CrossRef]
64. Rutledge, P.J.; Challis, G.L. Discovery of Microbial Natural Products by Activation of Silent Biosynthetic Gene Clusters. *Nat. Rev. Microbiol.* **2015**, *13*, 509–523. [CrossRef]
65. Xue, Y.; Braslavsky, I.; Quake, S.R. Temperature Effect on Polymerase Fidelity. *J. Biol. Chem.* **2021**, *297*, 101270. [CrossRef]
66. Gibson, D.G.; Young, L.; Chuang, R.-Y.; Venter, J.C.; Hutchison, C.A.; Smith, H.O. Enzymatic Assembly of DNA Molecules up to Several Hundred Kilobases. *Nat. Methods* **2009**, *6*, 343–345. [CrossRef]
67. Casini, A.; Storch, M.; Baldwin, G.S.; Ellis, T. Bricks and Blueprints: Methods and Standards for DNA Assembly. *Nat. Rev. Mol. Cell Biol.* **2015**, *16*, 568–576. [CrossRef]
68. Li, L.; Zhao, Y.; Ruan, L.; Yang, S.; Ge, M.; Jiang, W.; Lu, Y. A Stepwise Increase in Pristinamycin II Biosynthesis by *Streptomyces Pristinaespiralis* through Combinatorial Metabolic Engineering. *Metab. Eng.* **2015**, *29*, 12–25. [CrossRef]
69. Sharan, S.K.; Thomason, L.C.; Kuznetsov, S.G.; Court, D.L. Recombineering: A Homologous Recombination-Based Method of Genetic Engineering. *Nat. Protoc.* **2009**, *4*, 206–223. [CrossRef]
70. Fu, J.; Bian, X.; Hu, S.; Wang, H.; Huang, F.; Seibert, P.M.; Plaza, A.; Xia, L.; Müller, R.; Stewart, A.F.; et al. Full-Length RecE Enhances Linear-Linear Homologous Recombination and Facilitates Direct Cloning for Bioprospecting. *Nat. Biotechnol.* **2012**, *30*, 440–446. [CrossRef]
71. Kouprina, N.; Larionov, V. Transformation-Associated Recombination (TAR) Cloning for Genomics Studies and Synthetic Biology. *Chromosoma* **2016**, *125*, 621–632. [CrossRef]
72. Nagy, A. Cre Recombinase: The Universal Reagent for Genome Tailoring. *Genesis* **2000**, *26*, 99–109. [CrossRef]
73. Kuipers, A.; Wierenga, J.; Rink, R.; Kluskens, L.D.; Driessen, A.J.M.; Kuipers, O.P.; Moll, G.N. Sec-Mediated Transport of Posttranslationally Dehydrated Peptides in Lactococcus Lactis. *Appl. Environ. Microbiol.* **2006**, *72*, 7626–7633. [CrossRef]
74. Jiménez, J.J.; Diep, D.B.; Borrero, J.; Gútiez, L.; Arbulu, S.; Nes, I.F.; Herranz, C.; Cintas, L.M.; Hernández, P.E. Cloning Strategies for Heterologous Expression of the Bacteriocin Enterocin A by Lactobacillus Sakei Lb790, Lb. Plantarum NC8 and Lb. Casei CECT475. *Microb. Cell Factories* **2015**, *14*, 166. [CrossRef]
75. Li, X.; Yang, H.; Zhang, D.; Li, X.; Yu, H.; Shen, Z. Overexpression of Specific Proton Motive Force-Dependent Transporters Facilitate the Export of Surfactin in Bacillus Subtilis. *J. Ind. Microbiol. Biotechnol.* **2015**, *42*, 93–103. [CrossRef]
76. Kuipers, A.; de Boef, E.; Rink, R.; Fekken, S.; Kluskens, L.D.; Driessen, A.J.M.; Leenhouts, K.; Kuipers, O.P.; Moll, G.N. NisT, the Transporter of the Lantibiotic Nisin, Can Transport Fully Modified, Dehydrated, and Unmodified Prenisin and Fusions of the Leader Peptide with Non-Lantibiotic Peptides. *J. Biol. Chem.* **2004**, *279*, 22176–22182. [CrossRef]
77. Huo, L.; Rachid, S.; Stadler, M.; Wenzel, S.C.; Müller, R. Synthetic Biotechnology to Study and Engineer Ribosomal Bottromycin Biosynthesis. *Chem. Biol.* **2012**, *19*, 1278–1287. [CrossRef]
78. Havarstein, L.S.; Diep, D.B.; Nes, I.F. A Family of Bacteriocin ABC Transporters Carry out Proteolytic Processing of Their Substrates Concomitant with Export. *Mol. Microbiol.* **1995**, *16*, 229–240. [CrossRef]
79. Hegemann, J.D.; Jeanne Dit Fouque, K.; Santos-Fernandez, M.; Fernandez-Lima, F. A Bifunctional Leader Peptidase/ABC Transporter Protein Is Involved in the Maturation of the Lasso Peptide Cochonodin I from Streptococcus Suis. *J. Nat. Prod.* **2021**, *84*, 2683–2691. [CrossRef]
80. Rücker, E.; Schneider, G.; Steinhäuser, K.; Löwer, R.; Hauber, J.; Stauber, R.H. Rapid Evaluation and Optimization of Recombinant Protein Production Using GFP Tagging. *Protein Expr. Purif.* **2001**, *21*, 220–223. [CrossRef]
81. Fernandez, H.N.; Kretsch, A.M.; Kunakom, S.; Kadjo, A.E.; Mitchell, D.A.; Eustáquio, A.S. High-Yield Lasso Peptide Production in a Burkholderia Bacterial Host by Plasmid Copy Number Engineering. *ACS Synth. Biol.* **2024**, *13*, 337–350. [CrossRef]

82. Nguyen, N.A.; Cong, Y.; Hurrell, R.C.; Arias, N.; Garg, N.; Puri, A.W.; Schmidt, E.W.; Agarwal, V. A Silent Biosynthetic Gene Cluster from a Methanotrophic Bacterium Potentiates Discovery of a Substrate Promiscuous Proteusin Cyclodehydratase. *ACS Chem. Biol.* **2022**, *17*, 1577–1585. [CrossRef]
83. Precord, T.W.; Mahanta, N.; Mitchell, D.A. Reconstitution and Substrate Specificity of the Thioether-Forming Radical S-Adenosylmethionine Enzyme in Freyrasin Biosynthesis. *ACS Chem. Biol.* **2019**, *14*, 1981–1989. [CrossRef]
84. Burkhart, B.J.; Kakkar, N.; Hudson, G.A.; van der Donk, W.A.; Mitchell, D.A. Chimeric Leader Peptides for the Generation of Non-Natural Hybrid RiPP Products. *ACS Cent. Sci.* **2017**, *3*, 629–638. [CrossRef]
85. Jin, L.; Wu, X.; Xue, Y.; Jin, Y.; Wang, S.; Chen, Y. Mutagenesis of NosM Leader Peptide Reveals Important Elements in Nosiheptide Biosynthesis. *Appl. Environ. Microbiol.* **2017**, *83*, e02880-16. [CrossRef]
86. Liu, F.; van Heel, A.J.; Kuipers, O.P. Leader- and Terminal Residue Requirements for Circularin A Biosynthesis Probed by Systematic Mutational Analyses. *ACS Synth. Biol.* **2023**, *12*, 852–862. [CrossRef]
87. Levengood, M.R.; Patton, G.C.; van der Donk, W.A. The Leader Peptide Is Not Required for Post-Translational Modification by Lacticin 481 Synthetase. *J. Am. Chem. Soc.* **2007**, *129*, 10314–10315. [CrossRef]
88. Oman, T.J.; Knerr, P.J.; Bindman, N.A.; Velásquez, J.E.; van der Donk, W.A. An Engineered Lantibiotic Synthetase That Does Not Require a Leader Peptide on Its Substrate. *J. Am. Chem. Soc.* **2012**, *134*, 6952–6955. [CrossRef]
89. Patel, K.P.; Silsby, L.M.; Li, G.; Bruner, S.D. Structure-Based Engineering of Peptide Macrocyclases for the Chemoenzymatic Synthesis of Microviridins. *J. Org. Chem.* **2021**, *86*, 11212–11219. [CrossRef]
90. Reyna-González, E.; Schmid, B.; Petras, D.; Süssmuth, R.D.; Dittmann, E. Leader Peptide-Free In Vitro Reconstitution of Microviridin Biosynthesis Enables Design of Synthetic Protease-Targeted Libraries. *Angew. Chem. Int. Ed.* **2016**, *55*, 9398–9401. [CrossRef]
91. Koehnke, J.; Mann, G.; Bent, A.F.; Ludewig, H.; Shirran, S.; Botting, C.; Lebl, T.; Houssen, W.E.; Jaspars, M.; Naismith, J.H. Structural Analysis of Leader Peptide Binding Enables Leader-Free Cyanobactin Processing. *Nat. Chem. Biol.* **2015**, *11*, 558–563. [CrossRef]
92. Bosma, T.; Kuipers, A.; Bulten, E.; de Vries, L.; Rink, R.; Moll, G.N. Bacterial Display and Screening of Posttranslationally Thioether-Stabilized Peptides. *Appl. Environ. Microbiol.* **2011**, *77*, 6794–6801. [CrossRef]
93. Wang, X.S.; Chen, P.-H.C.; Hampton, J.T.; Tharp, J.M.; Reed, C.A.; Das, S.K.; Wang, D.-S.; Hayatshahi, H.S.; Shen, Y.; Liu, J.; et al. A Genetically Encoded, Phage-Displayed Cyclic-Peptide Library. *Angew. Chem. Int. Ed.* **2019**, *58*, 15904–15909. [CrossRef]
94. Urban, J.H.; Moosmeier, M.A.; Aumüller, T.; Thein, M.; Bosma, T.; Rink, R.; Groth, K.; Zulley, M.; Siegers, K.; Tissot, K.; et al. Phage Display and Selection of Lanthipeptides on the Carboxy-Terminus of the Gene-3 Minor Coat Protein. *Nat. Commun.* **2017**, *8*, 1500. [CrossRef]
95. Hetrick, K.J.; Walker, M.C.; van der Donk, W.A. Development and Application of Yeast and Phage Display of Diverse Lanthipeptides. *ACS Cent. Sci.* **2018**, *4*, 458–467. [CrossRef]
96. Gold, L. mRNA Display: Diversity Matters during in Vitro Selection. *Proc. Natl. Acad. Sci. USA* **2001**, *98*, 4825–4826. [CrossRef]
97. Bratkovič, T. Progress in Phage Display: Evolution of the Technique and Its Applications. *Cell. Mol. Life Sci.* **2010**, *67*, 749–767. [CrossRef]
98. Cwirla, S.E.; Peters, E.A.; Barrett, R.W.; Dower, W.J. Peptides on Phage: A Vast Library of Peptides for Identifying Ligands. *Proc. Natl. Acad. Sci. USA* **1990**, *87*, 6378–6382. [CrossRef]
99. Zade, H.M.; Keshavarz, R.; Shekarabi, H.S.Z.; Bakhshinejad, B. Biased Selection of Propagation-Related TUPs from Phage Display Peptide Libraries. *Amino Acids* **2017**, *49*, 1293–1308. [CrossRef]
100. Fields, S.; Sternglanz, R. The Two-Hybrid System: An Assay for Protein-Protein Interactions. *Trends Genet.* **1994**, *10*, 286–292. [CrossRef]

biomolecules

Review

LL-37: Structures, Antimicrobial Activity, and Influence on Amyloid-Related Diseases

Surajit Bhattacharjya [1,*], Zhizhuo Zhang [2] and Ayyalusamy Ramamoorthy [2,3,*]

[1] School of Biological Sciences, Nanyang Technological University, 60 Nanyang Drive, Singapore 637551, Singapore
[2] Department of Chemistry, Biomedical Engineering, Macromolecular Science and Engineering, Michigan Neuroscience Institute, The University of Michigan, Ann Arbor, MI 48109, USA; zhizhuoz@umich.edu
[3] National High Magnetic Field Laboratory, Department of Chemical and Biomedical Engineering, Florida State University, Tallahassee, FL 32310, USA
* Correspondence: surajit@ntu.edu.sg (S.B.); aramamoorthy@fsu.edu (A.R.)

Abstract: Antimicrobial peptides (AMPs), as well as host defense peptides (HDPs), constitute the first line of defense as part of the innate immune system. Humans are known to express antimicrobial precursor proteins, which are further processed to generate AMPs, including several types of α/β defensins, histatins, and cathelicidin-derived AMPs like LL37. The broad-spectrum activity of AMPs is crucial to defend against infections caused by pathogenic bacteria, viruses, fungi, and parasites. The emergence of multi-drug resistant pathogenic bacteria is of global concern for public health. The prospects of targeting antibiotic-resistant strains of bacteria with AMPs are of high significance for developing new generations of antimicrobial agents. The 37-residue long LL37, the only cathelicidin family of AMP in humans, has been the major focus for the past few decades of research. The host defense activity of LL37 is likely underscored by its expression throughout the body, spanning from the epithelial cells of various organs—testis, skin, respiratory tract, and gastrointestinal tract—to immune cells. Remarkably, apart from canonical direct killing of pathogenic organisms, LL37 exerts several other host defense activities, including inflammatory response modulation, chemo-attraction, and wound healing and closure at the infected sites. In addition, LL37 and its derived peptides are bestowed with anti-cancer and anti-amyloidogenic properties. In this review article, we aim to develop integrative, mechanistic insight into LL37 and its derived peptides, based on the known biophysical, structural, and functional studies in recent years. We believe that this review will pave the way for future research on the structures, biochemical and biophysical properties, and design of novel LL37-based molecules.

Keywords: antimicrobial peptides; host defense peptides; LL37; structure; biophysical; human antimicrobial peptides

Citation: Bhattacharjya, S.; Zhang, Z.; Ramamoorthy, A. LL-37: Structures, Antimicrobial Activity, and Influence on Amyloid-Related Diseases. *Biomolecules* **2024**, *14*, 320. https://doi.org/10.3390/biom14030320

Academic Editor: Annarita Falanga

Received: 20 January 2024
Revised: 1 March 2024
Accepted: 4 March 2024
Published: 8 March 2024

1. Introduction

Since the discovery of penicillin, antibiotics have saved millions of lives from infectious diseases. Antibiotics are still considered "magic bullets" and continue to serve as eminent drugs to reduce mortality from bacterial infections. However, as we note from the current affairs of antibiotics, these magic bullets are becoming less effective or sometimes even ineffective in curing patients in hospitals and in intensive care facilities [1–3]. At present, antibiotic resistance, or antimicrobial resistance (AMR), is increasing at a rapid rate across the globe, revealing serious consequences to human and animal health [4–6]. Notably, drug-resistant bacteria are responsible for most of the infections and deaths caused by AMR (*vide infra*). The Centers for Disease Control and Prevention (CDC), USA, published their first AMR threat report in 2013 that estimated that over 2 million people were infected by antibiotic-resistant bacteria, causing 23,000 deaths in the USA alone. In a more recent report, the CDC indicated that there are over 2.8 million antimicrobial-resistant infections and 35,000 human deaths every year [7]. In the year 2014, the government of the UK and the Welcome Trust jointly commissioned a review exercise to analyze the global economic impacts arising from AMR [8]. The landmark report of O'Neill made several vital recommendations to the international governments to tackle global AMR challenges [8]. The report also suggested that AMR could cause over 10 million deaths each year by 2050. A recent comprehensive report from the Antimicrobial Resistance Collaborators analyzed the worldwide occurrence of bacterial AMR for the year 2019 [9]. The study estimated a staggering number of deaths, 4.95 million, associated with bacterial AMR in that year. Notably, approximately 3.75 million mortalities associated with bacterial AMR were caused by the six bacterial pathogens, *Escherichia coli*, *Staphylococcus aureus*, *Klebsiella pneumoniae*, *Streptococcus pneumoniae*, *Acinetobacter baumannii*, and *Pseudomonas aeruginosa*. It is noteworthy that these bacteria are also included in the WHO-listed drug-resistant group of pathogens, ESKAPE (*Enterococcus faecium*, *Staphylococcus aureus*, *Klebsiella pneumoniae*, *Acinetobacter baumannii*, *Pseudomonas aeruginosa*, and *Enterobacter species*) [10].

To distinguish their pattern of susceptibility, antibiotic-resistant bacteria are categorized into three classes: multi-drug resistant (MDR), extremely drug resistant (XDR), and pan-drug resistant (PDR). MDR bacteria demonstrate resistance to at least one drug in three or more antimicrobial groups. The XDR group includes pathogens that are susceptible to only one or two categories of antibiotics. PDR bacteria have acquired resistance to all classes of antibiotics [11]. The AMR data analyses delineated that most of the deaths were caused by methicillin-resistant *S. aureus* and several MDR strains of Gram-negative bacteria, such as third-generation cephalosporin-resistant isolates of *E. coli* and *K. pneumoniae*, fluoroquinolone-resistant *E. coli*, and carbapenem-resistant strains of *A. baumannii* and *K. pneumoniae* [10]. In addition to these MDR strains of bacteria, the CDC of the USA has also indicated that drug-resistant strains of *Clostridioides difficile*, *Neisseria gonorrhoeae*, vancomycin-resistant *Enterococcus* (VRE), *Pseudomonas aeruginosa*, *Mycobacterium tuberculosis*, and *Salmonella* sp. are either urgent or serious threats.

Despite the rise of resistant strains of bacteria, the launch of new antibiotics that can be effective against multi-drug resistant pathogens from the major pharmaceutical industries has been extremely limited [12–14]. As a matter of fact, the introduction of any antibiotic is likely to be challenged by the development of resistance by the targeted bacteria. Therefore, new antimicrobial agents must be constantly developed to mitigate the acquisition of resistance among pathogenic bacteria [12–14]. For around four decades, the 1940s to the 1970s, pharmaceutical industries maintained a stable discovery pipeline in supplying new antibiotics. In that golden era, antibiotics were developed that could overcome the complications caused by bacterial resistance to earlier drugs. After that and in recent years, fewer antibiotics (quinupristin-dalfopristin, linezolid, and daptomycin) became available for the treatment of infections caused by MDR Gram-positive bacteria [15,16]. By contrast, there are now limited treatment options available to treat infections of MDR Gram-negative pathogens. In particular, infections caused by carbapenem-resistant Gram-negative bacteria are hard to treat with any another antibiotic [17,18]. To tackle these infections, an apparently nephrotoxic peptide antibiotic polymyxin B, or colistin, has been brought back for clinical usage [19,20].

2. Antimicrobial Peptides (AMPs) as Potential Alternatives to Antibiotic Resistance

Antimicrobial peptides (AMPs) are promising molecules of high translational potential against multi-drug resistant bacterial pathogens [21–24]. A PubMed search on "antimicrobial peptide" showed 52,404 results (Figure 1).

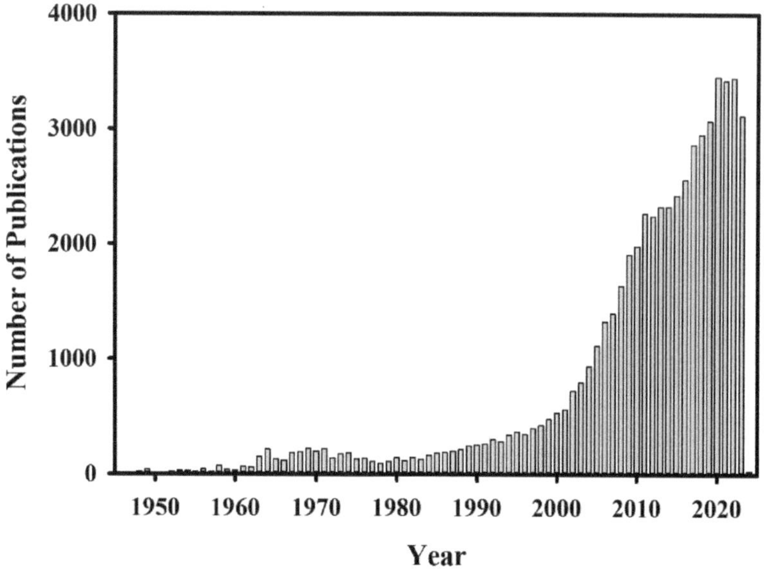

Figure 1. Bar diagram summarizing publications vs. years with "antimicrobial peptide" as the search option from the PubMed database.

The increasing number of scientific publications over the years asserts that AMPs can be valuable templates for the potential development of antibiotics. Ubiquitously found in all life forms, AMPs serve as an integral component of host innate immunity in multicellular organisms, including humans [25–27]. Many AMPs exert a broad spectrum of activity, killing bacteria, parasites, fungi, viruses, and cancer [28–31]. As a mode of action, amphipathic AMPs lyse bacterial cells by disrupting membranes following distinct mechanisms, e.g., barrel stave, toroidal pore, or carpet [32–34]; the non-membrane targeting mechanisms include the inhibition of cell division, protease activity, and biosynthesis of proteins and nucleic acids. Cationic AMPs preferentially interact with negatively charged bacterial cell membranes over zwitterionic or neutral membranes of host cell membranes [25–27]. Gram-negative bacteria are intrinsically more resistant to several frontline antibiotics that are extremely effective in killing Gram-positive bacteria [34,35]. The lipopolysaccharide (LPS) outer membrane (or LPS-OM) of Gram-negative bacteria serves as a permeability barrier that limits intra-cellular access of several antibiotics [35–38]. Interactions of cationic AMPs with anionic phosphates of LPS or lipid A can cause an efficient permeabilization of the LPS-OM barrier [39–42]. AMP-mediated disruption of the LPS-OM is pivotal in killing Gram-negative bacteria [39–42]. The ability of AMPs in killing drug-resistant bacteria, both Gram-positive and Gram-negative, has generated a strong interest in the development of antibiotics with novel modes of action [43–46]. More recent studies have demonstrated efficacy of several AMPs against MDR-resistant strains of Gram-negative bacteria in infected animal models with low host toxicity [47–50]. Notably, large-scale genomic data analyses have revealed that bacteria are less likely to develop resistance against AMPs compared to the conventional antibiotics [51,52]. These attributes of AMPs need to be exploited for the development of anti-infective agents to treat infections of the drug-resistant bacterial pathogens. Many studies have reported the antimicrobial activities of AMPs derived from amphibians, insects, mammals, microorganisms such as fungi and bacteria, and de novo design.

In humans, tissue-specific expressions of antimicrobial proteins and peptides constitute the innate immunity to eliminate invading pathogens [53–55]. Based on the Antimicrobial Peptide Database (APD), there are 153 host defense peptides in humans [56]. The well-characterized human AMPs include the defensins families, α and β, cathelicidin LL37, histatins, and dermcidin. In addition, a number of human proteins, e.g., multiple types of RNases, lysozyme, chemokines, and psoriasin, exhibit antimicrobial activities. Finally, proteolytic fragments of certain native proteins are bestowed with host defense activity [57–59]. Table 1 shows a selected list of AMPs identified in humans.

Table 1. A representative list of human antimicrobial peptides (AMPs) with antibacterial activity.

Name	Sequence	Net Change	Activity[@]	Ref.
LL37	LLGDFFRKSKEKIGKEFKRIVQRIKDFLRNLVPRTES	+6 (pI 10.6)	G+/G−	[60–62]
α-Defensin HNP-1	ACYCRIPACIAGERRYGTCIYQGRLWAFCC	+3 (pI 8.68)	G+/G−	[63]
α-Defensin HNP-2	CYCRIPACIAGERRYGTCIYQGRLWAFCC	+3 (pI 8.67)	G+/G−	[63]
α-Defensin HNP-3	DCYCRIPACIAGERRYGTCIYQGRLWAFCC	+2 (pI 8.33)	G+/G−	[63]
α-Defensin HNP-4	VCSCRLVFCRRTELRVGNCLIGGVSFTYCCTRV	+4 (pI 8.98)	G+/G−	[64]
α-Defensin HD-5	ATCYCRTGRCATRESLSGVCEISGRLYRLCCR	+4 (pI 8.96)	G+/G−	[65]
Histatin 3	DSHAKRHHGYKRKFHEKHHSHRGYRSNYLYDN	+5 (pI 9.9)	G+/G−	[66]
β-Defensin HBD-1	DHYNCVSSGGQCLYSACPIF TKIQGTCYRGKAKCCK	+4 (pI 8.87)	G+/G−	[67]
β-Defensin HBD-2	GIGDPVTCLKSGAICHPVFCP RRYKQIGTCGLPGTKCCKKP	+6 (pI 9.3)	G+/G−	[68]
β-Defensin HBD-3	GIINTLQKYYCRVRGGRCAVLSCLPKEEQ IGKCSTRGRKCCRRKK	+11 (pI 10)	G+/G−	[69]
β-Defensin HBD-4	FELDRICGYGTARCRKKCRSQEYRIGRCPNTYACCLRKW DESLLNRTKP	+7 (pI 9.45)	G+/G−	[70]
Dermcidin	SSLLEKGLDGAKKAVGGLGKLGKDAVEDLESVGKGAVHD VKDVLDSV	−2 (pI 5.07)	G+/G−	[71]
Granulysin	GRDYRTCLTIVQKLKKMVDKPTQRSVSNAATRVCRTGRSR WRDVCRNFMRRYQSRVTQGLVAGETAQQICEDLR	+11 (pI10.83)	G+/G−	[72]
Ubiquicidin	KVHGSLARAGKVRGQTPKVAKQEKKKKKTGRAKRRMQY NRRFVNVVPTFGKKKGPNANS	+19 (pI12.15)	G+/G−	[73]
Thrombocidin-1	AELRCMCIKTTSGIHPKNIQSLEVIGKGTHCNQVEVIATLKD GRKICLDPDAPRIKKIVQKKLAGDES	+4 (pI 9.05)	G+/G−	[74]
Hepcidin 25 (LEAP-1)	DTHFPICIFCCGCCHRSKCGMCCKT	+2 (pI 8.22)	G+/G−	[75]
Neuropeptide α-MSH	SYSMEHFRWGKPV	+1 (pI 8.33)	G+	[76]
PACAP Neuropeptide	HSDGIFTDSYSRYRKQMAVKKYLAAVLGKRYKQRVKNK	+9 (pI 10.41)	G+/G−	[77]
KDAMP	RAIGGGLSSVGGGSSTIKY	+2 (pI 9.99)	G−	[78]
DEFB114	DRCTKRYGRCKRDCLESEKQIDICSLPRKICCTEKLYEEDDMF	0 (pI 6.37)	G+/G−	[79]

[@]G+ and G− represent Gram-positive and Gram-negative bacteria, respectively.

3. Cathelicidin-Derived AMPs

Mainly found in higher organisms, including vertebrates and mammals, cathelicidin AMPs exert a broad spectrum of activity within the innate and adaptive host defense systems [80,81]. The cathelicidin family of AMPs are typically recognized by the presence of a conserved "cathelin" domain, ~14 KDa, in their precursor proteins [80,81]. The cathelin domain was first identified from analyses of proteolytic digestion of peptide fragments from pig leukocytes and was determined to be an inhibitor of the cysteine proteinase cathepsin L [82]. Structurally, the cathelin domain belongs to the cystatin superfamily of protease inhibitors, including cystatin (cysteine proteinase inhibitor), kininogen, and stefin proteins [82–85]. The cathelicidin protein is expressed as a precursor protein or a pre-protein that contains an N-terminal signal sequence followed by the cathelin domain and the C-terminus antimicrobial region [82–85]. The pre-protein undergoes multiple steps of proteolytic processing before cathelicidin AMP can be functionally activated [80,81]. The signal peptide is cleaved off, giving rise to the "holo-protein" during the translocation to an extra-cellular space or in zymogen granules. Further processing of the holo-protein to a pro-protein entails stabilization of the cathelin domain by the formation of two disulfide bonds. At the final stage of processing, the holo-protein is proteolytically cleaved, releasing the active forms of the antimicrobial region and the cathelin domain [80,81]. Although the cathelin domain is well conserved, the AMPs derived from cathelicidin proteins demonstrate great diversity in their amino acid sequence structure and activity [82–85]. The secondary structures of cathelicidin AMPs encompass amphipathic α-helix stabilized in the lipid membrane, disulfide bonded β-sheets, and AMPs rich in specific amino acid types [86–90]. In general, cathelicidin AMPs exhibit a broad spectrum of antimicrobial activity, although toxicity to cells and tissues in animal models has been observed [86–90]. Chicken cathelicidin AMPs or fowlicidins are extremely hemolytic although highly potent in killing wide-ranging pathogenic bacteria, including drug-resistant strains [91,92]. Table 2 summarizes a list of representative cathelicidin AMPs and their amino acid sequences, secondary structures, and activity profiles [86,87,89,93–107].

Table 2. A representative list of cathelicidin-derived AMPs across several species and structural classes.

Source	Name	Sequence	Net Charge	Sec. Structure	Antibacterial Activity$^{@}$	Toxicity	References
Human	LL37	^{1}LLGDFFRKSKEKIGKEFKRIV QRIKDFLRNLVPRTES^{37}	+6	Helix (NMR)	G+/G−	Hemolytic	[86]
Rhesus Monkey	RL37	^{1}RLGNFFRKVKEKIGGGLKKV GQKIKDFLGNLVPRTAS^{37}	+8	Helix (CD)	G+/G−	Hemolytic	[93]
Rabbit	CAP18	^{1}GLRKRLRKFRNKIKEKLKKIG QKIQGFVPKLAPRTDY^{37}	+12	Helix (CD)	G+/G−	Non-Hemolytic	[87]
Mice	CRAMP	^{1}GLLRKGGEKIGEKLKKIGQKI KNFFQKLVPQPEQ^{34}	+6	Helix (NMR)	G+/G−	Hemolytic	[94]
Guinea Pig	CAP11	^{1}GLRKKFRKTRKRIQKLGRKI GKTGRKVWKAWREYGQIPYPCRI^{43}-dimer -disulfide-linked	+16	ND	G+/G−	Hemolytic	[95]
Pig	Tritrpticin	^{1}VRRFPWWWPFLRR^{13}	+4	b-strand (NMR)	G+/G−	Hemolytic	[96]
Pig	Protegrin-1	^{1}RGGRLCYCRRRFCVCVGR^{18}	+7	b-sheet (NMR)	G+/G−	Hemolytic, cytotoxic	[97]
Pig	PMAP37	^{1}GLLSRLRDFLSDRGRRLGE KIERIGQKIKDLSEFFQS^{37}	+4	Helix (CD)	G+/G−	Hemolytic	[98]
Pig	PR39	^{1}RRRPRPPYLPRPRPPPFFP PRLPPRIPPGFPPRFPPRFP^{39}	+11	ND	G+/G−	ND	[99]
Bovine	Bactenecin	^{1}RLCRIVVIRVCR^{12}	+4	b-turn^{2}	G+/G−	Non-Hemolytic	[100]
Cattle	Indolicidin	^{1}ILPWKWPWWPWRR^{13}	+4	b-strand (NMR)	G+/G−	Non-Hemolytic	[89]
Sheep	SMAP29	^{1}RGLRRLGRKIAHGVKKY GPTVLRIIRIAG^{29}	+10	Helix (NMR)	G+/G	Hemolytic	[101]
Bovine	BMAP27	^{1}GRFKRFRKKFKKLFKKL SPVIPLLHLG^{27}	+10	Helix (NMR)	G+/G−	Non Hemolytic	[102]
Bovine	BMAP28	^{1}GGLRSLGRKILRAWKKY GPIIVPIIRIG^{28}	+7	Helix (NMR)	G+/G−	Hemolytic	[102]
Bovine	BMAP34	^{1}GLFRRLRDSIRRGQQKIL EKARRIGERIKDIFRG^{34}	+8	Helix (CD)	G+/G−	Non Hemolytic	[103]
Pig	PMAP23	^{1}RIIDLLWRVRRPQKPKFV TVWVR^{23}	+6	Helix (NMR)	G+/G−	Non Hemolytic	[98]
Pig	PMAP36	^{1}VGRFRRLRKKTRKRLKK IGKVLKWIPPIVGSIPLGCG^{37}	+13	ND	G+/G−	Hemolytic	[98]
Sheep	SMAP34	^{1}GLFGRLRDSLQRGGQKIL EKAERIWCKIKDIFR^{33}	+5	ND	G+/G−	Hemolytic	[104]
Equine	e-CATH1	^{1}KRFGRLAKSFLRMRILLP RRKILLAS^{26}	+9	Helix (CD)	G+/G−	Non Hemolytic	[105]
Chicken	Fowlicidin-1	^{1}RVKRVWPLVIRTVIAGY NLYRAIKKK^{26}	+8	Helix (NMR)	G+/G−	Hemolytic	[91]
Chicken	Fowlicidin-2	^{1}RFGRFLRKIRRFRPKVTI TIQGSARFG^{27}	+9	Helix (NMR)	G+/G−	Hemolytic	[91]
Chicken	Fowlicidin-3	^{1}RVKRFWPLVPVAINTVAA GINLYKAIRRK^{29}	+7	Helix (NMR)	G+/G−	Hemolytic	[91]
Hagfish	HFIAP-1	^{1}GFFKKAWRKVKHAGRRV LDTAKGVGRHYVNNWLNRYR^{37}	+10	ND	G+/G−	ND	[106]
Hagfish	HFIAP-3	^{1}GWFKKAWRKVKNAGRRV LKGVGIHYGVGLI^{30}	+8	ND	G+/G−	ND	[106]
Crocodile	As-CATH7	^{1}KRVNWRKVGRNTALGASYVLSFLG^{24}	+6	Helix (CD)	G+/G−	ND	[107]
Crocodile	As-CATH8	^{1}KRVNWAKVGRTALKLLPYIFG^{21}	+6	Helix (CD)	G+/G−	ND	[107]
Crocodile	Gg-CATH5	^{1}TRRKWWKKVLNGAIKIAPYILD^{22}	+6	Helix (CD)	G+/G−	ND	[107]
Crocodile	Gg-CATH7	^{1}KRVNWRKVGLGASYVMSWLG^{20}	+5	Helix (CD)	G+/G−	ND	[107]

$^{@}$G+ and G− represent Gram-positive and Gram-negative bacteria, respectively.

LL37 is the only cathelicidin-derived AMP in humans [86,108]. The 37-residue LL37 is linear in its amino acid sequence, without any disulfide bond, and helical in its structure [109–111]. These characteristics are widely different from disulfide-bonded β-sheet human defensin AMPs [112–114]. Towards the discovery of LL37, two independent studies were aimed to identify the cathelicidin gene(s) in humans using cDNA probes obtained from the homologous genes of pigs and rabbits [60,61]. Analyses of cDNA probes of pigs reported the existence of a human gene that may code for a putative 39-residue long peptide (or FALL39) as a part of a cathelin-like precursor protein [60]. The chemically synthesized FALL39 peptide demonstrated helical conformations and inhibited growth of bacterial strains of *E. coli* D21 and *B. megaterium* [60]. On the other hand, a cDNA probe based on the rabbit CAP18 gene has led to the characterization of the human CAP18 gene [61]. Western blot experiments have demonstrated the expression of CAP18 or 18 KDa precursor protein in granulocytes [61]. The 37-residue synthetic peptide of the C-terminus of CAP18 demonstrated high-affinity LPS binding and protected mice from LPS-induced endotoxic shock [62]. Another study isolated the LL37 precursor protein from human neutrophils and obtained its c-DNA clone from human myeloid cells [115]. Furthermore, analyses of total genomic DNA revealed the existence of only one cathelicidin gene in humans [115]. The 37-residue mature form of AMP of hCAP18 was isolated from granulocytes and was termed LL37, based on its first two Leu residues [115].

4. Importance of Structures of AMPs

AMPs are pivotal sources of natural arsenals that can be utilized to combat MDR infections [43–46]. Thus, the rational development of potent and selective antimicrobials from AMPs would require in-depth structure–activity relationship (SAR) studies. Traditionally, based on amphipathicity, AMPs are categorized as α-helix, β-sheet/β-hairpin, and non-random (no typical secondary structures). However, atomic-resolution structures of AMPs in a complex with bacterial targets are essential to generate SAR for novel antibiotics. Notably, three-dimensional structures of several AMPs are known to vary significantly when determined in cell membranes or membrane-mimicking environments [32,41,42]. In this regard, the atomic-resolution structures of several potent AMPs as a complex with an LPS outer membrane could be correlated with Gram-negative specific activity [116–123]. Cathelicidin-derived AMPs are found to be structurally diverse (Table 2). Atomic-resolution structures of several members of AMPs in the cathelicidin family have been determined in membranes or in membrane mimics (Table 2). NMR-derived structures of α-helical cathelicidin AMPs include LL37 [109–111], mice [124], pig [125], sheep [126], bovine [127], and fowlicidins [128–130]. The helical AMPs appear to be unstructured in a free solution and assume largely monomeric helical conformations in the solutions of membrane environments, e.g., detergent micelles, bicelles, nanodiscs, vesicles, or helix-promoting organic solvents. Interestingly, an oligomeric structure of fowlicidin-1, chicken cathelicidin, was determined in a solution of zwitterionic DPC detergent micelles [130]. Although the in-vivo concentrations for all AMPs are very low, the local population density is very high, enough to cause damage to the cell membrane. The lipids of the membrane have been shown to assist the self-assembly of the peptides to form an aggregate/oligomer, which is more potent in lysing bacterial cells. The oligomeric structure of fowlicidin-1 indicates membrane pore formation and cytotoxicity. The oligomerization and structures of protegrin-1, β-sheet cathelicidin from porcine, in membranes demonstrated mechanistic insights, cell selective activity, and SAR-based designs of analogs [131].

5. Biological Properties of LL37

LL-37, the only human cathelicidin-derived antimicrobial peptide, has long been a popular research subject because of its special abilities and vast applications. In the past 15 years, hundreds of papers have been published with LL-37 being their primary focus. Although minimal progress has been made on certain areas related to LL-37, such as the correlation between its high-resolution structure and activity, many multidisciplinary studies have shown LL-37 to be one of the most promising AMPs with a variety of applications. LL37's functional properties are summarized below.

5.1. Antimicrobial and Antiviral Activities of LL-37

LL-37, though it has been proven to be useful in many ways, is, in essence, an antimicrobial peptide that is primarily used by the body to fight microorganisms like bacteria and fungi. On top of that, the antiviral ability of LL-37 has also long been a popular topic. In the past 15 years, LL-37 has been considered as a promising candidate for the treatment of a number of diseases, with the majority of them being bacterial and some being viral. Table 3 summarizes some of the diseases that have been studied with LL-37. In the majority of the cases, treatments using LL-37 were found to have a positive effect, while in others, resistance to LL-37 was reported. Apart from the specific diseases, LL-37 has also been studied extensively with certain bacteria, especially the ones under the genera Burkholderia, Neisseria, Pseudomonas, Staphylococcus, and Streptococcus. The potential possibilities to treat diseases caused by microorganisms without leading to resistance make LL-37 a promising replacement for conventional antibiotics, which has been demonstrated in some cases. However, the resistance to LL37 noticed in some diseases points to the need for further studies before progressing to the next step towards drug development.

Table 3. Bacterial and viral diseases that have been studied with LL-37 in the past 15 years.

Disease Studied	General Conclusion	Ref.
Bacterial pneumonia	Possible candidate for treatment	[132–139]
COPD	Candidate for treatment, though it may also play a role in the pathogenesis process	[140–144]
Infected segmental bone defects	Possible candidate for treatment	[145]
Influenza A	Possible candidate for treatment	[146–151]
Gonorrhea	Possible candidate for treatment	[152,153]
Keratitis	Possible candidate for treatment	[154,155]
Leptospirosis	Bacteria inhibits LL-37	[156]
Lupus	Possible candidate for treatment	[157–160]
Meningitis	Candidate for treatment, though resistance to LL-37 has been reported	[161–163]
Periodontitis	Possible candidate for treatment	[164–168]
Psoriasis	LL-37 plays a role in the pathogenesis process but may still be used for therapeutic purposes.	[158,160,169–189]
Rheumatoid arthritis	LL-37 plays a role in the pathogenesis process but may still be used for therapeutic purposes.	[158,172–175]
Sepsis	Candidate for treatment, though significant possible side effects have been noted	[176–179]
Tuberculosis	Possible candidate for treatment	[134,180–183]
Ulcerative colitis	Possible candidate for treatment	[184]

Starting in 2008, a particular aspect of the antimicrobial activity of LL-37 has been investigated, which is its ability to inhibit the formation of bacterial biofilms [185]. A biofilm is an aggregate of bacterial cells that is covered by an extracellular polymeric substance (EPS) matrix. By forming biofilms, bacterial cells are able to protect themselves from harmful substances, such as attacks from the immune system and antibiotics. Like other antimicrobial agents, LL-37 is also prevented by bacterial biofilm from attacking the bacterial cells, which is why some bacteria exhibit resistance against LL-37. However, Overhage et al. noted that LL-37 is able to prevent the formation of biofilms through a series of mechanisms that have not yet been well understood [186]. Such mechanisms include biofilm gene suppression, bacteria adhesion inhibition, biofilm matrix degradation, bacteria cells elimination, and several other major or minor functions [185]. On the other hand, bacterial biofilms also have a variety of mechanisms that mediate the interference from LL-37, explaining why LL-37 has not yet been the solution to overcome biofilm-related challenges. That being said, certain ways to improve the antibiofilm ability of LL-37 have been proposed, such as using its synergy with other antimicrobial agents, indicating a possible therapeutic application in the future. Studies have also reported LL-37 degradation by the metalloprotease aureolysin, produced by *S. aureus* strains, suggesting the resistance of this pathogen correlating with the loss of LL-37's antibacterial activity. On the other hand, the fragment LL-17-37 produced due to the glutamyl endopeptidase V8 protease, exhibited antibacterial activity against *S. aureus* [187,188]. There are other studies that reported the inactivation of LL-37 [156,189–191].

5.2. Anticancer Activity of LL-37

Antimicrobial peptides have also been shown to exhibit anticancer activities [28,30,31,192–195]. Since cancer cells are anionic, the cationic AMPs exhibit selectivity in targeting cancer cells in a similar manner to their selective targeting of bacterial cells. While there is significant interest in designing anticancer peptides using AMPs, the LL-37 peptide has received special attention, as it is the only cathelicidin-derived human peptide. Although the chemotactic potential of LL-37 was noticed almost immediately upon its discovery, it was only beginning around 2005 that the anticancer potential became a noteworthy aspect of this AMP [196]. In recent years, more and more research has become oriented towards the influence of LL-37 on cancer, along with the rise of research interest in cancer in the biology field in general [197–199]. LL-37 has been found to have contrasting effects on different types of cancers: for certain cancers, such as breast, lung and ovary cancer, LL-37 is tumorigenic and facilitates the cancer formation process, while in other cancers, like colon and gastric cancer, LL-37 has been proven to be anticancer. Verjans et al. suggest that this result may be explained by the difference in receptors that respond to LL-37 in different cells [200]. Even though LL-37 is tumorigenic in some cases, it can still be used to help treat such cancer by acting as a biomarker [197]. In ovarian cancer, LL-37 has been found to be over-expressed, and it is able to facilitate cancer spread in many ways, like inducing cell proliferation and cell invasion. Similar results were found for lung, breast, and pancreas cancer and malignant melanoma, while the tumorigenic effect of LL-37 can also be extrapolated for prostate cancer and skin squamous cell carcinoma. In all these types of cancers, treatment of recombinant LL-37 has shown a positive correlation with tumor development. On the other hand, the over-expression of LL-37 is also observed in colon cancer, but it was also found in this case that LL-37 can lead to a decrease in cancer tissues. For gastric cancer, hematologic malignancy, and oral squamous cell carcinoma, a lower expression of LL-37 was found, and it has also been proven to down-regulate cancer development, showing an anticancer effect. More studies are needed to fully understand the mechanism behind LL-37's involvement in cancer growth, but current results do suggest some possible therapeutic applications of LL-37 in cancer treatments.

5.3. Other Functional Properties of LL-37

Another noteworthy aspect of LL-37 is its role in the human immune system [201–203]. LL-37 has been shown to be able to attract immune cells to fight microbial infection. The first group of cells attracted is the neutrophils, which form the first line of defense against infection. These cells can also produce more LL-37, leading to a positive feedback loop. Recent research has also noted that in the case of serum amyloid A inflammation and sepsis, LL-37 performs immunoregulatory functions by inhibiting neutrophil migration, which is another novel aspect of the immune activity of LL-37. In addition to neutrophils, LL-37 is also able to modulate monocytes, macrophages, and dendritic cells. Monocytes, sometimes referred to as adult stem cells, are able to differentiate into macrophages and dendritic cells, which are important components of the immune system that fights off infection. A crucial role of LL-37 in modulating the differentiation process, as well as regulating the immunological functions of macrophages and dendritic cells, has also been proven. Further immunoregulatory functions of LL-37 on lymphocytes, mast cells, and MSCs have also been noted, though minimal discoveries have been made. Another important function of

LL-37 in the immune system is its ability to neutralize lipopolysaccharides (LPSs), which can be crucial in bacterial infections.

The wound healing and angiogenesis ability of LL-37 has also been recognized for a long time [204]. This aspect of LL-37 may also act as a contributing factor in the curing of microbial diseases and cancer. Recently, Chinipardaz et al. also discovered a potentially important role of LL-37 in bone and periodontal regeneration [165]. This, combined with the wound healing ability of LL-37, may point to a potential application in treating oral cavity diseases. Furthermore, connections of LL-37 with amyloid proteins have also been reported in recent studies. Certain connections between LL-37 and beta-amyloid, which is a possible cause of Alzheimer's disease, have been proven, and the hypothesis that LL-37 may be involved in the pathogenesis of Alzheimer's disease has been proposed, with a need for further examination [205,206]. Similar connections between LL-37 and IAPP, which is linked with type 2 diabetes, have also been found, and follow-up studies in this area are also needed [207]. Overall, the vast function of LL-37 opens it up to a variety of therapeutic applications in many different fields, while an increasing number of studies are forthcoming.

6. Structures of LL-37

Ever since its discovery, LL-37 has been studied not only in its original monomeric form but also in more complex structures obtained under different conditions. Studies have found that when treated with detergents under certain conditions, LL-37 can form monomers as well as oligomerize into dimers and tetramers [111,208,209]. Furthermore, derivatives of LL-37, such as the core peptide (LL-3717-29) and KR-12 (LL-3717-29), have also been studied extensively [210,211]. These structures, each with unique features, can become useful for research purposes to better understand the different functional properties of LL-37 and its derivatives and also for further development towards pharmaceutical applications.

6.1. Monomeric Structures of LL-37

LL-37 has been shown to undergo a structural transition from an unstructured monomer in solution to a helical structure in any of the following conditions: (i) at high peptide concentrations, (ii) in the presence of salt, and (iii) in the presence of detergents or lipids [212]. Atomic-resolution three-dimensional structures of the LL-37 monomer have been reported under different environments with different detergents. A solution NMR study reported a helix-break-helix conformation for LL-37 reconstituted into dodecylphosphocholine (DPC) micelles [109]. This study also found that the unstructured N- and C-termini are solvent exposed, while the structured C-terminal helix is protected from the solvent, and the N-terminal helical domain is more dynamic. The peptide is bound to the surface of DPC micelles with the hydrophobic I13, F17, and I20 residues and a salt bridge between E16 and K12 stabilizing the break between the two helices.

Wang et al. reported a standard LL-37 monomer structure (PDB number 2K6O), obtained using a three-dimensional triple-resonance NMR technique [111]. The conditions used were 303 K and pH 5.4, and deuterated SDS (sodium dodecyl sulfate) detergent micelles were used. The structure that they determined, as shown below, is a curved alpha helix with a well-defined helical region covering residues 2–31, while the residues at the C-terminus appear to be disordered (Figure 2A). The structure also contains a notable bent located between residues 14–16, which is consistent with the helix-break-helix structure predicted in other publications. In addition, the LL-37 helix appears to be amphipathic, with about half of the residues, namely residues L2, F5, F6, I13, F17, I20, V21, I24, F27, L28, and L31, being hydrophobic and located on the concave side (Figure 2B). The hydrophilic residues are located on the other side, with the exception of residue S9, which is on the hydrophobic side and divides that region into two parts. The author also proposed that the helix-break-helix structure may be a result of the hydrophobic packing between residues I13 and F17, which are located next to each other with a bend in between.

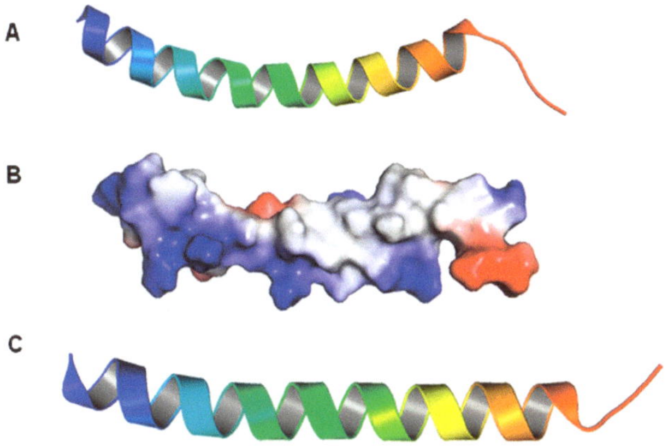

Figure 2. Structures of LL-37 monomers. (**A**) Structure of LL-37 monomer determined in deuterated SDS micelles (2K6O). (**B**) Electrostatic potential of LL-37 monomer in deuterated SDS micelles; blue represents positively charged residues, red represents negatively charged residues, and white represents hydrophobic residues. (**C**) Structure of LL-37 monomer determined in DPC micelles (5NMN).

In another study, an LL-37 structure determined from a different detergent, dioctanoylphosphatidylglycerol (D8PG) micelles, was reported, using the same technique and experimental conditions as described above. The obtained structure appears to be similar, if not identical, to the above-mentioned LL-37 structure determined for SDS micelles. However, because D8PG has the same head structure as many anionic phosphatidylglycerols, the author also used it to investigate the interaction between LL-37 and anionic PGs. Direct evidence for interactions between the aromatic rings of the phenylalanine residues as well as the arginine residues of LL-37 and the PGs was found. Sancho-Vaello et al. reported a monomeric LL-37 structure (5NMN), obtained with DPC micelles using X-ray crystallography, which also has similar features to the other structures determined from detergent micelles (Figure 2C) [208]. This structure is less bent compared to the structure determined in SDS micelles, with residues 35–37 missing on the model, possibly because they are disordered and cannot be detected by the X-ray diffraction technique.

6.2. *Oligomeric Structures of LL-37*

In addition to the structure of the LL-37 monomer, the structures of the oligomers of LL-37 are important to better understand the stability of the peptide against enzymatic degradation. LL-37 has been shown to form aggregates at high peptide concentrations in solution [212–215]. Sancho-Vaello et al. also explored the structure of LL-37 dimers in a detergent-free environment (5NNM), as well as in DPC (5NNT) and LDAO (5NNK) micelles [208]. When there is no detergent present, the dimeric LL-37 appears to be an antiparallel dimer made from two alpha helices without supercoiling (Figure 3A). The two monomers are similar to the monomer obtained in DPC (5NMN), especially since there is very little bending compared to the SDS and D8PG ones. Each helix in this dimer extends to around 5 nm, with approximately two turns shifted at each terminus, leading to a 3.5 nm interface. The hydrophilic interactions that link the two dimers are formed by the residues S9, K12, and E16 of the two monomers, whereas intermolecular stabilization is mainly provided by the H-bond and four salt bridges. In addition, the hydrophobic residues at the interface form a hydrophobic core in the dimer that extends to the C-terminus, which also contributes to the high stability of the dimer. The authors also noted a discontinuity in the hydrophobic region, which is the positively charged residue K10. The opposite side of the dimer is dominated by the hydrophilic residues, with 20 of those being positively charged and eight being negatively charged, leading to a +12 overall charge. Another point worth noting is that like the DPC monomer described above, eight of the 74 residues are not present in the structure, indicating a disordered region at the C-terminus. The same applies for the two other dimers made in detergents.

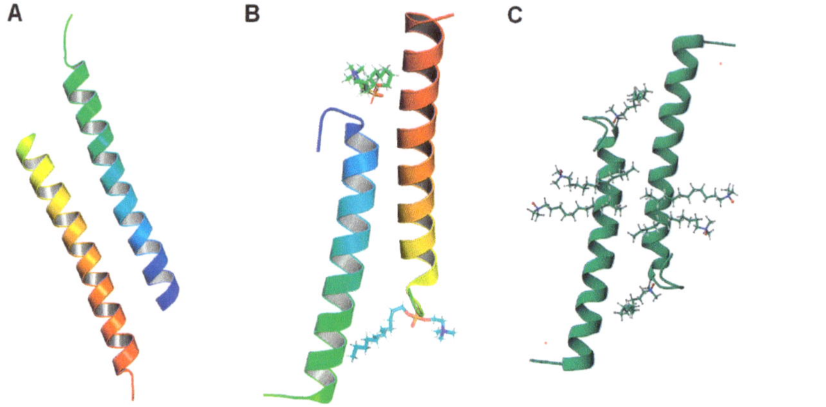

Figure 3. Structures of LL-37 dimers. (**A**) LL-37 dimer structure in detergent-free environment (5NNM). (**B**) LL-37 dimer structure in DPC micelles (5NNT). (**C**) LL-37 dimer structure in LDAO micelles (5NNK).

The dimer structures obtained in DPC and LDAO micelles are highly similar antiparallel dimers, but they differ strongly from the one obtained in a detergent-free environment (Figure 3B,C). The authors found that only the core region of the two dimers can align with the detergent-free dimer as a result of the structural remodeling caused by detergents. Specifically, the remodeling at the N-terminus shortens each monomer to about 4 nm and the interface to 2.5 nm. The residues L1 to R7 at the N-terminus, unlike in the dimer obtained without detergents, appear to be randomly coiling. This remodeling allows residues F5 and F6 to be exposed so that they can form hydrophobic contacts with the alkyl chains of the detergents, which is assisted by residues I24 and F27 of the second monomer. This conformation is further stabilized by the H bond between residue K10 and residues G3 and F5. Further conformational changes at residues L1, I13, and I17 can also be attributed to the influence of the detergent. The residues at the C-terminus also experience a shift in conformation, though not as significant as the remodeling at the N-terminus. Because of the change in structure, the bond that connects the two monomers in this case is formed by residue S9 on one monomer and residue E16 on the other. The authors also found that these dimer structures can also form tetramers and other fiber-like oligomers with a head-to-tail arrangement. The oligomers are primarily stabilized by residues F5, F6, and F27, which form hydrophobic scaffolds to embed detergent molecules. The exact structure of the tetramer (7PDC) is documented in another paper written by the same group of authors.

The LL-37 tetramer structure was also obtained with DPC micelles and modeled using a crystallization technique (7PDC) [209]. The tetramer is made by two asymmetric dimers, each containing two antiparallel monomers (Figure 4A). This structure is a narrow tetrameric channel with a 4 nm length, and its monomers are similar to those in the DPC dimers (5NNT) and the DPC monomer (5NMN). Disordered residues are observed at both termini, leaving a well-defined helical region between residues 6 and 30. However, the dimer structure seen in this tetramer is very different from the dimers described above, and the new structure seems to provide a better structural fit. The tetramer appears to be asymmetrical, but the structure does form a continuous and positively charged inner cavity. As a result of this asymmetric structure, there exist three interfaces, with one being hydrophobic and the others being charged and polar (Figure 4B). These interfaces are stabilized by salt bridges and hydrophilic contacts. The authors also suggested that the influence of the three interfaces might be the cause of this unique conformation, as opposed to being caused by detergents like the dimers described above. In the center of the tetramer, there is a chlorine ion trapped by two R23 residues and coordinated by two water molecules. The core itself is stabilized by many hydrogen bond interactions as well as 15 water molecules that are also found within the channel, while no water molecules are present in the surrounding of the tetramer. The authors also noted two aromatic grindles on the tetramer, each formed by two F17 and two F27 residues, which indicate the membrane integration potential of this structure. With follow-up tests, the presence of this tetramer in membrane-like environments is confirmed in the paper, as well as the conductivity of the channel to pass molecules into cells.

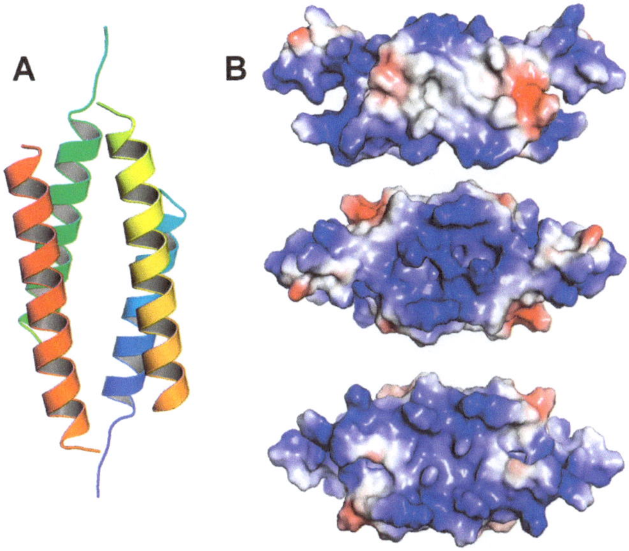

Figure 4. The structures of LL-37 tetramer. (**A**) LL-37 tetramer structure in DPC micelles (7PDC). (**B**) The three interfaces of the tetramer, with the first one being hydrophobic and the other two being polar.

7. LL-37 Derivatives

7.1. Core Peptide and Related Fragments

Because LL-37 has been studied extensively in the past two decades, its original structure and the structures of its many derivatives have been explored in great detail. One of the first derivatives that draws a lot of attention is its core peptide, LL-3717-29. The core peptide is 13 residues long, and it is referred to in such a way because it was thought at the time to be the smallest fragment that exhibits AMP properties [210]. Li et al. studied the structure of the LL-37 core peptide with solution NMR under a 298 K temperature 5.4 pH and using both D8PG and deuterated SDS as detergents (2FBS). The structure obtained is an amphipathic alpha helix, which appears to be the same under the two detergent environments (Figure 5A). The authors found that about half of the residues are located on the hydrophobic surface, while the other half are on the hydrophilic one. For the hydrophilic surface, it is evident that the positively charged residues dominate the region, just like in many other LL-37 structures, and this suggests that the peptide is more ideal for targeting negatively charged membranes. The authors also noted an analogical structure to the core peptide, aurein 1.2, which also has antimicrobial and anticancer properties. By studying these two peptides along with a bacterial membrane anchor, the authors proposed that hydrophobic clusters that involve aromatic rings might be crucial for membrane binding. Apart from the core peptide, the article also reported two other derivatives of LL-37, which are the N-terminal fragment (LL-37_{1-12}) and the C-terminal fragment (LL-$37_{13–37}$). The N-terminal fragment (2FBU) obtained appears to be disordered for the most part, with only a one-turn helix covering residues 3–7 present (Figure 5B). For this peptide, only 62% of the backbone angles are located in the most favored region, in contrast to the result of 100% for the core peptide. The backbone angles in the less favored region are located in the disordered region, namely residues 8–12. The authors also focused on the hydrophobic clusters that involve aromatic–aromatic interaction, just like that noted in the core peptide. It was found that a single hydrophobic cluster created by the aromatic rings on P5 and P6 as well as the side chain of L2 leads to the poor hydrophobicity of the peptide, which could be the reason for this fragment's poor AMP and anticancer ability. In addition to that, this cluster may also play a role in the oligomerization of LL-37, as described in the last section. The C-terminal fragment (2FCG) contains a well-defined alpha-helical structure between residues 17–29, corresponding perfectly to the core peptide (). The rest of the fragment, residues 13–16 and 30–37, appears to be disordered, and their backbone angles are also located in less favored regions similar to that of the N-terminal fragment. A weaker AMP ability of this fragment compared to the core peptide and the whole peptide was also noted, which may as well be a result of the interference of this poorly defined region with membrane binding.

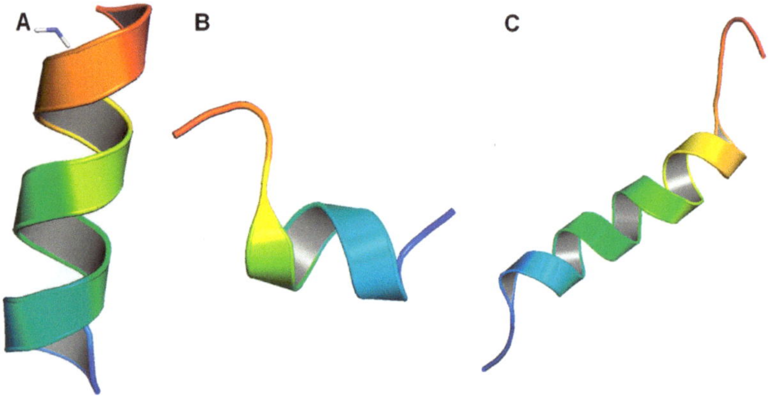

Figure 5. The structures of LL-37 core peptide and other fragments. (**A**) LL-37 core peptide structure in D8PG and deuterated SDS (2FBS). (**B**) LL-37 N-terminal fragment structure in D8PG and deuterated SDS (2FBU). (**C**) LL-37 C-terminal fragment structure in D8PG and deuterated SDS (2FCG).

Li et al. also reported the structure of the retro core peptide of LL-37 (2F3A) [216], which was investigated as an analog of aurein 1.2. Obtained in the presence of SDS and D8PG, the structure appears to be alpha-helical with a well-defined helix covering residues 2–12 (Figure 6A). Similar to all LL-37 related peptides, the retro core peptide is also amphipathic with hydrophobic residues on one side and hydrophilic residues on the other. One interesting feature of this peptide is that the aromatic rings on residues F3 and F13 are located in the same chemical environment in SDS and D8PG. Because F13 penetrates the micelles deeper than F3 and the NOE pattern of F3 is similar to what is found in bacterial membrane anchors, it was concluded that F3 might also be serving the same purpose in this case. Engelberg and Landau further explored the structure of fibrils formed by LL-37 core peptides (6S6M) using crystallization techniques [7,217]. In a detergent-free environment with sodium acetate used as salt, the core peptides assemble into a densely packed hexameric fibrous structure with a central pore, composed of numerous four-helix bundles as the building unit (Figure 6B,C). These bundles, each containing a hydrophobic core that provides stabilization for the structure, are highly positively charged. The polar interactions between the bundles, especially the salt bridge formed by adjacent helices, allow the formation of the hexameric fibrils. The resulting fibrils are found to be highly stable and are capable of interacting with bacterial membranes. In another article, Engelberg et al. also reported a mutant of the core peptide, I24C (7NPQ) (Figure 6D) [8,218]. This mutant is found initially as dimers connected by a disulfide bond at the C24 residue, but they can further assemble to form fibrils using a network of interaction, particularly salt bridges, as a stabilizing factor. The fibrils contain a hydrophobic core, which extends through the structure.

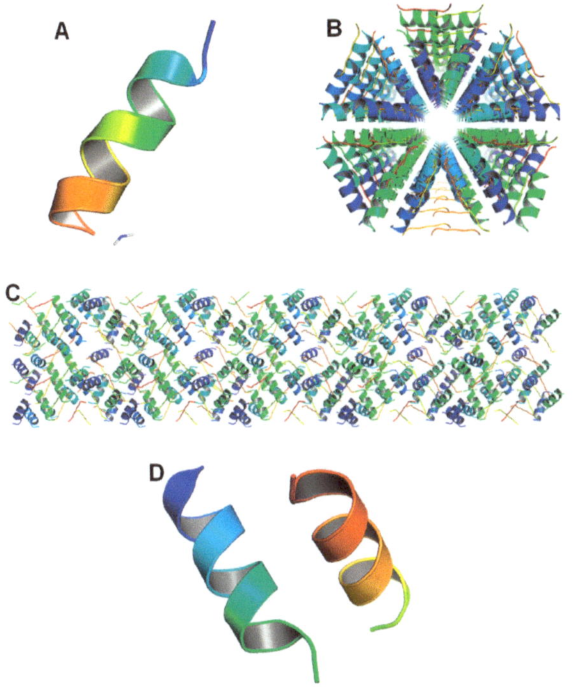

Figure 6. The structures of LL-37 core peptide variations. (**A**) LL-37 retro core peptide structure in D8PG and SDS (2F3A). (**B**) LL-37 core peptide fiber structure, viewed from the top (6S6M). (**C**) LL-37 core peptide fiber structure, viewed from the side (6S6M). (**D**) LL-37 core peptide I24C mutant structure in sodium acetate (7NPQ).

7.2. *KR-12 Based Peptides*

KR-12 (LL-$37_{18\text{-}29}$) is one of the most important derivatives of LL-37 because of its outstanding AMP properties and low toxicity to human cells. Gunasekera et al. studied the structure of KR-12 (2NA3) and retro KR-12 (2NAL) using solution NMR with lysophosphatidylglycerol and SDS as the detergents [211]. KR-12 is in the form of an alpha helix, with a clear helical structure between residues 3–11 (Figure 7A). Like the other peptides, KR-12 has the charged and hydrophilic residues on one side and the hydrophobic ones on the other, while having a net positive charge. The overall structure is not much different from the core peptide, which is only one residue more than KR-12. However, it was noticed that KR-12 can form cyclic dimers that possess enhanced AMP ability, although the dimer structure was not reported on the PDB. The retro KR-12, being simply the reverse of KR-12, shows a very similar structure to the KR-12 structure (Figure 7B). The only noticeable difference between the two is the marginally decreased AMP ability seen in retro KR-12 compared to KR-12. Yun et al. also found an analog of KR-12 (6M0Y) in another article, which may have the potential to become a cosmetic product [219].

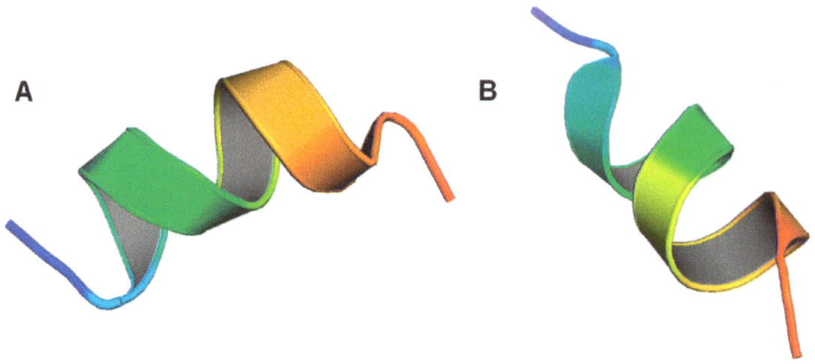

Figure 7. The structures of LL-37 derivative KR-12. (**A**) LL-37 KR-12 structure in lysophosphatidylglycerol and SDS (2NA3). (**B**) LL-37 retro KR-12 structure in lysophosphatidylglycerol and SDS (2NAL).

8. Solid-State NMR Studies on the Mechanism of Membrane Disruption by LL-37

A complete understanding of the function of an antimicrobial peptide can only be accomplished by determining the atomic-resolution three-dimensional structure, dynamics, and membrane folding/topology of the peptide in a lipid membrane environment. A detergent micelle is not a suitable membrane mimetic to study antimicrobial peptides because of the following reasons: (i) it does not have an appropriate hydrophobic membrane core to enable native folding of the hydrophobic domains (like the transmembrane domain) of the peptide, and (ii) its curvature can distort the overall shape of the amphipathic structural regions, such as by bending the helix. In addition, the absence of native-like lipid–peptide interactions both with the head groups and hydrophobic acyl chains is unlikely to allow the self-assembly of peptides and oligomer formation to occur. Therefore, it is essential to use a better membrane mimetic. A lipid bilayer is considered to be a better mimetic, and the feasibility to alter the lipid/membrane composition to mimic bacterial versus mammalian cell membrane is an added advantage. Since lipid bilayers are fluid and dynamic but an isotropic phase, they pose challenges for atomic-resolution structural studies. On the other hand, solid-state NMR techniques are well-suited to studying such dynamic systems [220–225].

Solid-state NMR is a technique used to determine the structure and dynamics of a variety of solids and semi-solids (examples include liquid crystalline systems), and it is an ideal approach to investigate biological membranes that are difficult to study with other biophysical techniques like solution NMR or crystallization techniques [226–230]. In the case of LL-37, solid-state NMR experiments were used to determine the backbone conformation, dynamics, and membrane orientation in order to determine the mechanism of lipid membrane disruption by LL-37. The cell membrane disruption process by a peptide or protein has been broadly defined using three possible mechanisms: the barrel-stave, detergent-like, and toroidal-pore mechanisms. Henzler-Wildman et al. used synthetic LL-37 peptides selectively labeled with ^{15}N and/or ^{13}C isotopes and model membranes composed of a combination of synthetic lipids [212]. The backbone conformation of LL-37 associated with a lipid bilayer was found to be helical using ^{13}C CP-MAS (cross-polarization magic angle spinning) solid-state NMR experiments, which was found to be in excellent agreement with CD experiments. Then, using static cross-polarization solid-state NMR experiments performed on mechanically aligned lipid bilayers containing site-specifically ^{15}N-labeled LL-37, the helix was found to be oriented nearly parallel to the bilayer surface (or nearly perpendicular to the bilayer normal) (Figure 8). This observation ruled out the barrel-stave mechanism of membrane disruption for which the peptide should be assembled to form channel-like structures with the helical axis oriented parallel to the bilayer normal (or transmembrane topology). Then, to measure the LL-37-induced perturbation of the lipid bilayer structure, static ^{31}P NMR experiments were carried out on mechanically aligned lipid bilayers and also on multilamellar vesicles. The observed ^{31}P NMR spectra revealed the absence of isotropic peaks that would arise from the peptide-induced fragmentation and formation of any small "micellar-like" lipid aggregates, which ruled out a detergent-like membrane of membrane disruption. The observed aligned, anisotropic ^{31}P NMR spectral line shapes were consistent with a carpet/toroidal-type mechanism in which the bilayer surface association of LL-37 disrupted the head group region of lipids. Differential scanning calorimetry (DSC) experiments revealed LL-37's ability to induce positive curvature on the lipid bilayer, which is indicative of a toroidal pore-type mechanism. Taken together, these NMR and DSC experimental results indicated that a toroidal pore-type membrane disruption is the likely possibility. Mechanisms of membrane interaction and disruption by LL-37 have also been investigated by other approaches [86,110,214,231–236].

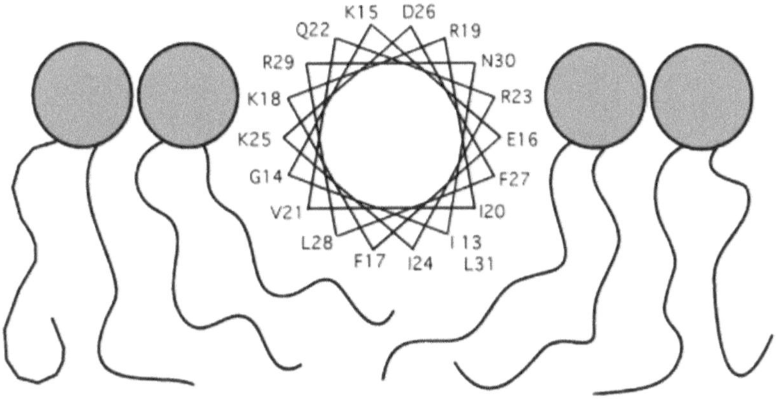

Figure 8. Cartoon showing the orientation of helical LL-37 peptide with respect to the lipid bilayer. As mentioned in the text, magic angle spinning (MAS) solid-state NMR of LL-37 reconstituted in a lipid bilayer, solution NMR of LL-37 in detergent micelles, and circular dichroism (CD) experiments on micelles or lipid vesicles containing LL-37 revealed the amphipathic helical structure of LL-37 [109,207] The use of static solid-state NMR experiments on mechanically aligned lipid bilayers containing ^{15}N-labeled LL-37 rendered the in-plane orientation of the peptide [212]. The figure is reprinted with copyright permission from Ref. [212].

To investigate the mechanism by which LL-37 perturbs the hydrophobic core of the lipid bilayer, a series of static 2H solid-state NMR and DSC experiments were carried out on lipid vesicles [237]. The 2H quadrupole couplings measured from 2H-labeled lipids were used to determine an LL-37-induced disorder of the acyl chains of lipids. The peptide-induced disorder of the hydrophobic core of the lipid bilayer was found to be maximal for the lower-order carbons of the lipid acyl chains. These results along with the above-mentioned NMR findings confirmed that amphipathic helices of LL-37 associate with the lipid bilayer surface through electrostatic interactions and inserts into the hydrophobic region of the membrane stabilized via hydrophobic interactions with lipid acyl chains. These interactions act together to cause membrane disruption (Figure 9). Further evidence showed that LL-37 insertion also alters the material properties of the membrane and that the order of the bilayer influences the depth of the insertion, as well as the effectiveness of the disruption.

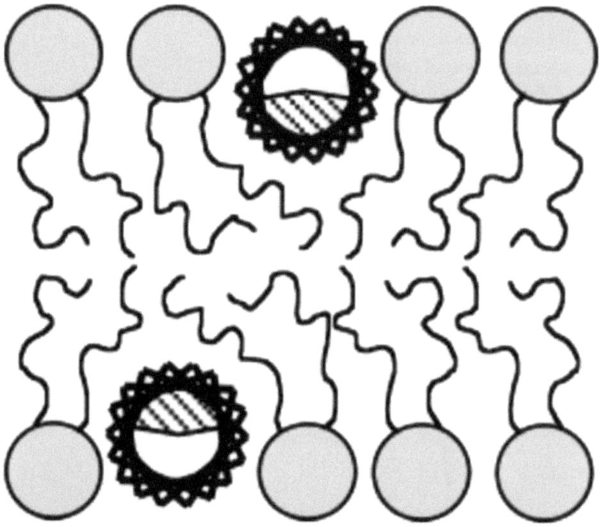

Figure 9. Cartoon showing the insertion of LL-37 helices into the lipid membrane bilayer with the hydrophobic region of the helix shown as shaded [237]. In addition to the solid-state NMR experiments used to determine the membrane orientation of LL-37 (see Figure 8), ^{2}H solid-state NMR experiments on vesicles containing deuterated lipids and LL-37 were used to determine the peptide-induced disorder of the acyl chains of lipids, as shown [237]. The figure is reprinted with copyright permission from Ref. [237].

9. Influence of LL-37 on Amyloid Aggregation

With many properties of LL-37 being uncovered over the past decades, its interactions with amyloid β (Aβ) have also been investigated. Studies have reported the misfolding, aggregation, oligomer formation, and fibril formation of an intrinsically disordered peptide Aβ [238]. These properties of Aβ have been shown to be associated with the pathogenesis of Alzheimer's disease (AD). Studies have reported the aggregation-induced oligomer formation and membrane-disrupting properties of Aβ peptides [239–250]. Studies have also reported the interaction between beta-amyloid and LL-37 peptides [205]. In addition, recent studies have also reported neuroinflammation and a variety of in vivo properties of LL-37 [251,252]. De Lorenzi et al. explored the possible influence of LL-37 on the amyloid aggregation of the Aβ42 isomer [205]. Through surface plasmon resonance imaging (SPRi) in vitro experiments, De Lorenzi et al. found evidence showing that LL-37 binds specifically to Aβ. Transmission electron microscopy (TEM) analysis of the aggregates showed that LL-37 inhibits Aβ42's ability to form amyloid fibril structures, which is associated with the pathogenesis of AD. Circular dichroism (CD) spectroscopy also showed that LL-37 directly interacts with Aβ42 to prevent the formation of a β-sheet secondary structure and therefore the fibril formation. It was also found that when allowed to interact with each other, the toxicities of LL-37 and Aβ42 to neurons were both significantly reduced. Based on these findings, it is proposed that the AD pathogenesis may be associated with the expression of LL-37 and its balance with Aβ42. As De Lorenzi et al. pointed out, this finding only marks the starting point of research regarding the interaction between LL-37 and Aβ42. More investigations and evidence are needed to fully understand this relationship between the two peptides (Figure 10).

LL-37 cathelicidin peptide:
LLGDFFRKSKEKIGKEFKRIVQRIKDFLRNLVPRTES

$A\beta_{42}$ pro-amyloid peptide:
DAEFRHDSGYEVHHQKLVFFAEDVGSNKGAIIGLMVGGVVIA

Blue: positively charged; Red: negatively charged; Purple: aromatic hydrophobic; Green: aliphatic hydrophobic

Figure 10. Amino acid sequences of LL-37 and $A\beta_{42}$ with charges and aromatic and aliphatic amino acids identified.

A 37-residue human hormone amylin (also called IAPP, islet amyloid polypeptide) aggregates to form amyloid fibrils in the pancreatic islet cells [253–256]. The self-assembly of IAPP results in the formation of oligomeric intermediates that are shown to exhibit major cell toxicity. Therefore, there is significant interest in the development of inhibitors of IAPP's aggregation [257–261]. Remarkably, nanomolar affinity of LL-37 binding with IAPP (islet amyloid polypeptide) has been shown to effectively suppress the amyloid aggregation of IAPP and its cell toxicity [207].

10. Summary and Future Directions

There is considerable interest and an urgent need for the development of novel compounds to overcome the increasing bacterial resistance. While antimicrobial peptides have been thought to be promising candidates, and significant research progress has been reported towards understanding their mechanisms of action, there are very few peptide-based compounds that have successfully become pharmaceutical compounds. On the other hand, studies have explored other types of biological activities for AMPs. For example, the only type of cathelicidin-derived AMP in humans, LL-37, has drawn much attention due to its numerous biological activities, including antimicrobial activities, LPS-neutralizing activities, and modulation of immune and inflammatory pathways [262–266]. While LL-37's mechanisms of antibacterial activity have been reasonably well investigated through biophysical studies, further studies to better understand its other biological roles, such as its effects on immune system function, are essential to fully exploit its potential therapeutic applications and side effects. In addition, LL-37's interference with other biological processes such as protein misfolding and aggregation and biocondensation is an exciting area for future research. In particular, further studies to fully understand the effects of LL-37 on the molecular processes underlying amyloid aggregation, membrane disruption, oligomer formation, and neuronal cell toxicity associated with the pathology of Alzheimer's disease would be useful.

Funding: Research in the Ramamoorthy lab has been supported by funds from the National Institutes of Health (DK132214 and GM084018 to A.R.). Research from the Bhattacharjya lab has been supported by funds from the Biomedical Research Council (BMRC) and Ministry of Education (MOE), Singapore. A.R. and S.B. acknowledge excellent contributions from students, post-doctoral fellows, and collaborators to the topics reported in this article.

Conflicts of Interest: The authors have no conflict of interest.

References

1. Taubes, G. The Bacteria Fight Back. *Science* **2008**, *321*, 356–361. [CrossRef] [PubMed]
2. Kupferschmidt, K. Resistance Fighters. *Science* **2016**, *352*, 758–761. [CrossRef] [PubMed]
3. Ikuta, K.S.; Swetschinski, L.R.; Robles Aguilar, G.; Sharara, F.; Mestrovic, T.; Gray, A.P.; Davis Weaver, N.; Wool, E.E.; Han, C.; Gershberg Hayoon, A. Global Mortality Associated with 33 Bacterial Pathogens in 2019: A Systematic Analysis for the Global Burden of Disease Study 2019. *Lancet* **2022**, *400*, 2221–2248. [CrossRef] [PubMed]

4. Morrison, L.; Zembower, T.R. Antimicrobial Resistance. *Gastrointest. Endosc. Clin. N. Am.* **2020**, *30*, 619–635. [CrossRef] [PubMed]
5. Hutchings, M.I.; Truman, A.W.; Wilkinson, B. Antibiotics: Past, present and future. *Curr. Opin. Microbiol.* **2019**, *51*, 72–80. [CrossRef]
6. Wang, Z.; Koirala, B.; Hernandez, Y.; Zimmerman, M.; Park, S.; Perlin, D.S.; Brady, S.F. A Naturally Inspired Antibiotic to Target Multidrug-resistant Pathogens. *Nature* **2022**, *601*, 606–611. [CrossRef]
7. *Antibiotic Resistance Threats in the United States*; CDC: Atlanta, GA, USA, 2019.
8. O'Neill, J. *Tackling Drug-Resistant Infections Globally: Final Report and Recommendations*; Government of the United Kingdom: London, UK, 2016.
9. Murray, C.J.L.; Ikuta, K.S.; Sharara, F.; Swetschinski, L.; Robles Aguilar, G.; Gray, A.; Han, C.; Bisignano, C.; Rao, P.; Wool, E. Global Burden of Bacterial Antimicrobial Resistance in 2019: A Systematic Analysis. *Lancet* **2022**, *399*, 629–655. [CrossRef]
10. De Oliveira, D.M.P.; Forde, B.M.; Kidd, T.J.; Harris, P.N.A.; Schembri, M.A.; Beatson, S.A.; Paterson, D.L.; Walker, M.J. Antimicrobial Resistance in ESKAPE Pathogens. *Clin. Microbiol. Rev.* **2020**, *33*, 10–1128. [CrossRef]
11. Magiorakos, A.-P.; Srinivasan, A.; Carey, R.B.; Carmeli, Y.; Falagas, M.E.; Giske, C.G.; Harbarth, S.; Hindler, J.F.; Kahlmeter, G.; Olsson-Liljequist, B. Multidrug-resistant, Extensively Drug-resistant and Pandrug-resistant Bacteria: An International Expert Proposal for Interim Standard Definitions for Acquired Resistance. *Clin. Microbiol. Infect.* **2012**, *18*, 268–281. [CrossRef]
12. May, M. Drug Development: Time for Teamwork. *Nature* **2014**, *509*, S4–S5. [CrossRef]
13. Smith, P.A.; Koehler, M.F.T.; Girgis, H.S.; Yan, D.; Chen, Y.; Chen, Y.; Crawford, J.J.; Durk, M.R.; Higuchi, R.I.; Kang, J. Optimized Arylomycins Are a New Class of Gram-negative Antibiotics. *Nature* **2018**, *561*, 189–194. [CrossRef] [PubMed]
14. Hegemann, J.D.; Birkelbach, J.; Walesch, S.; Müller, R. Current developments in antibiotic discovery: Global microbial diversity as a source for evolutionary optimized anti-bacterials: Global microbial diversity as a source for evolutionary optimized anti-bacterials. *EMBO Rep.* **2023**, *24*, e56184. [CrossRef]
15. Madden, J.; Outterson, K. Trends in the Global Antibiotics Market. *Nat. Rev. Drug Discov.* **2023**, *22*, 174. [CrossRef] [PubMed]
16. Hashemian, S.M.; Farhadi, T.; Ganjparvar, M. Linezolid: A Review of Its Properties, Function, and Use in Critical Care. *Drug Des. Dev. Ther.* **2018**, *12*, 1759–1767. [CrossRef] [PubMed]
17. Adams-Sapper, S.; Nolen, S.; Donzelli, G.F.; Lal, M.; Chen, K.; Justo Da Silva, L.H.; Moreira, B.M.; Riley, L.W. Rapid Induction of High-level Carbapenem Resistance in Heteroresistant Kpc-producing Klebsiella Pneumoniae. *Antimicrob. Agents Chemother.* **2015**, *59*, 3281–3289. [CrossRef] [PubMed]
18. Balm, M.N.D.; La, M.-V.; Krishnan, P.; Jureen, R.; Lin, R.T.P.; Teo, J.W.P. Emergence of Klebsiella Pneumoniae Co-producing Ndm-type and OXA-181 Carbapenemases. *Clin. Microbiol. Infect.* **2013**, *19*, E421–E423. [CrossRef] [PubMed]
19. Rabanal, F.; Cajal, Y. Recent Advances and Perspectives in the Design and Development of Polymyxins. *Nat. Prod. Rep.* **2017**, *34*, 886–908. [CrossRef]
20. Brown, P.; Dawson, M.J. Development of New Polymyxin Derivatives for Multi-drug Resistant Gram-negative Infections. *J. Antibiot.* **2017**, *70*, 386–394. [CrossRef]
21. Lazzaro, B.P.; Zasloff, M.; Rolff, J. Antimicrobial peptides: Application informed by evolution. *Science* **2020**, *368*, eaau5480. [CrossRef]
22. Magana, M.; Pushpanathan, M.; Santos, A.L.; Leanse, L.; Fernandez, M.; Ioannidis, A.; Giulianotti, M.A.; Apidianakis, Y.; Bradfute, S.; Ferguson, A.L.; et al. The value of antimicrobial peptides in the age of resistance. *Lancet Infect. Dis.* **2020**, *20*, e216–e230. [CrossRef]
23. Zasloff, M. Antimicrobial Peptides of Multicellular Organisms: My Perspective. *Adv. Exp. Med. Biol.* **2019**, *1117*, 3–6. [CrossRef]
24. Bhattacharjya, S.; Straus, S.K. Design, Engineering and Discovery of Novel α-Helical and β-Boomerang Antimicrobial Peptides against Drug Resistant Bacteria. *Int. J. Mol. Sci.* **2020**, *21*, 5773. [CrossRef]
25. Haney, E.F.; Straus, S.K.; Hancock, R.E.W. Reassessing the Host Defense Peptide Landscape. *Front. Chem.* **2019**, *7*, 43. [CrossRef] [PubMed]
26. Boman, H.G. Antibacterial peptides: Basic facts and emerging concepts. *J. Intern. Med.* **2003**, *254*, 197–215. [CrossRef]
27. Torres, M.D.T.; Sothiselvam, S.; Lu, T.K.; de la Fuente-Nunez, C. Peptide Design Principles for Antimicrobial Applications. *J. Mol. Biol.* **2019**, *43*, 3547–3567. [CrossRef] [PubMed]
28. Hoskin, D.W.; Ramamoorthy, A. Studies on anticancer activities of antimicrobial peptides. *Biochim. Biophys. Acta* **2008**, *1778*, 357–375. [CrossRef]
29. Tornesello, A.L.; Borrelli, A.; Buonaguro, L.; Buonaguro, F.M.; Tornesello, M.L. Antimicrobial Peptides as Anticancer Agents: Functional Properties and Biological Activities. *Molecules* **2020**, *25*, 2850. [CrossRef]
30. Kardani, K.; Bolhassani, A. Antimicrobial/anticancer peptides: Bioactive molecules and therapeutic agents. *Immunotherapy* **2021**, *13*, 669–684. [CrossRef] [PubMed]
31. Madera, L.; Hoskin, D.W. Protocols for Studying Antimicrobial Peptides (AMPs) as Anticancer Agents. In *Methods in Molecular Biology*; Springer: Berlin/Heidelberg, Germany, 2017; pp. 331–343.
32. Nguyen, L.T.; Haney, E.F.; Vogel, H.J. The expanding scope of antimicrobial peptide structures and their modes of action. *Trends Biotechnol.* **2011**, *29*, 464–472. [CrossRef]
33. Shai, Y. Mode of action of membrane active antimicrobial peptides. *Biopolymers* **2002**, *66*, 236–248. [CrossRef]
34. Matsuzaki, K. Why and how are peptide-lipid interactions utilized for self defence? *Biochem. Soc. Trans.* **2001**, *29*, 598–601. [CrossRef] [PubMed]

35. Theuretzbacher, U. Global antimicrobial resistance in Gram-negative pathogens and clinical need. *Curr. Opin. Microbiol.* **2017**, *39*, 106–112. [CrossRef] [PubMed]
36. Brown, D. Antibiotic Resistance Breakers: Can Repurposed Drugs Fill the Antibiotic Discovery Void? *Nat. Rev. Drug Discov.* **2015**, *14*, 821–832. [CrossRef] [PubMed]
37. Payne, D.J.; Gwynn, M.N.; Holmes, D.J.; Pompliano, D.L. Drugs for Bad Bugs: Confronting the Challenges of Antibacterial Discovery. *Nat. Rev. Drug Discov.* **2007**, *6*, 29–40. [CrossRef] [PubMed]
38. Willyard, C. The Drug-resistant Bacteria That Pose the Greatest Health Threats. *Nature* **2017**, *543*, 15. [CrossRef] [PubMed]
39. Nikaido, H. Molecular Basis of Bacterial Outer Membrane Permeability Revisited. *Microbiol. Mol. Biol. Rev.* **2003**, *67*, 593–656. [CrossRef]
40. Zgurskaya, H.I.; López, C.A.; Gnanakaran, S. Permeability Barrier of Gram-negative Cell Envelopes and Approaches to Bypass It. *ACS Infect. Dis.* **2015**, *1*, 512–522. [CrossRef]
41. Bhattacharjya, S. NMR Structures and Interactions of Antimicrobial Peptides with Lipopolysaccharide: Connecting Structures to Functions. *Curr. Top. Med. Chem.* **2015**, *16*, 4–15. [CrossRef]
42. Bhattacharjya, S.; Mohid, S.A.; Bhunia, A. Atomic-resolution Structures and Mode of Action of Clinically Relevant Antimicrobial Peptides. *Lancet Infect. Dis.* **2022**, *23*, 4558. [CrossRef]
43. Luther, A.; Urfer, M.; Zahn, M.; Müller, M.; Wang, S.-Y.; Mondal, M.; Vitale, A.; Hartmann, J.-B.; Sharpe, T.; Monte, F.L. Chimeric Peptidomimetic Antibiotics Against Gram-negative Bacteria. *Nature* **2019**, *576*, 452–458. [CrossRef]
44. Nicolas, I.; Bordeau, V.; Bondon, A.; Baudy-Floc'H, M.; Felden, B. Novel Antibiotics Effective Against Gram-positive and -negative Multi-resistant Bacteria with Limited Resistance. *PLoS Biol.* **2019**, *17*, e3000337. [CrossRef]
45. Chen, C.H.; Bepler, T.; Pepper, K.; Fu, D.; Lu, T.K. Synthetic molecular evolution of antimicrobial peptides. *Curr. Opin. Biotechnol.* **2022**, *75*, 102718. [CrossRef]
46. Shelburne, C.E.; An, F.Y.; Dhople, V.; Ramamoorthy, A.; Lopatin, D.E.; Lantz, M.S. The spectrum of antimicrobial activity of bacteriocin subtilosin A. *J. Antimicrob. Chemother.* **2007**, *59*, 297–300. [CrossRef] [PubMed]
47. Mishra, B.; Lakshmaiah Narayana, J.; Lushnikova, T.; Wang, X.; Wang, G. Low Cationicity Is Important for Systemic in Vivo Efficacy of Database-derived Peptides Against Drug-resistant Gram-positive Pathogens. *Proc. Natl. Acad. Sci. USA* **2019**, *116*, 13517–13522. [CrossRef] [PubMed]
48. Schuster, M.; Brabet, E.; Oi, K.K.; Desjonquères, N.; Moehle, K.; Le Poupon, K.; Hell, S.; Gable, S.; Rithié, V.; Dillinger, S. Peptidomimetic Antibiotics Disrupt the Lipopolysaccharide Transport Bridge of Drug-resistant Enterobacteriaceae. *Sci. Adv.* **2023**, *9*, eadg3683. [CrossRef] [PubMed]
49. Dash, R.; Bhattacharjya, S. Thanatin: An Emerging Host Defense Antimicrobial Peptide with Multiple Modes of Action. *Lancet Infect. Dis.* **2021**, *22*, 1522. [CrossRef]
50. Nyembe, P.L.; Ntombela, T.; Makatini, M.M. Review: Structure-activity Relationship of Antimicrobial Peptoids. *Pharmaceutics* **2023**, *15*, 1506. [CrossRef]
51. Spohn, R.; Daruka, L.; Lázár, V.; Martins, A.; Vidovics, F.; Grézal, G.; Méhi, O.; Kintses, B.; Számel, M.; Jangir, P.K. Integrated Evolutionary Analysis Reveals Antimicrobial Peptides with Limited Resistance. *Nat. Commun.* **2019**, *10*, 4538. [CrossRef]
52. Lázár, V.; Martins, A.; Spohn, R.; Daruka, L.; Grézal, G.; Fekete, G.; Számel, M.; Jangir, P.K.; Kintses, B.; Csörgő, B. Antibiotic-resistant Bacteria Show Widespread Collateral Sensitivity to Antimicrobial Peptides. *Nat. Microbiol.* **2018**, *3*, 718–731. [CrossRef]
53. Gschwandtner, M.; Zhong, S.; Tschachler, A.; Mlitz, V.; Karner, S.; Elbe-Bürger, A.; Mildner, M. Fetal Human Keratinocytes Produce Large Amounts of Antimicrobial Peptides: Involvement of Histone-methylation Processes. *J. Investig. Dermatol.* **2014**, *134*, 2192–2201. [CrossRef]
54. Underwood, M.; Bakaletz, L. Innate Immunity and the Role of Defensins in Otitis Media. *Curr. Allergy Asthma Rep.* **2011**, *11*, 499–507. [CrossRef]
55. Jones, D.E.; Bevins, C.L. Defensin-6 Mrna in Human Paneth Cells: Implications for Antimicrobia Peptides in Host Defense of the Human Bowel. *FEBS Lett.* **1993**, *315*, 187–192. [CrossRef]
56. Wang, G.; Li, X.; Wang, Z. APD3: The Antimicrobial Peptide Database as a Tool for Research and Education. *Nucleic Acids Res.* **2016**, *44*, D1087–D1093. [CrossRef] [PubMed]
57. Ibrahim, H.R.; Thomas, U.; Pellegrini, A. A Helix-loop-helix Peptide at the Upper Lip of the Active Site Cleft of Lysozyme Confers Potent Antimicrobial Activity with Membrane Permeabilization Action. *J. Biol. Chem.* **2001**, *276*, 43767–43774. [CrossRef] [PubMed]
58. Pane, K.; Sgambati, V.; Zanfardino, A.; Smaldone, G.; Cafaro, V.; Angrisano, T.; Pedone, E.; Di Gaetano, S.; Capasso, D.; Haney, E.F. A New Cryptic Cationic Antimicrobial Peptide from Human Apolipoprotein E with Antibacterial Activity and Immunomodulatory Effects on Human Cells. *FEBS J.* **2016**, *283*, 2115–2131. [CrossRef]
59. Sinha, S.; Harioudh, M.K.; Dewangan, R.P.; Ng, W.J.; Ghosh, J.K.; Bhattacharjya, S. Cell-selective Pore Forming Antimicrobial Peptides of the Prodomain of Human Furin: A Conserved Aromatic/cationic Sequence Mapping, Membrane Disruption, and Atomic-resolution Structure and Dynamics. *ACS Omega* **2018**, *3*, 14650–14664. [CrossRef]
60. Agerberth, B.; Gunne, H.; Odeberg, J.; Kogner, P.; Boman, H.G.; Gudmundsson, G.H. FALL-39, a Putative Human Peptide Antibiotic, Is Cysteine-free and Expressed in Bone Marrow and Testis. *Proc. Natl. Acad. Sci. USA* **1995**, *92*, 195–199. [CrossRef] [PubMed]

61. Larrick, J.W.; Hirata, M.; Balint, R.F.; Lee, J.; Zhong, J.; Wright, S.C. Human CAP18: A Novel Antimicrobial Lipopolysaccharide-binding Protein. *Infect. Immun.* **1995**, *63*, 1291–1297. [CrossRef]
62. Cowland, J.B.; Johnsen, A.H.; Borregaard, N. Hcap-18, a Cathelin/pro-bactenecin-like Protein of Human Neutrophil Specific Granules. *FEBS Lett.* **1995**, *368*, 173–176. [CrossRef]
63. Selsted, M.E.; Harwig, S.S.; Ganz, T.; Schilling, J.W.; Lehrer, R.I. Primary Structures of Three Human Neutrophil Defensins. *J. Clin. Investig.* **1985**, *76*, 1436–1439. [CrossRef]
64. Wilde, C.G.; Griffith, J.E.; Marra, M.N.; Snable, J.L.; Scott, R.W. Purification and characterization of human neutrophil peptide 4, a novel member of the defensin family. *J. Biol. Chem.* **1989**, *264*, 11200–11203. [CrossRef]
65. Jones, D.E.; Bevins, C.L. Paneth cells of the human small intestine express an antimicrobial peptide gene. *J. Biol. Chem.* **1992**, *267*, 23216–23225. [CrossRef]
66. Oppenheim, F.G.; Xu, T.; McMillian, F.M.; Levitz, S.M.; Diamond, R.D.; Offner, G.D.; Troxler, R.F. Histatins, a novel family of histidine-rich proteins in human parotid secretion. Isolation, characterization, primary structure, and fungistatic effects on *Candida albicans*. *J. Biol. Chem.* **1988**, *263*, 7472–7477. [CrossRef]
67. Bensch, K.W.; Raida, M.; Mägert, H.-J.; Schulz-Knappe, P.; Forssmann, W.-G. Hbd-1: A Novel Β-defensin from Human Plasma. *FEBS Lett.* **1995**, *368*, 331–335. [CrossRef]
68. Harder, J.; Bartels, J.; Christophers, E.; Schröder, J.-M. A Peptide Antibiotic from Human Skin. *Nature* **1997**, *387*, 861. [CrossRef] [PubMed]
69. Harder, J.; Bartels, J.; Christophers, E.; Schröder, J.-M. Isolation and Characterization of Human Μ-defensin-3, a Novel Human Inducible Peptide Antibiotic. *J. Biol. Chem.* **2001**, *276*, 5707–5713. [CrossRef] [PubMed]
70. García, J.R.; Krause, A.; Schulz, S.; Rodríguez-Jiménez, F.J.; Klüver, E.; Adermann, K.; Forssmann, U.; Frimpong-Boateng, A.; Bals, R.; Forssmann, W.G. Human beta-defensin 4: A novel inducible peptide with a specific salt-sensitive spectrum of antimicrobial activity. *FASEB J.* **2001**, *15*, 1819–1821. [CrossRef] [PubMed]
71. Schittek, B.; Hipfel, R.; Sauer, B.; Bauer, J.; Kalbacher, H.; Stevanovic, S.; Schirle, M.; Schroeder, K.; Blin, N.; Meier, F. Dermcidin: A Novel Human Antibiotic Peptide Secreted by Sweat Glands. *Nat. Immunol.* **2001**, *2*, 1133–1137. [CrossRef] [PubMed]
72. Stenger, S.; Hanson, D.A.; Teitelbaum, R.; Dewan, P.; Niazi, K.R.; Froelich, C.J.; Ganz, T.; Thoma-Uszynski, S.; Melián, A.; Bogdan, C.; et al. An antimicrobial activity of cytolytic T cells mediated by granulysin. *Science* **1998**, *282*, 121–125. [CrossRef] [PubMed]
73. Hieshima, K.; Ohtani, H.; Shibano, M.; Izawa, D.; Nakayama, T.; Kawasaki, Y.; Shiba, F.; Shiota, M.; Katou, F.; Saito, T.; et al. CCL28 has dual roles in mucosal immunity as a chemokine with broad-spectrum antimicrobial activity. *J. Immunol.* **2003**, *170*, 1452–1461. [CrossRef] [PubMed]
74. Krijgsveld, J.; Zaat, S.A.J.; Meeldijk, J.; Van Veelen, P.A.; Fang, G.; Poolman, B.; Brandt, E.; Ehlert, J.E.; Kuijpers, A.J.; Engbers, G.H.M. Thrombocidins, Microbicidal Proteins from Human Blood Platelets, Are C-terminal Deletion Products of CXC Chemokines. *J. Biol. Chem.* **2000**, *275*, 20374–20381. [CrossRef] [PubMed]
75. Krause, A.; Neitz, S.; Mägert, H.-J.; Schulz, A.; Forssmann, W.-G.; Schulz-Knappe, P.; Adermann, K. LEAP-1, a Novel Highly Disulfide-bonded Human Peptide, Exhibits Antimicrobial Activity. *FEBS Lett.* **2000**, *480*, 147–150. [CrossRef] [PubMed]
76. Cutuli, M.; Cristiani, S.; Lipton, J.M.; Catania, A. Antimicrobial Effects of Α-msh Peptides. *J. Leukoc. Biol.* **2000**, *67*, 233–239. [CrossRef] [PubMed]
77. Lee, E.Y.; Chan, L.C.; Wang, H.; Lieng, J.; Hung, M.; Srinivasan, Y.; Wang, J.; Waschek, J.A.; Ferguson, A.L.; Lee, K.-F. PACAP Is a Pathogen-inducible Resident Antimicrobial Neuropeptide Affording Rapid and Contextual Molecular Host Defense of the Brain. *Proc. Natl. Acad. Sci. USA* **2021**, *118*, e1917623117. [CrossRef]
78. Tam, C.; Mun, J.J.; Evans, D.J.; Fleiszig, S.M.J. Cytokeratins Mediate Epithelial Innate Defense Through Their Antimicrobial Properties. *J. Clin. Investig.* **2012**, *122*, 3665–3677. [CrossRef]
79. Tollner, T.L.; Yudin, A.I.; Tarantal, A.F.; Treece, C.A.; Overstreet, J.W.; Cherr, G.N. Beta-defensin 126 on the Surface of Macaque Sperm Mediates Attachment of Sperm to Oviductal Epithelia1. *Biol. Reprod.* **2008**, *78*, 400–412. [CrossRef]
80. Kościuczuk, E.M.; Lisowski, P.; Jarczak, J.; Strzałkowska, N.; Jóźwik, A.; Horbańczuk, J.; Krzyżewski, J.; Zwierzchowski, L.; Bagnicka, E. Cathelicidins: Family of Antimicrobial Peptides. A Review. *Mol. Biol. Rep.* **2012**, *39*, 10957–10970. [CrossRef]
81. Zanetti, M. Cathelicidins, multifunctional peptides of the innate immunity. *J. Leukoc. Biol.* **2004**, *75*, 39–48. [CrossRef]
82. Lenarčič, B.; Ritonja, A.; Dolenc, I.; Stoka, V.; Berbič, S.; Pungerčar, J.; Štrukelj, B.; Turk, V. Pig Leukocyte Cysteine Proteinase Inhibitor (PLCPI), a New Member of the Stefin Family. *FEBS Lett.* **1993**, *336*, 289–292. [CrossRef] [PubMed]
83. Ritonja, A.; Kopitar, M.; Jerala, R.; Turk, V. Primary Structure of a New Cysteine Proteinase Inhibitor from Pig Leucocytes. *FEBS Lett.* **1989**, *255*, 211–214. [CrossRef] [PubMed]
84. Storici, P.; Tossi, A.; Lenarčič, B.; Romeo, D. Purification and Structural Characterization of Bovine Cathelicidins, Precursors of Antimicrobial Peptides. *Eur. J. Biochem.* **1996**, *238*, 769–776. [CrossRef] [PubMed]
85. Scocchi, M.; Wang, S.; Zanetti, M. Structural Organization of the Bovine Cathelicidin Gene Family and Identification of a Novel Member1. *FEBS Lett.* **1997**, *417*, 311–315. [CrossRef] [PubMed]
86. Johansson, J.; Gudmundsson, G.H.; Rottenberg, M.E.; Berndt, K.D.; Agerberth, B. Conformation-dependent Antibacterial Activity of the Naturally Occurring Human Peptide LL-37. *J. Biol. Chem.* **1998**, *273*, 3718–3724. [CrossRef] [PubMed]
87. Chen, C.; Brock, R.; Luh, F.; Chou, P.-J.; Larrick, J.W.; Huang, R.-F.; Huang, T.-H. The Solution Structure of the Active Domain of CAP18—A Lipopolysaccharide Binding Protein from Rabbit Leukocytes. *FEBS Lett.* **1995**, *370*, 46–52. [CrossRef] [PubMed]

88. Mani, R.; Cady, S.D.; Tang, M.; Waring, A.J.; Lehrer, R.I.; Hong, M. Membrane-dependent Oligomeric Structure and Pore Formation of a B-hairpin Antimicrobial Peptide in Lipid Bilayers from Solid-state NMR. *Proc. Natl. Acad. Sci. USA* **2006**, *103*, 16242–16247. [CrossRef] [PubMed]
89. Rozek, A.; Friedrich, C.L.; Hancock, R.E. Structure of the bovine antimicrobial peptide indolicidin bound to dodecylphosphocholine and sodium dodecyl sulfate micelles. *Biochemistry* **2000**, *39*, 15765–15774. [CrossRef] [PubMed]
90. Ramanathan, B.; Davis, E.G.; Ross, C.R.; Blecha, F. Cathelicidins: Microbicidal activity, mechanisms of action, and roles in innate immunity. *Microbes Infect.* **2002**, *4*, 361–372. [CrossRef]
91. Xiao, Y.; Cai, Y.; Bommineni, Y.R.; Fernando, S.C.; Prakash, O.; Gilliland, S.E.; Zhang, G. Identification and Functional Characterization of Three Chicken Cathelicidins with Potent Antimicrobial Activity. *J. Biol. Chem.* **2006**, *281*, 2858–2867. [CrossRef]
92. Bhunia, A.; Mohanram, H.; Bhattacharjya, S. Lipopolysaccharide bound structures of the active fragments of fowlicidin-1, a cathelicidin family of antimicrobial and antiendotoxic peptide from chicken, determined by transferred nuclear Overhauser effect spectroscopy. *Biopolymers* **2009**, *92*, 9–22. [CrossRef]
93. Bals, R.; Lang, C.; Weiner, D.J.; Vogelmeier, C.; Welsch, U.; Wilson, J.M. Rhesus monkey (*Macaca mulatta*) mucosal antimicrobial peptides are close homologues of human molecules. *Clin. Diagn. Lab. Immunol.* **2001**, *9*, 370–375. [CrossRef]
94. Gallo, R.L.; Kim, K.J.; Bernfield, M.; Kozak, C.A.; Zanetti, M.; Merluzzi, L.; Gennaro, R. Identification of CRAMP, a Cathelin-related Antimicrobial Peptide Expressed in the Embryonic and Adult Mouse. *J. Biol. Chem.* **1997**, *272*, 13088–13093. [CrossRef]
95. Nagaoka, I.; Tsutsumi-Ishii, Y.; Yomogida, S.; Yamashita, T. Isolation of Cdna Encoding Guinea Pig Neutrophil Cationic Antibacterial Polypeptide of 11 Kda (CAP11) and Evaluation of CAP11 Mrna Expression During Neutrophil Maturation. *J. Biol. Chem.* **1997**, *272*, 22742–22750. [CrossRef]
96. Lawyer, C.; Pai, S.; Watabe, M.; Borgia, P.; Mashimo, T.; Eagleton, L.; Watabe, K. Antimicrobial Activity of a 13 Amino Acid Tryptophan-rich Peptide Derived from a Putative Porcine Precursor Protein of a Novel Family of Antibacterial Peptides. *FEBS Lett.* **1996**, *390*, 95–98. [CrossRef] [PubMed]
97. Gidalevitz, D.; Ishitsuka, Y.; Muresan, A.S.; Konovalov, O.; Waring, A.J.; Lehrer, R.I.; Lee, K.Y.C. Interaction of Antimicrobial Peptide Protegrin with Biomembranes. *Proc. Natl. Acad. Sci. USA* **2003**, *100*, 6302–6307. [CrossRef]
98. Tossi, A.; Scocchi, M.; Zanetti, M.; Storici, P.; Gennaro, R. PMAP-37, a Novel Antibacterial Peptide from Pig Myeloid Cells. Cdna Cloning, Chemical Synthesis and Activity. *Eur. J. Biochem.* **1995**, *228*, 941–946. [CrossRef] [PubMed]
99. Agerberth, B.; Lee, J.; Bergman, T.; Carlquist, M.; Boman, H.G.; Mutt, V.; Jörnvall, H. Amino Acid Sequence of PR-39. *Eur. J. Biochem.* **1991**, *202*, 849–854. [CrossRef] [PubMed]
100. Romeo, D.; Skerlavaj, B.; Bolognesi, M.; Gennaro, R. Structure and bactericidal activity of an antibiotic dodecapeptide purified from bovine neutrophils. *J. Biol. Chem.* **1988**, *263*, 9573–9575. [CrossRef] [PubMed]
101. Bagella, L.; Scocchi, M.; Zanetti, M. Cdna Sequences of Three Sheep Myeloid Cathelicidins. *FEBS Lett.* **1995**, *376*, 225–228. [CrossRef] [PubMed]
102. Skerlavaj, B.; Gennaro, R.; Bagella, L.; Merluzzi, L.; Risso, A.; Zanetti, M. Biological Characterization of Two Novel Cathelicidin-derived Peptides and Identification of Structural Requirements for Their Antimicrobial and Cell Lytic Activities. *J. Biol. Chem.* **1996**, *271*, 28375–28381. [CrossRef]
103. Thennarasu, S.; Tan, A.; Penumatchu, R.; Shelburne, C.E.; Heyl, D.L.; Ramamoorthy, A. Antimicrobial and membrane disrupting activities of a peptide derived from the human cathelicidin antimicrobial peptide LL-37. *Biophys. J.* **2010**, *98*, 248–257. [CrossRef]
104. Travis, S.M.; Anderson, N.N.; Forsyth, W.R.; Espiritu, C.; Conway, B.D.; Greenberg, E.P.; Mccray, P.B.; Lehrer, R.I.; Welsh, M.J.; Tack, B.F. Bactericidal Activity of Mammalian Cathelicidin-derived Peptides. *Infect. Immun.* **2000**, *68*, 2748–2755. [CrossRef]
105. Schlusselhuber, M.; Torelli, R.; Martini, C.; Leippe, M.; Cattoir, V.; Leclercq, R.; Laugier, C.; Grötzinger, J.; Sanguinetti, M.; Cauchard, J. The Equine Antimicrobial Peptide Ecath1 Is Effective Against the Facultative Intracellular Pathogen Rhodococcus Equi in Mice. *Antimicrob. Agents Chemother.* **2013**, *57*, 4615–4621. [CrossRef]
106. Uzzell, T.; Stolzenberg, E.D.; Shinnar, A.E.; Zasloff, M. Hagfish intestinal antimicrobial peptides are ancient cathelicidins. *Peptides* **2003**, *24*, 1655–1667. [CrossRef]
107. Santana, F.L.; Estrada, K.; Alford, M.A.; Wu, B.C.; Dostert, M.; Pedraz, L.; Akhoundsadegh, N.; Kalsi, P.; Haney, E.F.; Straus, S.K. Novel Alligator Cathelicidin As-cath8 Demonstrates Anti-infective Activity Against Clinically Relevant and Crocodylian Bacterial Pathogens. *Antibiotics* **2022**, *11*, 1603. [CrossRef]
108. Dürr, U.H.; Sudheendra, U.S.; Ramamoorthy, A. LL-37, the only human member of the cathelicidin family of antimicrobial peptides. *Biochim. Biophys. Acta Biomembr.* **2006**, *1758*, 1408–1425. [CrossRef] [PubMed]
109. Porcelli, F.; Verardi, R.; Shi, L.; Henzler-Wildman, K.A.; Ramamoorthy, A.; Veglia, G. NMR Structure of the Cathelicidin-derived Human Antimicrobial Peptide LL-37 in Dodecylphosphocholine Micelles. *Biochemistry* **2008**, *47*, 5565–5572. [CrossRef] [PubMed]
110. Ding, B.; Soblosky, L.; Nguyen, K.; Geng, J.; Yu, X.; Ramamoorthy, A.; Chen, Z. Physiologically-relevant Modes of Membrane Interactions by the Human Antimicrobial Peptide, LL-37, Revealed by SFG Experiments. *Sci. Rep.* **2013**, *3*, srep01854. [CrossRef] [PubMed]
111. Wang, G. Structures of Human Host Defense Cathelicidin LL-37 and Its Smallest Antimicrobial Peptide KR-12 in Lipid Micelles. *J. Biol. Chem.* **2008**, *283*, 32637–32643. [CrossRef] [PubMed]
112. Valore, E.V.; Park, C.H.; Quayle, A.J.; Wiles, K.R.; Mccray, P.B.; Ganz, T. Human Beta-defensin-1: An Antimicrobial Peptide of Urogenital Tissues. *J. Clin. Investig.* **1998**, *101*, 1633–1642. [CrossRef] [PubMed]

113. Dhople, V.; Krukemeyer, A.; Ramamoorthy, A. The human beta-defensin-3, an antibacterial peptide with multiple biological functions. *Biochim. Biophys. Acta* **2006**, *1758*, 1499–1512. [CrossRef] [PubMed]
114. Lehrer, R.I.; Lichtenstein, A.K.; Ganz, T. Defensins: Antimicrobial and cytotoxic peptides of mammalian cells. *Annu. Rev. Immunol.* **1993**, *11*, 105–128. [CrossRef]
115. Gudmundsson, G.H.; Agerberth, B.; Odeberg, J.; Bergman, T.; Olsson, B.; Salcedo, R. The Human Gene FALL39 and Processing of the Cathelin Precursor to the Antibacterial Peptide LL-37 in Granulocytes. *Eur. J. Biochem.* **1996**, *238*, 325–332. [CrossRef]
116. Sinha, S.; Zheng, L.; Mu, Y.; Ng, W.J.; Bhattacharjya, S. Structure and Interactions of A Host Defense Antimicrobial Peptide Thanatin in Lipopolysaccharide Micelles Reveal Mechanism of Bacterial Cell Agglutination. *Sci. Rep.* **2017**, *7*, 17795. [CrossRef] [PubMed]
117. Domadia, P.N.; Bhunia, A.; Ramamoorthy, A.; Bhattacharjya, S. Structure, interactions, and antibacterial activities of MSI-594 derived mutant peptide MSI-594F5A in lipopolysaccharide micelles: Role of the helical hairpin conformation in outer-membrane permeabilization. *J. Am. Chem. Soc.* **2010**, *132*, 18417–18428. [CrossRef] [PubMed]
118. Bhunia, A.; Mohanram, H.; Domadia, P.N.; Torres, J.; Bhattacharjya, S. Designed B-boomerang Antiendotoxic and Antimicrobial Peptides. *J. Biol. Chem.* **2009**, *284*, 21991–22004. [CrossRef] [PubMed]
119. Ilyas, H.; Kim, J.; Lee, D.; Malmsten, M.; Bhunia, A. Structural Insights into the Combinatorial Effects of Antimicrobial Peptides Reveal a Role of Aromatic–aromatic Interactions in Antibacterial Synergism. *J. Biol. Chem.* **2019**, *294*, 14615–14633. [CrossRef] [PubMed]
120. Datta, A.; Jaiswal, N.; Ilyas, H.; Debnath, S.; Biswas, K.; Kumar, D.; Bhunia, A. Glycine-Mediated Short Analogue of a Designed Peptide in Lipopolysaccharide Micelles: Correlation Between Compact Structure and Anti-Endotoxin Activity. *Biochemistry* **2017**, *56*, 1348–1362. [CrossRef]
121. Jakubec, M.; Rylandsholm, F.G.; Rainsford, P.; Silk, M.; Bril'Kov, M.; Kristoffersen, T.; Juskewitz, E.; Ericson, J.U.; Svendsen, J.S.M. Goldilocks Dilemma: LPS Works Both as the Initial Target and a Barrier for the Antimicrobial Action of Cationic Amps on E. Coli. *Biomolecules* **2023**, *13*, 1155. [CrossRef]
122. Mares, J.; Kumaran, S.; Gobbo, M.; Zerbe, O. Interactions of Lipopolysaccharide and Polymyxin Studied by NMR Spectroscopy. *J. Biol. Chem.* **2009**, *284*, 11498–11506. [CrossRef]
123. Swarbrick, J.D.; Karas, J.A.; Li, J.; Velkov, T. Structure of Micelle Bound Cationic Peptides by NMR Spectroscopy Using a Lanthanide Shift Reagent. *Chem. Commun.* **2020**, *56*, 2897–2900. [CrossRef]
124. Yu, K.; Park, K.; Kang, S.W.; Shin, S.Y.; Hahm, K.S.; Kim, Y. Solution structure of a cathelicidin-derived antimicrobial peptide, CRAMP as determined by NMR spectroscopy. *J. Pept. Res.* **2002**, *60*, 1–9. [CrossRef]
125. Park, K.; Oh, D.; Shin, S.Y.; Hahm, K.S.; Kim, Y. Structural studies of porcine myeloid antibacterial peptide PMAP-23 and its analogues in DPC micelles by NMR spectroscopy. *Biochem. Biophys. Res. Commun.* **2002**, *290*, 204–212. [CrossRef]
126. Tack, B.F.; Sawai, M.V.; Kearney, W.R.; Robertson, A.D.; Sherman, M.A.; Wang, W.; Hong, T.; Boo, L.M.; Wu, H.; Waring, A.J. SMAP-29 Has Two Lps-binding Sites and a Central Hinge. *Eur. J. Biochem.* **2002**, *269*, 1181–1189. [CrossRef]
127. Yang, S.; Lee, C.W.; Kim, H.J.; Jung, H.H.; Kim, J.I.; Shin, S.Y.; Shin, S.H. Structural analysis and mode of action of BMAP-27, a cathelicidin-derived antimicrobial peptide. *Peptides* **2019**, *118*, 170106. [CrossRef]
128. Xiao, Y.; Dai, H.; Bommineni, Y.R.; Soulages, J.L.; Gong, Y.; Prakash, O.; Zhang, G. Structure–activity Relationships of Fowlicidin-1, a Cathelicidin Antimicrobial Peptide in Chicken. *FEBS J.* **2006**, *273*, 2581–2593. [CrossRef]
129. Bommineni, Y.R.; Dai, H.; Gong, Y.X.; Soulages, J.L.; Fernando, S.C.; Desilva, U.; Prakash, O.; Zhang, G. Fowlicidin-3 is an alpha-helical cationic host defense peptide with potent antibacterial and lipopolysaccharide-neutralizing activities. *FEBS J.* **2007**, *274*, 418–428. [CrossRef]
130. Saravanan, R.; Bhattacharjya, S. Oligomeric structure of a cathelicidin antimicrobial peptide in dodecylphosphocholine micelle determined by NMR spectroscopy. *Biochim. Biophys. Acta Biomembr.* **2011**, *1808*, 369–381. [CrossRef]
131. Chen, J.; Falla, T.J.; Liu, H.; Hurst, M.A.; Fujii, C.A.; Mosca, D.A.; Embree, J.R.; Loury, D.J.; Radel, P.A.; Cheng Chang, C.; et al. Development of protegrins for the treatment and prevention of oral mucositis: Structure-activity relationships of synthetic protegrin analogues. *Biopolymers* **2000**, *55*, 88–98. [CrossRef]
132. Hou, M.; Zhang, N.; Yang, J.; Meng, X.; Yang, R.; Li, J.; Sun, T. Antimicrobial Peptide LL-37 and IDR-1 Ameliorate MRSA Pneumonia in Vivo. *Cell. Physiol. Biochem.* **2013**, *32*, 614–623. [CrossRef]
133. Aronen, M.; Viikari, L.; Langen, H.; Kohonen, I.; Wuorela, M.; Vuorinen, T.; Söderlund-Venermo, M.; Viitanen, M.; Camargo, C.A.; Vahlberg, T. The Long-term Prognostic Value of Serum 25(OH)D, Albumin, and LL-37 Levels in Acute Respiratory Diseases Among Older Adults. *BMC Geriatr.* **2022**, *22*, 146. [CrossRef]
134. Zhu, C.; Zhou, Y.; Zhu, J.; Liu, Y.; Sun, M. Proteína 3 Contendo Um Domínio NACHT, Porção C-terminal Rica Em Repetições De Leucina E De Domínio Pirina E LL-37: Valor Prognóstico De Novos Biomarcadores Em Pneumonia Adquirida Na Comunidade. *J. Bras. Pneumol.* **2019**, *45*, e20190001. [CrossRef]
135. Majewski, K.; Żelechowska, P.; Brzezińska-Błaszczyk, E. Circulating Cathelicidin LL-37 in Adult Patients with Pulmonary Infectious Diseases. *Clin. Investig. Med.* **2017**, *40*, 34. [CrossRef]
136. Kozłowska, E.; Wysokiński, A.; Majewski, K.; Agier, J.; Margulska, A.; Brzezińska-Błaszczyk, E. Human Cathelicidin LL-37—Does It Influence the Homeostatic Imbalance in Mental Disorders? *J. Biosci.* **2018**, *43*, 321–327. [CrossRef]
137. Majewski, K.; Kozłowska, E.; Żelechowska, P.; Brzezińska-Błaszczyk, E. Serum Concentrations of Antimicrobial Peptide Cathelicidin LL-37 in Patients with Bacterial Lung Infections. *Cent. Eur. J. Immunol.* **2018**, *43*, 453–457. [CrossRef] [PubMed]

138. Krasnodembskaya, A.; Song, Y.; Fang, X.; Gupta, N.; Serikov, V.; Lee, J.-W.; Matthay, M.A. Antibacterial Effect of Human Mesenchymal Stem Cells Is Mediated in Part from Secretion of the Antimicrobial Peptide LL-37. *Stem Cells* **2010**, *28*, 2229–2238. [CrossRef] [PubMed]
139. Mücke, P.-A.; Maaß, S.; Kohler, T.P.; Hammerschmidt, S.; Becher, D. Proteomic Adaptation of Streptococcus Pneumoniae to the Human Antimicrobial Peptide LL-37. *Microorganisms* **2020**, *8*, 413. [CrossRef] [PubMed]
140. Pouwels, S.D.; Hesse, L.; Wu, X.; Allam, V.S.R.R.; Van Oldeniel, D.; Bhiekharie, L.J.; Phipps, S.; Oliver, B.G.; Gosens, R.; Sukkar, M.B. LL-37 and HMGB1 Induce Alveolar Damage and Reduce Lung Tissue Regeneration via RAGE. *Am. J. Physiol. -Lung Cell. Mol. Physiol.* **2021**, *321*, L641–L652. [CrossRef] [PubMed]
141. Tatsuta, M.; Kan-o, K.; Ishii, Y.; Yamamoto, N.; Ogawa, T.; Fukuyama, S.; Ogawa, A.; Fujita, A.; Nakanishi, Y.; Matsumoto, K. Effects of Cigarette Smoke on Barrier Function and Tight Junction Proteins in the Bronchial Epithelium: Protective Role of Cathelicidin LL-37. *Respir. Res.* **2019**, *20*, 251. [CrossRef] [PubMed]
142. Uysal, P.; Simsek, G.; Durmus, S.; Sozer, V.; Aksan, H.; Yurt, S.; Cuhadaroglu, C.; Kosar, F.; Gelisgen, R.; Uzun, H. evaluation of Plasma Antimicrobial Peptide LL-37 and Nuclear Factor-kappab Levels in Stable Chronic Obstructive Pulmonary Disease. *Int. J. Chronic Obstr. Pulm. Dis.* **2019**, *14*, 321–330. [CrossRef] [PubMed]
143. Jiang, Y.-Y.; Xiao, W.; Zhu, M.-X.; Yang, Z.-H.; Pan, X.-J.; Zhang, Y.; Sun, C.-C.; Xing, Y. The Effect of Human Antibacterial Peptide LL-37 in the Pathogenesis of Chronic Obstructive Pulmonary Disease. *Respir. Med.* **2012**, *106*, 1680–1689. [CrossRef] [PubMed]
144. Sun, C.; Zhu, M.; Yang, Z.; Pan, X.; Zhang, Y.; Wang, Q.; Xiao, W. LL-37 Secreted by Epithelium Promotes Fibroblast Collagen Production: A Potential Mechanism of Small Airway Remodeling in Chronic Obstructive Pulmonary Disease. *Lab. Investig.* **2014**, *94*, 991–1002. [CrossRef]
145. Li, X.; Huang, X.; Li, L.; Wu, J.; Yi, W.; Lai, Y.; Qin, L. Ll-37-coupled Porous Composite Scaffold for the Treatment of Infected Segmental Bone Defect. *Pharmaceutics* **2022**, *15*, 88. [CrossRef]
146. Barlow, P.G.; Svoboda, P.; Mackellar, A.; Nash, A.A.; York, I.A.; Pohl, J.; Davidson, D.J.; Donis, R.O. Antiviral Activity and Increased Host Defense Against Influenza Infection Elicited by the Human Cathelicidin LL-37. *PLoS ONE* **2011**, *6*, e25333. [CrossRef]
147. Tripathi, S.; Tecle, T.; Verma, A.; Crouch, E.; White, M.; Hartshorn, K.L. The Human Cathelicidin LL-37 Inhibits Influenza A Viruses Through a Mechanism Distinct from That of Surfactant Protein D or Defensins. *J. Gen. Virol.* **2013**, *94*, 40–49. [CrossRef] [PubMed]
148. White, M.R.; Tripathi, S.; Verma, A.; Kingma, P.; Takahashi, K.; Jensenius, J.; Thiel, S.; Wang, G.; Crouch, E.C.; Hartshorn, K.L. Collectins, H-ficolin and LL-37 Reduce Influence Viral Replication in Human Monocytes and Modulate Virus-induced Cytokine Production. *Innate Immun.* **2017**, *23*, 77–88. [CrossRef]
149. Lee, I.H.; Jung, Y.-J.; Cho, Y.G.; Nou, I.S.; Huq, M.A.; Nogoy, F.M.; Kang, K.-K. SP-LL-37, Human Antimicrobial Peptide, Enhances Disease Resistance in Transgenic Rice. *PLoS ONE* **2017**, *12*, e0172936. [CrossRef] [PubMed]
150. Palusinska-Szysz, M.; Jurak, M.; Gisch, N.; Waldow, F.; Zehethofer, N.; Nehls, C.; Schwudke, D.; Koper, P.; Mazur, A. The human LL-37 peptide exerts antimicrobial activity against Legionella micdadei interacting with membrane phospholipids. *Biochim. Biophys. Acta Mol. Cell. Biol. Lipids* **2022**, *1867*, 159138. [CrossRef]
151. Tripathi, S.; Wang, G.; White, M.; Rynkiewicz, M.; Seaton, B.; Hartshorn, K. Identifying the Critical Domain of LL-37 Involved in Mediating Neutrophil Activation in the Presence of Influenza Virus: Functional and Structural Analysis. *PLoS ONE* **2015**, *10*, e0133454. [CrossRef] [PubMed]
152. Hu, L.I.; Stohl, E.A.; Seifert, H.S. The Neisseria Gonorrhoeae Type IV Pilus Promotes Resistance to Hydrogen Peroxide- and Ll-37-mediated Killing by Modulating the Availability of Intracellular, Labile Iron. *PLoS Pathog.* **2022**, *18*, e1010561. [CrossRef] [PubMed]
153. Kiattiburut, W.; Zhi, R.; Lee, S.G.; Foo, A.C.; Hickling, D.R.; Keillor, J.W.; Goto, N.K.; Li, W.; Conlan, W.; Angel, J.B. Antimicrobial Peptide LL-37 and Its Truncated Forms, GI-20 and GF-17, Exert Spermicidal Effects and Microbicidal Activity Against Neisseria Gonorrhoeae. *Hum. Reprod.* **2018**, *33*, 2175–2183. [CrossRef]
154. Pashapour, A.; Sardari, S.; Ehsani, P. In Silicodesign and in Vitro Evaluation of Some Novel Amps Derived from Human LL-37 as Potential Antimicrobial Agents for Keratitis. *Iran. J. Pharm. Res.* **2022**, *21*, e124017. [CrossRef]
155. Sharma, P.; Sharma, N.; Mishra, P.; Joseph, J.; Mishra, D.K.; Garg, P.; Roy, S. Differential Expression of Antimicrobial Peptides in Streptococcus Pneumoniae Keratitis and Stat3-dependent Expression of LL-37 by Streptococcus Pneumoniae in Human Corneal Epithelial Cells. *Pathogens* **2019**, *8*, 31. [CrossRef]
156. Oliveira, P.N.; Courrol, D.S.; Chura-Chambi, R.M.; Morganti, L.; Souza, G.O.; Franzolin, M.R.; Wunder, E.A., Jr.; Heinemann, M.B.; Barbosa, A.S. Inactivation of the antimicrobial peptide LL-37 by pathogenic leptospira. *Microb. Pathog.* **2021**, *150*, 104704. [CrossRef] [PubMed]
157. Moreno-Angarita, A.; Aragón, C.C.; Tobón, G.J. Cathelicidin ll-37: A new important molecule in the pathophysiology of systemic lupus erythematosus. *J. Transl. Autoimmun.* **2020**, *3*, 100029. [CrossRef] [PubMed]
158. Kahlenberg, J.M.; Kaplan, M.J. Little Peptide, Big Effects: The Role of LL-37 in Inflammation and Autoimmune Disease. *J. Immunol.* **2013**, *191*, 4895–4901. [CrossRef] [PubMed]
159. Lande, R.; Ganguly, D.; Facchinetti, V.; Frasca, L.; Conrad, C.; Gregorio, J.; Meller, S.; Chamilos, G.; Sebasigari, R.; Riccieri, V. Neutrophils Activate Plasmacytoid Dendritic Cells by Releasing Self-dna–peptide Complexes in Systemic Lupus Erythematosus. *Sci. Transl. Med.* **2011**, *3*, 73ra19. [CrossRef] [PubMed]

160. Pahar, B.; Madonna, S.; Das, A.; Albanesi, C.; Girolomoni, G. Immunomodulatory Role of the Antimicrobial LL-37 Peptide in Autoimmune Diseases and Viral Infections. *Vaccines* **2020**, *8*, 517. [CrossRef] [PubMed]
161. Jones, A.; Geörg, M.; Maudsdotter, L.; Jonsson, A.-B. Endotoxin, Capsule, and Bacterial Attachment Contribute to Neisseria Meningitidis Resistance to the Human Antimicrobial Peptide LL-37. *J. Bacteriol.* **2009**, *191*, 3861–3868. [CrossRef]
162. Zughaier, S.M.; Svoboda, P.; Pohl, J.; Stephens, D.S.; Shafer, W.M. The Human Host Defense Peptide LL-37 Interacts with Neisseria Meningitidis Capsular Polysaccharides and Inhibits Inflammatory Mediators Release. *PLoS ONE* **2010**, *5*, e13627. [CrossRef]
163. Seib, K.L.; Serruto, D.; Oriente, F.; Delany, I.; Adu-Bobie, J.; Veggi, D.; Aricò, B.; Rappuoli, R.; Pizza, M. Factor H-binding Protein Is Important for Meningococcal Survival in Human Whole Blood and Serum and in the Presence of the Antimicrobial Peptide LL-37. *Infect. Immun.* **2009**, *77*, 292–299. [CrossRef]
164. Gutner, M.; Chaushu, S.; Balter, D.; Bachrach, G. Saliva Enables the Antimicrobial Activity of LL-37 in the Presence of Proteases of Porphyromonas Gingivalis. *Infect. Immun.* **2009**, *77*, 5558–5563. [CrossRef]
165. Chinipardaz, Z.; Zhong, J.M.; Yang, S. Regulation of LL-37 in Bone and Periodontium Regeneration. *Life* **2022**, *12*, 1533. [CrossRef]
166. Tada, H.; Shimizu, T.; Matsushita, K.; Takada, H. Porphyromonas Gingivalisinduced IL-33 Down-regulates Hcap-18/Il-37 Production in Human Gingival Epithelial cells. *Biomed. Res.* **2017**, *38*, 167–173. [CrossRef]
167. Bedran, T.B.L.; Mayer, M.P.A.; Spolidorio, D.P.; Grenier, D. Synergistic Anti-inflammatory Activity of the Antimicrobial Peptides Human Beta-defensin-3 (hbd-3) and Cathelicidin (LL-37) in a Three-dimensional Co-culture Model of Gingival Epithelial Cells and Fibroblasts. *PLoS ONE* **2014**, *9*, e106766. [CrossRef] [PubMed]
168. Puklo, M.; Guentsch, A.; Hiemstra, P.S.; Eick, S.; Potempa, J. Analysis of Neutrophil-derived Antimicrobial Peptides in Gingival Crevicular Fluid Suggests Importance of Cathelicidin LL-37 in the Innate Immune Response Against Periodontogenic Bacteria. *Oral Microbiol. Immunol.* **2008**, *23*, 328–335. [CrossRef]
169. Lao, J.; Xie, Z.; Qin, Q.; Qin, R.; Li, S.; Yuan, Y. Serum LL-37 and Inflammatory Cytokines Levels in Psoriasis. *Immun. Inflamm. Dis.* **2023**, *11*, e802. [CrossRef]
170. Dombrowski, Y.; Schauber, J. Cathelicidin LL-37: A Defense Molecule with a Potential Role in Psoriasis Pathogenesis. *Exp. Dermatol.* **2012**, *21*, 327–330. [CrossRef]
171. Morizane, S.; Yamasaki, K.; Mühleisen, B.; Kotol, P.F.; Murakami, M.; Aoyama, Y.; Iwatsuki, K.; Hata, T.; Gallo, R.L. Cathelicidin Antimicrobial Peptide LL-37 in Psoriasis Enables Keratinocyte Reactivity Against TLR9 Ligands. *J. Investig. Dermatol.* **2012**, *132*, 135–143. [CrossRef] [PubMed]
172. Hoffmann, M.H.; Bruns, H.; Bäckdahl, L.; Neregård, P.; Niederreiter, B.; Herrmann, M.; Catrina, A.I.; Agerberth, B.; Holmdahl, R. The Cathelicidins LL-37 and Rcramp Are Associated with Pathogenic Events of Arthritis in Humans and Rats. *Ann. Rheum. Dis.* **2013**, *72*, 1239–1248. [CrossRef] [PubMed]
173. Cheah, C.W.; Al-Maleki, A.R.; Vaithilingam, R.D.; Vadivelu, J.; Sockalingam, S.; Baharuddin, N.A.; Bartold, P.M. Associations Between Inflammation-related LL-37 with Subgingival Microbial Dysbiosis in Rheumatoid Arthritis Patients. *Clin. Oral Investig.* **2022**, *26*, 4161–4172. [CrossRef]
174. Chow, L.N.Y.; Choi, K.-Y.; Piyadasa, H.; Bossert, M.; Uzonna, J.; Klonisch, T.; Mookherjee, N. Human Cathelicidin Ll-37-derived Peptide IG-19 Confers Protection in a Murine Model of Collagen-induced Arthritis. *Mol. Immunol.* **2014**, *57*, 86–92. [CrossRef]
175. Kuensaen, C.; Chomdej, S.; Kongdang, P.; Sirikaew, N.; Jaitham, R.; Thonghoi, S.; Ongchai, S. LL-37 Alone and in Combination with IL17A Enhances Proinflammatory Cytokine Expression in Parallel with Hyaluronan Metabolism in Human Synovial Sarcoma Cell Line SW982—A Step Toward Understanding the Development of Inflammatory Arthritis. *PLoS ONE* **2019**, *14*, e0218736. [CrossRef] [PubMed]
176. Koziel, J.; Bryzek, D.; Sroka, A.; Maresz, K.; Glowczyk, I.; Bielecka, E.; Kantyka, T.; Pyrć, K.; Svoboda, P.; Pohl, J.; et al. Citrullination Alters Immunomodulatory Function of LL-37 Essential for Prevention of Endotoxin-Induced Sepsis. *J. Immunol.* **2014**, *192*, 5363–5372. [CrossRef] [PubMed]
177. Leite, M.L.; Duque, H.M.; Rodrigues, G.R.; da Cunha, N.B.; Franco, O.L. The LL-37 domain: A clue to cathelicidin immunomodulatory response? *Peptide* **2023**, *165*, 171011. [CrossRef]
178. Hu, Z.; Murakami, T.; Suzuki, K.; Tamura, H.; Kuwahara-Arai, K.; Iba, T.; Nagaoka, I. Antimicrobial Cathelicidin Peptide LL-37 Inhibits the Lps/atp-induced Pyroptosis of Macrophages by Dual Mechanism. *PLoS ONE* **2014**, *9*, e85765. [CrossRef]
179. Nagaoka, I.; Tamura, H.; Reich, J. Therapeutic Potential of Cathelicidin Peptide LL-37, an Antimicrobial Agent, in a Murine Sepsis Model. *Lancet Infect. Dis.* **2020**, *21*, 5973. [CrossRef]
180. Rivas-Santiago, B.; Hernandez-Pando, R.; Carranza, C.; Juarez, E.; Contreras, J.L.; Aguilar-Leon, D.; Torres, M.; Sada, E. Expression of Cathelicidin LL-37 Duringmycobacterium Tuberculosisinfection in Human Alveolar Macrophages, Monocytes, Neutrophils, and Epithelial Cells. *Infect. Immun.* **2008**, *76*, 935–941. [CrossRef] [PubMed]
181. Rekha, R.S.; Rao Muvva, S.J.; Wan, M.; Raqib, R.; Bergman, P.; Brighenti, S.; Gudmundsson, G.H.; Agerberth, B. Phenylbutyrate Induces Ll-37-dependent Autophagy and Intracellular Killing of Mycobacterium Tuberculosis in Human Macrophages. *Autophagy* **2015**, *11*, 1688–1699. [CrossRef]
182. Torres-Juarez, F.; Cardenas-Vargas, A.; Montoya-Rosales, A.; González-Curiel, I.; Garcia-Hernandez, M.H.; Enciso-Moreno, J.A.; Hancock, R.E.W.; Rivas-Santiago, B. LL-37 Immunomodulatory Activity During Mycobacterium Tuberculosis Infection in Macrophages. *Infect. Immun.* **2015**, *83*, 4495–4503. [CrossRef]

183. Dhiman, A.; Talukdar, S.; Chaubey, G.K.; Dilawari, R.; Modanwal, R.; Chaudhary, S.; Patidar, A.; Boradia, V.M.; Kumbhar, P.; Raje, C.I. Regulation of Macrophage Cell Surface GAPDH Alters LL-37 Internalization and Downstream Effects in the Cell. *J. Innate Immun.* **2023**, *15*, 581–598. [CrossRef]
184. Duan, Z.; Fang, Y.; Sun, Y.; Luan, N.; Chen, X.; Chen, M.; Han, Y.; Yin, Y.; Mwangi, J.; Niu, J.; et al. Antimicrobial peptide LL-37 forms complex with bacterial DNA to facilitate blood translocation of bacterial DNA and aggravate ulcerative colitis. *Sci. Bull.* **2018**, *63*, 1364–1375. [CrossRef]
185. Memariani, H.; Memariani, M. Antibiofilm Properties of Cathelicidin LL-37: An In-depth Review. *World J. Microbiol. Biotechnol.* **2023**, *39*, 99. [CrossRef]
186. Overhage, J.; Campisano, A.; Bains, M.; Torfs, E.C.W.; Rehm, B.H.A.; Hancock, R.E.W. Human Host Defense Peptide LL-37 Prevents Bacterial Biofilm Formation. *Infect. Immun.* **2008**, *76*, 4176–4182. [CrossRef]
187. Schmidtchen, A.; Frick, I.; Andersson, E.; Tapper, H.; Björck, L. Proteinases of Common Pathogenic Bacteria Degrade and Inactivate the Antibacterial Peptide LL-37. *Mol. Microbiol.* **2002**, *46*, 157–168. [CrossRef]
188. Sieprawska-Lupa, M.; Mydel, P.; Krawczyk, K.; Wójcik, K.; Puklo, M.; Lupa, B.; Suder, P.; Silberring, J.; Reed, M.; Pohl, J. Degradation of Human Antimicrobial Peptide LL-37 by *Staphylococcus Aureus* -derived Proteinases. *Antimicrob. Agents Chemother.* **2004**, *48*, 4673–4679. [CrossRef] [PubMed]
189. Koziel, J.; Karim, A.Y.; Przybyszewska, K.; Ksiazek, M.; Rapala-Kozik, M.; Nguyen, K.-A.; Potempa, J. Proteolytic Inactivation of LL-37 by Karilysin, a Novel Virulence Mechanism of *Tannerella forsythia*. *J. Innate Immun.* **2010**, *2*, 288–293. [CrossRef] [PubMed]
190. Thomassin, J.-L.; Brannon, J.R.; Gibbs, B.F.; Gruenheid, S.; Le Moual, H. Ompt Outer Membrane Proteases of Enterohemorrhagic and Enteropathogenic Escherichia Coli Contribute Differently to the Degradation of Human LL-37. *Infect. Immun.* **2012**, *80*, 483–492. [CrossRef] [PubMed]
191. Brannon, J.R.; Thomassin, J.-L.; Desloges, I.; Gruenheid, S.; Le Moual, H. Role of Uropathogenicescherichia Coliompt in the Resistance Against Human Cathelicidin LL-37. *FEMS Microbiol. Lett.* **2013**, *345*, 64–71. [CrossRef]
192. Papo, N.; Shahar, M.; Eisenbach, L.; Shai, Y. A Novel Lytic Peptide Composed of Dl-amino Acids Selectively Kills Cancer Cells in Culture and in Mice. *J. Biol. Chem.* **2003**, *278*, 21018–21023. [CrossRef] [PubMed]
193. Makovitzki, A.; Fink, A.; Shai, Y. Suppression of Human Solid Tumor Growth in Mice by Intratumor and Systemic Inoculation of Histidine-rich and Ph-dependent Host Defense–like Lytic Peptides. *Cancer Res.* **2009**, *69*, 3458–3463. [CrossRef]
194. Kamarajan, P.; Hayami, T.; Matte, B.; Liu, Y.; Danciu, T.; Ramamoorthy, A.; Worden, F.; Kapila, S.; Kapila, Y. Nisin ZP, a Bacteriocin and Food Preservative, Inhibits Head and Neck Cancer Tumorigenesis and Prolongs Survival. *PLoS ONE* **2015**, *10*, e0131008. [CrossRef]
195. Wang, G.; Vaisman, I.I.; Van Hoek, M.L. Machine Learning Prediction of Antimicrobial Peptides. In *Single Cell Analysis*; Springer: Berlin/Heidelberg, Germany, 2022; pp. 1–37.
196. Heilborn, J.D.; Nilsson, M.F.; Jimenez, C.I.C.; Sandstedt, B.; Borregaard, N.; Tham, E.; Sørensen, O.E.; Weber, G.; Ståhle, M. Antimicrobial Protein Hcap18/Il-37 Is Highly Expressed in Breast Cancer and Is a Putative Growth Factor for Epithelial Cells. *Int. J. Cancer* **2005**, *114*, 713–719. [CrossRef] [PubMed]
197. Chen, X.; Zou, X.; Qi, G.; Tang, Y.; Guo, Y.; Si, J.; Liang, L. Roles and Mechanisms of Human Cathelicidin LL-37 in Cancer. *Cell. Physiol. Biochem.* **2018**, *47*, 1060–1073. [CrossRef] [PubMed]
198. Piktel, E.; Niemirowicz, K.; Wnorowska, U.; Wątek, M.; Wollny, T.; Głuszek, K.; Góźdź, S.; Levental, I.; Bucki, R. The Role of Cathelicidin LL-37 in Cancer Development. *Arch. Immunol. Ther. Exp.* **2016**, *64*, 33–46. [CrossRef] [PubMed]
199. Wu, W.K.K.; Wang, G.; Coffelt, S.B.; Betancourt, A.M.; Lee, C.W.; Fan, D.; Wu, K.; Yu, J.; Sung, J.J.Y.; Cho, C.H. Emerging Roles of the Host Defense Peptide LL-37 in Human Cancer and Its Potential Therapeutic Applications. *Int. J. Cancer* **2010**, *127*, 1741–1747. [CrossRef]
200. Verjans, E.T.; Zels, S.; Luyten, W.; Landuyt, B.; Schoofs, L. Molecular mechanisms of LL-37-induced receptor activation: An overview. *Peptides* **2016**, *85*, 16–26. [CrossRef] [PubMed]
201. Doss, M.; White, M.R.; Tecle, T.; Hartshorn, K.L. Human Defensins and LL-37 in Mucosal Immunity. *J. Leukoc. Biol.* **2009**, *87*, 79–92. [CrossRef]
202. Wang, G.; Narayana, J.L.; Mishra, B.; Zhang, Y.; Wang, F.; Wang, C.; Zarena, D.; Lushnikova, T.; Wang, X. Design of Antimicrobial Peptides: Progress Made with Human Cathelicidin LL-37. In *Advances in Experimental Medicine and Biology*; Springer: Berlin/Heidelberg, Germany, 2019; pp. 215–240.
203. Yang, B.; Good, D.; Mosaiab, T.; Liu, W.; Ni, G.; Kaur, J.; Liu, X.; Jessop, C.; Yang, L.; Fadhil, R. Significance of LL-37 on Immunomodulation and Disease Outcome. *BioMed Res. Int.* **2020**, *2020*, 8349712. [CrossRef]
204. Bucki, R.; Leszczyńska, K.; Namiot, A.; Sokołowski, W. Cathelicidin LL-37: A Multitask Antimicrobial Peptide. *Arch. Immunol. Ther. Exp.* **2010**, *58*, 15–25. [CrossRef]
205. De Lorenzi, E.; Chiari, M.; Colombo, R.; Cretich, M.; Sola, L.; Vanna, R.; Gagni, P.; Bisceglia, F.; Morasso, C.; Lin, J.S. Evidence That the Human Innate Immune Peptide LL-37 May Be a Binding Partner of Amyloid-β and Inhibitor of Fibril Assembly. *J. Alzheimer's Dis.* **2017**, *59*, 1213–1226. [CrossRef]
206. Chen, X.; Deng, S.; Wang, W.; Castiglione, S.; Duan, Z.; Luo, L.; Cianci, F.; Zhang, X.; Xu, J.; Li, H. Human Antimicrobial Peptide LL-37 Contributes to Alzheimer's Disease Progression. *Mol. Psychiatry* **2022**, *27*, 4790–4799. [CrossRef] [PubMed]

207. Armiento, V.; Hille, K.; Naltsas, D.; Lin, J.S.; Barron, A.E.; Kapurniotu, A. The Human Host-defense Peptide Cathelicidin LL-37 Is a Nanomolar Inhibitor of Amyloid Self-assembly of Islet Amyloid Polypeptide (IAPP). *Angew. Chem. Int. Ed.* **2020**, *59*, 12837–12841. [CrossRef]
208. Sancho-Vaello, E.; François, P.; Bonetti, E.-J.; Lilie, H.; Finger, S.; Gil-Ortiz, F.; Gil-Carton, D.; Zeth, K. Structural Remodeling and Oligomerization of Human Cathelicidin on Membranes Suggest Fibril-like Structures as Active Species. *Sci. Rep.* **2017**, *7*, 15371. [CrossRef] [PubMed]
209. Sancho-Vaello, E.; Gil-Carton, D.; François, P.; Bonetti, E.-J.; Kreir, M.; Pothula, K.R.; Kleinekathöfer, U.; Zeth, K. The Structure of the Antimicrobial Human Cathelicidin LL-37 Shows Oligomerization and Channel Formation in the Presence of Membrane Mimics. *Sci. Rep.* **2020**, *10*, 17356. [CrossRef] [PubMed]
210. Li, X.; Li, Y.; Han, H.; Miller, D.W.; Wang, G. Solution Structures of Human LL-37 Fragments and NMR-Based Identification of a Minimal Membrane-Targeting Antimicrobial and Anticancer Region. *J. Am. Chem. Soc.* **2006**, *128*, 5776–5785. [CrossRef]
211. Gunasekera, S.; Muhammad, T.; Strömstedt, A.A.; Rosengren, K.J.; Göransson, U. Backbone Cyclization and Dimerization of Ll-37-derived Peptides Enhance Antimicrobial Activity and Proteolytic Stability. *Front. Microbiol.* **2020**, *11*, 168. [CrossRef]
212. Henzler Wildman, K.A.; Lee, D.K.; Ramamoorthy, A. Mechanism of bilayer disruption by the human antimicrobial peptide, LL-37. *Biochemistry* **2003**, *42*, 6545–6558. [CrossRef]
213. Nielsen, J.E.; Alford, M.A.; Yung, D.B.Y.; Molchanova, N.; Fortkort, J.A.; Lin, J.S.; Diamond, G.; Hancock, R.E.W.; Jenssen, H.; Pletzer, D. Self-assembly of Antimicrobial Peptoids Impacts Their Biological Effects on ESKAPE Bacterial Pathogens. *ACS Infect. Dis.* **2022**, *8*, 533–545. [CrossRef]
214. Jiang, X.; Yang, C.; Qiu, J.; Ma, D.; Xu, C.; Hu, S.; Han, W.; Yuan, B.; Lu, Y. Nanomolar LL-37 Induces Permeability of a Biomimetic Mitochondrial Membrane. *Nanoscale* **2022**, *14*, 17654–17660. [CrossRef]
215. Mitra, A.; Paul, S. Pathways of hLL-37_{17-29} Aggregation Give Insight into the Mechanism of α-Amyloid Formation. *J. Phys. Chem. B* **2023**, *127*, 8162–8175. [CrossRef]
216. Li, X.; Li, Y.; Peterkosfsky, A.; Wang, G. NMR studies of aurein 1.2 analogs. *Biochim. Biophys. Acta Biomembr.* **2006**, *1758*, 1203–1214. [CrossRef]
217. Engelberg, Y.; Landau, M. The Human LL-37(17-29) Antimicrobial Peptide Reveals a Functional Supramolecular Structure. *Nat. Commun.* **2020**, *11*, 3894. [CrossRef]
218. Engelberg, Y.; Ragonis-Bachar, P.; Landau, M. Rare by Natural Selection: Disulfide-bonded Supramolecular Antimicrobial Peptides. *Biomacromolecules* **2022**, *23*, 926–936. [CrossRef] [PubMed]
219. Yun, H.; Min, H.J.; Lee, C.W. NMR Structure and Bactericidal Activity of KR-12 Analog Derived from Human LL-37 as a Potential Cosmetic Preservative. *J. Anal. Sci. Technol.* **2020**, *11*, 14. [CrossRef]
220. Shcherbakov, A.A.; Spreacker, P.J.; Dregni, A.J.; Henzler-Wildman, K.A.; Hong, M. High-ph Structure of Emre Reveals the Mechanism of Proton-coupled Substrate Transport. *Nat. Commun.* **2022**, *13*, 991. [CrossRef] [PubMed]
221. Nishiyama, Y.; Hou, G.; Agarwal, V.; Su, Y.; Ramamoorthy, A. Ultrafast Magic Angle Spinning Solid-State NMR Spectroscopy: Advances in Methodology and Applications. *Chem. Rev.* **2023**, *123*, 918–988. [CrossRef]
222. Hellmich, U.A.; Lyubenova, S.; Kaltenborn, E.; Doshi, R.; van Veen, H.W.; Prisner, T.F.; Glaubitz, C. Probing the ATP Hydrolysis Cycle of the ABC Multidrug Transporter LmrA by Pulsed EPR Spectroscopy. *J. Am. Chem. Soc.* **2013**, *134*, 5857–5862. [CrossRef]
223. Rogawski, R.; MecDermott, A.E. New NMR tools for protein structure and function: Spin tags for dynamic nuclear polarization solid state NMR. *Arch. Biochem. Biophys.* **2017**, *628*, 102–113. [CrossRef] [PubMed]
224. Reif, B.; Ashbrook, S.E.; Emsley, L.; Hong, M. Solid-state NMR Spectroscopy. *Nat. Rev. Methods Primers* **2021**, *1*, 2. [CrossRef]
225. Gopinath, T.; Weber, D.; Wang, S.; Larsen, E.; Veglia, G. Solid-State NMR of Membrane Proteins in Lipid Bilayers: To Spin or Not to Spin? *Acc. Chem. Res.* **2021**, *54*, 1430–1439. [CrossRef]
226. Roversi, D.; Troiano, C.; Salnikov, E.; Giordano, L.; Riccitelli, F.; De Zotti, M.; Casciaro, B.; Loffredo, M.R.; Park, Y.; Formaggio, F.; et al. Effects of antimicrobial peptides on membrane dynamics: A comparison of fluorescence and NMR experiments. *Biophys. Chem.* **2023**, *300*, 107060. [CrossRef]
227. Salnikov, E.; Aisenbrey, C.; Bechinger, B. Lipid saturation and head group composition have a pronounced influence on the membrane insertion equilibrium of amphipathic helical polypeptides. *Biochim. Biophys. Acta Biomembr.* **2022**, *1864*, 183844. [CrossRef] [PubMed]
228. Schweigardt, F.; Strandberg, E.; Wadhwani, P.; Reichert, J.; Bürck, J.; Cravo, H.L.P.; Burger, L.; Ulrich, A.S. Membranolytic Mechanism of Amphiphilic Antimicrobial Β-stranded [kl]n Peptides. *Biomedicines* **2022**, *10*, 2071. [CrossRef] [PubMed]
229. Ramamoorthy, A. Beyond NMR Spectra of Antimicrobial Peptides: Dynamical Images at Atomic Resolution and Functional Insights. *Solid State Nucl. Magn. Reson.* **2009**, *35*, 201–207. [CrossRef]
230. Mihailescu, M.; Sorci, M.; Seckute, J.; Silin, V.I.; Hammer, J.; Perrin, B.S.; Hernandez, J.I.; Smajic, N.; Shrestha, A.; Bogardus, K.A. Structure and Function in Antimicrobial Piscidins: Histidine Position, Directionality of Membrane Insertion, and Ph-dependent Permeabilization. *J. Am. Chem. Soc.* **2019**, *141*, 9837–9853. [CrossRef] [PubMed]
231. Xhindoli, D.; Morgera, F.; Zinth, U.; Rizzo, R.; Pacor, S.; Tossi, A. New Aspects of the Structure and Mode of Action of the Human Cathelicidin LL-37 Revealed by the Intrinsic Probe P-cyanophenylalanine. *Biochem. J.* **2015**, *465*, 443–457. [CrossRef]
232. Oren, Z.; Lerman, J.C.; Gudmundsson, G.H.; Agerberth, B.; Shai, Y. Structure and Organization of the Human Antimicrobial Peptide LL-37 in Phospholipid Membranes: Relevance to the Molecular Basis for Its Non-cell-selective Activity. *Biochem. J.* **1999**, *341*, 501–513. [CrossRef]

233. Sood, R.; Domanov, Y.; Pietiäinen, M.; Kontinen, V.P.; Kinnunen, P.K. Binding of LL-37 to model biomembranes: Insight into target vs host cell recognition. *Biochim. Biophys. Acta* **2008**, *1778*, 983–996. [CrossRef]
234. Liu, C.; Henning-Knechtel, A.; Österlund, N.; Wu, J.; Wang, G.; Gräslund, R.A.O.; Kirmizialtin, S.; Luo, J. Oligomer Dynamics of LL-37 Truncated Fragments Probed by A-hemolysin Pore and Molecular Simulations. *Small* **2023**, *19*, e2206232. [CrossRef] [PubMed]
235. Zeth, K.; Sancho-Vaello, E. The Human Antimicrobial Peptides Dermcidin and LL-37 Show Novel Distinct Pathways in Membrane Interactions. *Front. Chem.* **2017**, *5*, 86. [CrossRef] [PubMed]
236. Xhindoli, D.; Pacor, S.; Benincasa, M.; Scocchi, M.; Gennaro, R.; Tossi, A. The human cathelicidin LL-37—A pore-forming antibacterial peptide and host-cell modulator. *Biochim. Biophys. Acta* **2016**, *1858*, 546–566. [CrossRef]
237. Henzler-Wildman, K.A.; Martinez, G.V.; Brown, M.F.; Ramamoorthy, A. Perturbation of the hydrophobic core of lipid bilayers by the human antimicrobial peptide LL-37. *Biochemistry* **2004**, *43*, 8459–8469. [CrossRef] [PubMed]
238. Hardy, J.; Selkoe, D.J. The amyloid hypothesis of Alzheimer's disease: Progress and problems on the road to therapeutics. *Science* **2002**, *297*, 353–356. [CrossRef] [PubMed]
239. Michele; Samuel; Jeffrey; Chen, J.; Lee, D.-K.; Ramamoorthy, A. Two-step Mechanism of Membrane Disruption by Aβ Through Membrane Fragmentation and Pore Formation. *Biophys. J.* **2012**, *103*, 702–710. [CrossRef]
240. Kotler, S.A.; Brender, J.R.; Vivekanandan, S.; Suzuki, Y.; Yamamoto, K.; Monette, M.; Krishnamoorthy, J.; Walsh, P.; Cauble, M.; Holl, M.M.B. High-resolution NMR Characterization of Low Abundance Oligomers of Amyloid-β Without Purification. *Sci. Rep.* **2015**, *5*, 11811. [CrossRef]
241. Colombo, L.; Gamba, A.; Cantù, L.; Salmona, M.; Tagliavini, F.; Rondelli, V.; Del Favero, E.; Brocca, P. Pathogenic Aβ A2V Versus Protective Aβ A2T Mutation: Early Stage Aggregation and Membrane Interaction. *Biophys. Chem.* **2017**, *229*, 11–18. [CrossRef]
242. Ma, L.; Li, X.; Peterson, R.B.; Peng, A.; Huang, K. Probing the interactions between amyloidogenic proteins and bio-membranes. *Biophys. Chem.* **2023**, *296*, 106984. [CrossRef] [PubMed]
243. Fatafta, H.; Kav, B.; Bundschuh, B.F.; Loschwitz, J.; Strodel, B. Disorder-to-order transition of the amyloid-β peptide upon lipid binding. *Biophys. Chem.* **2022**, *280*, 106700. [CrossRef] [PubMed]
244. Zambrano, P.; Jemiola-Rzeminska, M.; Muñoz-Torrero, D.; Suwalsky, M.; Strzalka, K. A rhein-huprine hybrid protects erythrocyte membrane integrity against Alzheimer's disease related Aβ(1-42) peptide. *Biophys. Chem.* **2023**, *300*, 107061. [CrossRef]
245. Nicastro, M.C.; Spigolon, D.; Librizzi, F.; Moran, O.; Ortore, M.G.; Bulone, D.; Biagio, P.L.; Carrotta, R. Amyloid β-peptide insertion in liposomes containing GM1-cholesterol domains. *Biophys. Chem.* **2016**, *208*, 9–16. [CrossRef]
246. Saha, J.; Ford, B.J.; Wang, X.; Boyd, S.; Morgan, S.E.; Rangachari, V. Sugar distributions on gangliosides guide the formation and stability of amyloid-β oligomers. *Biophys. Chem.* **2023**, *300*, 197073. [CrossRef]
247. Kenyaga, J.M.; Oteino, S.A.; Sun, Y.; Qiang, W. In-cell 31P solid-state NMR measurements of the lipid dynamics and influence of exogeneous β-amyloid peptides on live neuroblastoma neuro-2a cells. *Biophys. Chem.* **2023**, *297*, 107008. [CrossRef] [PubMed]
248. Morita, M.; Vestergaard, M.; Hamada, T.; Takagi, M. Real-time observation of model membrane dynamics induced by Alzheimer's amyloid beta. *Biophys. Chem.* **2009**, *147*, 81–86. [CrossRef] [PubMed]
249. Kumar, M.; Ivanova, M.I.; Ramamoorthy, A. Non-micellar ganglioside GM1 induces an instantaneous conformational change in Aβ42 leading to the modulation of the peptide amyloid-fibril pathway. *Biophys. Chem.* **2023**, *301*, 107091. [CrossRef]
250. Kumar, M.; I Ivanova, M.; Ramamoorthy, A. Ganglioside GM1 Produces Stable, Short, and Cytotoxic Aβ40 Protofibrils. *Chem. Commun.* **2023**, *59*, 7040–7043. [CrossRef]
251. Lee, M.; Shi, X.; Barron, A.E.; McGeer, E.; McGeer, P.L. Human antimicrobial peptide LL-37 induces glial-mediated neuroinflammation. *Biochem. Pharmacol.* **2015**, *94*, 130–141. [CrossRef]
252. Fülöp, T.; Itzhaki, R.F.; Balin, B.J.; Miklossy, J.; Barron, A.E. Role of Microbes in the Development of Alzheimer's Disease: State of the Art—An International Symposium Presented at the 2017 IAGG Congress in San Francisco. *Front. Genet.* **2018**, *9*, 362. [CrossRef]
253. Betsholtz, C.; Johnson, K.H.; Westermark, P. 'amylin' Hormone. *Nature* **1989**, *338*, 211. [CrossRef] [PubMed]
254. Westermark, G.T.; Westermark, P. Islet amyloid polypeptide and diabetes. *Curr. Protein Pept. Sci.* **2013**, *14*, 330–337. [CrossRef]
255. Westermark, P.; Andersson, A.; Westermark, G.T. Is Aggregated IAPP a Cause of Beta-cell Failure in Transplanted Human Pancreatic Islets? *Curr. Diabetes Rep.* **2005**, *5*, 184–188. [CrossRef] [PubMed]
256. Milardi, D.; Gazit, E.; Radford, S.E.; Xu, Y.; Gallardo, R.U.; Caflisch, A.; Westermark, G.T.; Westermark, P.; Rosa, C.L.; Ramamoorthy, A. Proteostasis of Islet Amyloid Polypeptide: A Molecular Perspective of Risk Factors and Protective Strategies for Type II Diabetes. *Chem. Rev.* **2021**, *121*, 1845–1893. [CrossRef]
257. Pithadia, A.; Brender, J.R.; Fierke, C.A.; Ramamoorthy, A. Inhibition of IAPP Aggregation and Toxicity by Natural Products and Derivatives. *J. Diabetes Res.* **2016**, *2016*, 2046327. [CrossRef]
258. Sciacca, M.F.M.; Chillemi, R.; Sciuto, S.; Greco, V.; Messineo, C.; Kotler, S.A.; Lee, D.; Brender, J.R.; Ramamoorthy, A.; Rosa, C.L.; et al. A blend of two resveratrol derivatives abolishes hIAPP amyloid growth and membrane damage. *Biochim. Biophys. Acta Biomembr.* **2018**, *1860*, 1793–1802. [CrossRef]
259. Cox, S.J.; Rodriguez Camargo, D.C.; Lee, Y.-H.; Dubini, R.C.A.; Rovó, P.; Ivanova, M.I.; Padmini, V.; Reif, B.; Ramamoorthy, A. Small Molecule Induced Toxic Human-iapp Species Characterized by NMR. *Chem. Commun.* **2020**, *56*, 13129–13132. [CrossRef]
260. Tsai, H.; Huang, C.; Tu, L. TPE conjugated islet amyloid polypeptide probe for detection of peptide oligomers. *Biophys. Chem.* **2024**, *304*, 107129. [CrossRef]

261. Yu, F.; Teng, Y.; Yang, S.; He, Y.; Zhang, Z.; Yang, H.; Ding, C.; Zhou, P. The thermodynamic and kinetic mechanisms of a Ganoderma lucidum proteoglycan inhibiting hIAPP amyloidosis. *Biophys. Chem.* **2022**, *280*, 106702. [CrossRef]
262. Nireeksha; Hegde, M.N.; Kumari, N.S. Potential Role of Salivary Vitamin D Antimicrobial Peptide LL-37 and Interleukins in Severity of Dental Caries: An Exvivo Study. *BMC Oral Health* **2024**, *24*, 79. [CrossRef]
263. Juszczak, M.; Zawrotniak, M.; Rapala-Kozik, M. Complexation of Fungal Extracellular Nucleic Acids by Host LL-37 Peptide Shapes Neutrophil Response to Candida Albicans Biofilm. *Front. Immunol.* **2024**, *15*, 1295168. [CrossRef] [PubMed]
264. Song, Y.; Zhang, S.; Zhao, N.; Nong, C.; He, Y.; Bao, R. Pseudomonas Aeruginosa Two-component System Cprrs Regulates Higba Expression and Bacterial Cytotoxicity in Response to LL-37 Stress. *PLoS Pathog.* **2024**, *20*, e1011946. [CrossRef] [PubMed]
265. Zhang, Y.; Bharathi, V.; Dokoshi, T.; De Anda, J.; Ursery, L.T.; Kulkarni, N.N.; Nakamura, Y.; Chen, J.; Luo, E.W.C.; Wang, L. Viral Afterlife: SARS-CoV-2 as a Reservoir of Immunomimetic Peptides That Reassemble into Proinflammatory Supramolecular Complexes. *Proc. Natl. Acad. Sci. USA* **2024**, *121*, e2300644120. [CrossRef] [PubMed]
266. Lei, R.; Yang, C.; Sun, Y.; Li, D.; Hao, L.; Li, Y.; Wu, S.; Li, H.; Lan, C.; Fang, X. Turning Cationic Antimicrobial Peptide KR-12 into Self-assembled Nanobiotics with Potent Bacterial Killing and LPS Neutralizing Activities. *Nanoscale* **2024**, *16*, 887–902. [CrossRef] [PubMed]

biomolecules

MDPI

Article

A Novel Dimeric Short Peptide Derived from α-Defensin-Related Rattusin with Improved Antimicrobial and DNA-Binding Activities

Gwansik Park [1,†], Hyosuk Yun [1,†], Hye Jung Min [2,*] and Chul Won Lee [1,*]

1 Department of Chemistry, Chonnam National University, Gwangju 61186, Republic of Korea; lineageyapo@naver.com (G.P.); 5300747yun@hanmail.net (H.Y.)
2 Department of Cosmetic Science, Gwangju Women's University, Gwangju 62396, Republic of Korea
* Correspondence: sarock@kwu.ac.kr (H.J.M.); cwlee@jnu.ac.kr (C.W.L.)
† These authors contributed equally to this work.

Abstract: Rattusin, an α-defensin-related antimicrobial peptide isolated from the small intestine of rats, has been previously characterized through NMR spectroscopy to elucidate its three-dimensional structure, revealing a C2 homodimeric scaffold stabilized by five disulfide bonds. This study aimed to identify the functional region of rattusin by designing and synthesizing various short analogs, subsequently leading to the development of novel peptide-based antibiotics. The analogs, designated as F1, F2, F3, and F4, were constructed based on the three-dimensional configuration of rattusin, among which F2 is the shortest peptide and exhibited superior antimicrobial efficacy compared to the wild-type peptide. The central cysteine residue of F2 prompted an investigation into its potential to form a dimer at neutral pH, which is critical for its antimicrobial function. This activity was abolished upon the substitution of the cysteine residue with serine, indicating the necessity of dimerization for antimicrobial action. Further, we synthesized β-hairpin-like analogs, both parallel and antiparallel, based on the dimeric structure of F2, which maintained comparable antimicrobial potency. In contrast to rattusin, which acts by disrupting bacterial membranes, the F2 dimer binds directly to DNA, as evidenced by fluorescence assays and DNA retardation experiments. Importantly, F2 exhibited negligible cytotoxicity up to 515 μg/mL, assessed via hemolysis and MTT assays, underscoring its potential as a lead compound for novel peptide-based antibiotic development.

Keywords: antimicrobial peptide; rattusin; antibiotics; DNA binding; cytotoxicity

Citation: Park, G.; Yun, H.; Min, H.J.; Lee, C.W. A Novel Dimeric Short Peptide Derived from α-Defensin-Related Rattusin with Improved Antimicrobial and DNA-Binding Activities. *Biomolecules* **2024**, *14*, 659. https://doi.org/10.3390/biom14060659

Academic Editor: Annarita Falanga

Received: 30 April 2024
Revised: 24 May 2024
Accepted: 4 June 2024
Published: 5 June 2024

1. Introduction

The discovery of antibiotics marked a revolution in medical treatment, offering a means to effectively combat bacterial infections through various mechanisms, such as the inhibition of cell wall synthesis by penicillin and vancomycin [1,2], DNA synthesis by rifampicin, and protein synthesis by streptomycin [3–5]. These antimicrobial agents have saved countless lives and are critical to modern medicine. However, the widespread and often indiscriminate use of antibiotics has led to an unintended consequence: the emergence and proliferation of antibiotic-resistant bacteria. These bacteria have evolved through mechanisms such as the modification of target molecules, the enzymatic degradation or alteration of antibiotics, and changes in membrane permeability to evade the effects of antibiotics. The rise of antibiotic-resistant strains, such as vancomycin-resistant *Enterococcus* (VRE) [6,7], methicillin-resistant *Staphylococcus aureus* (MRSA) [8,9], and multidrug-resistant *Acinetobacter baumannii* (MRAB) [10,11], represents a growing public health crisis, with infections from resistant strains leading to increased morbidity and mortality rates worldwide.

The escalating challenge of antibiotic resistance has spurred a global effort to discover new antimicrobial strategies that can circumvent these resistance mechanisms. In this context, antimicrobial peptides (AMPs) have emerged as a particularly promising avenue of research [12,13]. AMPs, a diverse class of molecules integral to the innate immune systems of all life forms, exhibit broad-spectrum activity against bacteria, viruses, fungi, and even cancer cells [14–16]. Their mode of action, typically involving the disruption of microbial membranes through electrostatic interactions, differs fundamentally from that of traditional antibiotics, thus offering a potential solution to the problem of resistance. Moreover, AMPs are less likely to induce resistance due to their mechanism of action and the high cost to the organism of altering membrane composition [17–19].

Recent advances in genomics, proteomics, and computational biology have enabled the identification and characterization of AMPs from a wide range of organisms, from humans to plants and insects [20–22]. This has led to the development of novel AMPs through bioengineering and synthetic chemistry, aimed at enhancing their stability, efficacy, and specificity while reducing toxicity toward human cells [23,24]. The design of shorter peptides by identifying and optimizing the active regions of naturally occurring AMPs has become a focal point of this research. Shorter peptides not only offer practical advantages in terms of synthesis and cost but also often exhibit improved antimicrobial activity and reduced immunogenicity [25–27].

Rattusin, an α-defensin-related antimicrobial peptide isolated from the rat small intestine, stands at the forefront of this research [28]. The defensins, to which rattusin is related, represent a well-studied class of AMPs noted for their potent antimicrobial activity and role in mammalian innate immunity. The unique structure of rattusin, a C2 homodimeric scaffold formed by five disulfide bonds, contributes to its antimicrobial properties, which include activity against a broad spectrum of pathogens, such as Gram-negative and Gram-positive bacteria, and notably, strains resistant to conventional antibiotics. Previous studies have elucidated the three-dimensional structure of rattusin via NMR spectroscopy, providing a blueprint for the design of analogs with potentially enhanced antimicrobial properties [29,30].

Building on these foundations, the current study seeks to explore the functional regions of rattusin by employing a strategy of sequence dissection and analog design. By focusing on the hairpin loop region, we have identified a peptide fragment that not only demonstrates enhanced antimicrobial efficacy compared to the wild-type peptide but also exhibits significantly lower cytotoxicity toward mammalian cells. These findings highlight the potential of rattusin derivatives as a new class of peptide-based antibiotics, offering hope in the fight against antibiotic-resistant bacterial infections.

2. Materials and Methods

2.1. Materials and Reagents

The materials used included Rink amide 4-methylbenzhydrylamine (MBHA) resin, 9-Fluorenylmethoxycarbonyl (Fmoc) amino acids and amide resin (GL Biochem, Shanghai, China), 1-hydroxybenzotriazole (HOBt), Diisopropylcarbodiimide (DIC), Trifluoroacetic acid (TFA, Sigma Aldrich, St. Louis, MO, USA), HPLC grade Acetonitrile (ACN, Merck, Darmstadt, Germany), 1,2-Ethanedithiol (EDT), Thioanisole, Dichloromethane (DCM, DAEJUNG, Siheung-si, Republic of Korea), N,N-dimethylformamide (DMF, DAEJUNG, Siheung-si, Republic of Korea), Sodium phosphate (NaH_2PO_4, Na_2HPO_4), Peptone, NaCl (JUNSEI, 4-4-16 Nihonbashi-honcho, Chuo-ku, Tokyo, Japan), Phosphate buffer saline (PBS), N-(2-Hydroxyethyl)piperazine-N′-(2-ethanesulfonic acid) (HEPES), *o*-nitrophenyl-β-galactoside (ONPG), Dimethyl sulfoxide (DMSO), 3-(4,5-dimethlythiazol-2-yl)-2,5-diphenyltetrazolium bromide (MTT Sigma Aldrich, St. Louis, MO, USA), Dulbecco's modified eagle medium (DMEM, Gibco, Waltham, MA, USA), Fetal bovine serum (FBS, Capricorn, Shanghai, China), 2,2,2-trifluoroethanol (TFE), 3,3′-Dipropylthiadicarbocyanine iodide ($DiSC_3$-(5)), and Fluorescein isothiocyanate (FITC, Sigma Aldrich, St. Louis, MO, USA).

2.2. Peptide Synthesis

Rattusin analogs were synthesized using the solid-phase peptide synthesis (SPPS) method. The Fmoc-Rink Amide resin capacity was approximately 0.6–0.7 mmol/g, and the synthesis was conducted on a 0.1 mmol scale. A 20% solution of piperidine in N,N-dimethylformamide (DMF) served as the deprotecting agent to remove the Fmoc protecting group, while dichloromethane (DCM) and DMF were employed for resin washing steps. The amino acid coupling reaction was facilitated by 1-hydroxybenzotriazole (HOBt) and diisopropylcarbodiimide (DIC), each used at two equivalents (eq), and the reaction was allowed to proceed for 2 to 3 h. Following peptide synthesis, cleavage of the peptide from the resin and deprotection of sidechain protecting groups were achieved using a cleavage cocktail of trifluoroacetic acid (TFA), water, thioanisole, and 1,2-ethanedithiol (EDT) in a volume/volume ratio of 87.5:5:5:2.5 at room temperature. The crude synthetic peptide was subsequently lyophilized and stored at −20 °C until purification.

2.3. HPLC and LC-MS Analysis

The synthesized peptides were purified by reversed-phase high-performance liquid chromatography (RP-HPLC, Shimadzu, Kyoto, Japan) using a Shim-pack C18 column (20 mm × 250 mm, 5 μm particle size) with detection at 230 nm using a UV detector. The mobile phases consisted of 100% H_2O with 0.05% trifluoroacetic acid (TFA) as solvent A and 100% acetonitrile (ACN) with 0.05% TFA as solvent B. The molecular weight and purity of the purified peptides were determined using liquid chromatography–mass spectrometry (LC-MS, API2000, AB SCIEX, Framingham, MA, USA).

2.4. Disulfide Bond Formation

The rattusin fragments F2, F4, F2-AH, and F2-PH contain one or two cysteine residues that can form a disulfide bond. The F2 peptide was incubated in 50 mM sodium phosphate buffer (pH 7) for 24 h at 4 °C. Similarly, the F2-AH and F2-PH peptides were refolded by air oxidation to form intramolecular disulfide bonds under the same conditions. The reaction progress was monitored using liquid chromatography–mass spectrometry (LC-MS) and quenched by the addition of trifluoroacetic acid (TFA).

2.5. Antimicrobial Activity

The minimal inhibitory concentrations (MICs) of the peptides were determined following the broth microdilution method recommended by the Clinical and Laboratory Standards Institute (CLSI). Briefly, bacteria in their mid-logarithmic growth phase were diluted in Mueller–Hinton broth (MHB) (Difco, Franklin Lakes, NJ, USA) and aliquoted into a 96-well microtiter plate at a density of 4×10^6 CFU/well. The assay included both Gram-negative bacteria (*Escherichia coli, Salmonella typhimurium, and Pseudomonas aeruginosa*) and Gram-positive bacteria (*Bacillus subtilis, Staphylococcus aureus, and Staphylococcus epidermidis*), as well as methicillin-resistant *Staphylococcus aureus* strains (MRSA: CCARM 3089, CCARM 3090, CCARM 3095). The samples were subjected to a two-fold serial dilution before being added to the wells, and the plate was incubated at 37 °C for 24 h. The MIC was defined as the lowest peptide concentration that prevented visible bacterial growth. All experiments were conducted in triplicate and included appropriate growth and sterility controls.

2.6. Membrane Depolarization Assay

The cytoplasmic membrane depolarization activity of the peptides was assessed using the membrane-potential-sensitive dye DiSC3-(5), following methodologies previously described in the literature. *Staphylococcus aureus* was cultured in Luria–Bertani (LB) broth at 37 °C until reaching an optical density (O.D.) at 600 nm of 0.3–0.4, indicative of mid-logarithmic phase growth. The cells were then washed with a buffer containing 20 mM glucose and 5 mM HEPES, and the cell suspension was diluted to an O.D. 600 of 0.05 in the same buffer. Potassium chloride (KCl) was added to achieve a final concentration of 100 mM to equilibrate potassium ion levels. The concentrations used for each peptide in our membrane depolarization assays were based on their respective MICs: 32 μM for F2, 4 μM for Melittin, and 16 μM for Buferin-2.

Fluorescence was monitored using an F-4500 FL fluorescence spectrophotometer (Shimadzu, Kyoto, Japan) with excitation and emission wavelengths set at 622 nm and 670 nm, respectively. Melittin, known for its membrane-disrupting properties, served as a positive control, while buforin-2, which translocates across membranes without causing depolarization, acted as a negative control. Both melittin and buforin-2 were tested at concentrations twice their minimal inhibitory concentration (MIC) levels.

2.7. SYTOX Green Uptake Assay

The membrane permeabilization activity of the peptides was determined using the SYTOX Green uptake assay, as described previously. *S. aureus* was cultured in LB broth at 37 °C until it reached an optical density (O.D.) at 600 nm of 0.4, indicative of the mid-logarithmic phase. The cells were then washed and diluted to an O.D. 600 of 0.05 using 1× PBS buffer. The dye (SYTOX Green nucleic acid stain) was added to the bacterial suspension at a concentration of 1 mM, and the mixture was incubated at 4 °C for 18 h with agitation in the dark. The SYTOX Green-treated bacteria were placed in a quartz cell, where they were simultaneously exposed to the positive control melittin (2× MIC), the negative control buforin-2 (2× MIC), and the F2 dimer (2× MIC). An F-4500 FL fluorescence spectrophotometer (Shimadzu, Kyoto, Japan) was used to monitor fluorescence (excitation 485 nm, emission 520 nm).

2.8. ONPG Hydrolysis Assay

The internal membrane permeability was assessed using the ONPG hydrolysis assay, as described previously. *E. coli* ML-35p, which constitutively expresses cytoplasmic β-galactosidase and periplasmic β-lactamase, is resistant to ampicillin and deficient in lactose permease. *E. coli* ML-35 was incubated in LB broth containing ampicillin at 37 °C until the optical density (O.D.) at 600 nm reached 1.0. The cells were then washed with a buffer consisting of 97% 1× PBS and 3% LB and diluted to an O.D. 600 of 0.4 in the same buffer. A mixture of 50 µL of serially diluted peptide and 20 µL of dye (ONPG, final concentration 3 mM) was added to 100 µL of the bacterial suspension in a sterilized 96-well plate. Melittin served as a positive control, while buforin-2 was used as a negative control. The hydrolysis of ONPG was measured using a PHOMO Elisa reader (Autobio, Zhengzhou, China) at 405 nm for each time period.

2.9. DNA-Binding Assay

We evaluated the DNA-binding ability of F2 and F2 (C4S) monomeric peptides using gel retardation experiments. The concentration of plasmid DNA (pHIS2) was fixed at 145 µg/mL. The peptide was serially diluted in a binding buffer consisting of 10 mM Tris-HCl (pH 8.0), 5% glucose, 50 µg/mL BSA, 1 mM EDTA, and 20 mM KCl. This solution was then mixed with the DNA and incubated at 37 °C for 1 h. After incubation, the DNA–peptide mixture was stained with DNA gel loading dye. The samples were analyzed using 1% agarose gel electrophoresis in 0.5× TAE buffer. Plasmid bands were detected with a UV illuminator (Bio-Rad, Hercules, CA, USA).

2.10. Hemolysis Assay

Sheep red blood cells (RBCs) were used to assess the hemolytic activity of F2. Fresh blood was gently washed with 1× PBS and centrifuged for 5 min at 3000 rpm to obtain purified RBCs, which were then resuspended in 1× PBS to achieve a 4% RBC solution. Each well of a sterilized 96-well plate received 100 µL of the serially diluted peptide and 4% RBCs, and the mixture was incubated at 37 °C for 1 h at 60 rpm. Subsequently, the plates were centrifuged at 1200 rpm for 5 min, and the supernatant was transferred to a new 96-well plate. The absorbance of the transferred supernatant was measured at 405 nm using a PHOMO Elisa reader (Autobio, China). The hemolytic activity was calculated as the percentage of hemolysis, determined by subtracting the absorbance of the negative control (containing only PBS buffer) from the absorbance of the peptide-treated samples. This value was then divided by the result obtained by subtracting the absorbance of the negative control from the absorbance of a 1% Triton X-100 solution, which served as a positive control indicating 100% hemolysis. The final value was multiplied by 100 to express the hemolytic activity as a percentage.

2.11. MTT Assay

An MTT assay was performed to evaluate cytotoxicity. Normal cells (Hs68) and cancer cells (HeLa) were each seeded in sterile 96-well plates using a 150 µL mixture of DMEM and 10% FBS and cultured for 24 h at 37 °C in a 5% CO_2 atmosphere. Serial dilutions of the F2 dimer were administered to the cultured cells, which were then incubated for an additional 24 h. Subsequently, 20 µL of MTT solution (5 mg/mL in PBS buffer) was added to each well, and the plates were incubated for 4 h at 37 °C before the media were removed. The precipitated MTT formazan crystals were dissolved in 100 µL of DMSO for 5 min. Absorbance at 550 nm was measured using a PHOMO Elisa reader (Autobio, China). Cell viability was calculated by dividing the absorbance value (A550) of cells treated with the peptide by that of cells treated with buffer only, and the result was expressed as a percentage.

3. Results

3.1. Design of Rattusin Fragments

Rattusin is characterized by its homodimeric structure, which is stabilized by five disulfide bonds, yet it exhibits relatively low antimicrobial activity considering the complexity of its structure. To pinpoint the functional region and identify the minimal peptide fragment derived from rattusin, we segmented the rattusin sequence into four distinct fragments: F1, F2, F3, and F4, as illustrated in Figure 1.

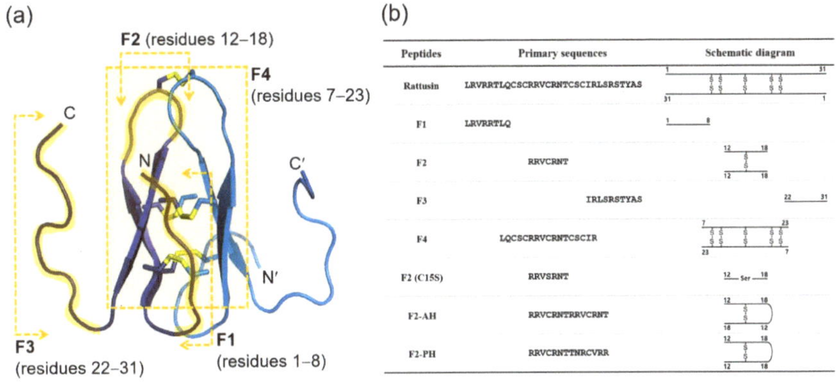

Figure 1. The design and sequences of rattusin fragments based on its three-dimensional structure. (**a**) The identification of fragment regions in the rattusin structure, with F1 (residues 1–8), F2 (residues 12–18), F3 (residues 22–31), and F4 (residues 7–23) highlighted in the full rattusin tertiary structure. The N-terminus (N) and C-terminus (C) are indicated for each fragment. (**b**) The primary sequences of the rattusin fragments alongside schematic diagrams representing the amino acid sequences and positions. Each fragment is depicted with its corresponding segment of the rattusin molecule, with disulfide bonds illustrated by lines connecting the cysteine residues.

F1 corresponds to the N-terminal segment, spanning residues 1 to 8 (8-mer). F2 encompasses the dimeric hairpin loop region, which includes residues 12 to 18 and features a cysteine at position 15 (7-mer). F3 comprises the C-terminal segment, covering residues 22 to 31 (10-mer). F4 represents the dimeric core region, which is refolded by five disulfide bonds and comprises residues 7 to 23 (17-mer). Additionally, we synthesized the F2 (C15S) peptide, which was designed to prevent dimerization by substituting the cysteine at position 15. Furthermore, to elucidate the impact of F2 dimerization on its activity, we designed analogs of the F2 dimer: the antiparallel hairpin-like F2 (F2-AH) and the parallel hairpin-like F2 (F2-PH).

3.2. Preparation of Rattusin Fragments

Peptide fragments derived from the dimeric structure of rattusin were synthesized using solid-phase peptide synthesis (SPPS). Following synthesis, they were purified by RP-HPLC and characterized by LC-MS. Fragments F2, F4, F2-AH, and F2-PH, which contain either intra- or inter-disulfide bonds, underwent air oxidative refolding processes to achieve their oxidized forms. The purity of these peptides was confirmed to be greater than 95%, as evidenced by HPLC and LC-MS analyses (Table S1 and Figure S1).

3.3. Antimicrobial Activity of Fragments

The antimicrobial activities of the four fragments (F1, F2, F3, and F4) were initially evaluated against *E. coli* and *S. aureus*, with comparisons made to the activity of rattusin (Table 1). The MIC values obtained were consistent across all replicates, showing no deviations. The minimum inhibitory concentration (MIC) for rattusin was established at 58 μg/mL. Notably, F3 exhibited no antimicrobial activity at concentrations up to 590 μg/mL.

Table 1. Comparative minimal inhibitory concentrations (MICs) of rattusin and derived fragments against *E. coli* and *S. aureus* (μg/mL).

Bacteria	Rattusin	F1	F2	F3	F4
Escherichia coli	58	67	15	>590	32
Staphylococcus aureus	117	>500	58	>590	64

In contrast, F1 and F4 demonstrated MIC values that were either comparable to or slightly lower than that of rattusin. Remarkably, F2 displayed an MIC of 15 μg/mL, indicating antimicrobial activity fourfold greater than that of rattusin.

To elucidate the detailed structure–activity relationships of F2, we designed, synthesized, and tested various F2 analogs for their antimicrobial activity against nine different bacterial strains, including MRSA (Table 2). Among these, the F2 (C15S) variant, unable to form a dimer due to the absence of a cysteine residue, showed no antibacterial activity up to an MIC of 227 μg/mL. This observation underscores the critical role of dimer formation in the antimicrobial efficacy of F2. Furthermore, we developed the F2-AH and F2-PH analogs, characterized by continuously connected F2 sequences. Both analogs exhibited MIC values of 15 μg/mL, equivalent to that of the F2.

Table 2. MICs of F2 derivative peptides against Gram-negative and Gram-positive bacteria, including methicillin-resistant *S. aureus* (MRSA) (μg/mL).

Bacteria	F2	F2 (C15S)	F2-AH	F2-PH
Gram-negative				
Escherichia coli	15	>227	15	15
Salmonella typhimurium	15	>227	15	15
Pseudomonas aeruginosa	15	>227	15	15
Gram-positive				
Staphylococcus aureus	58	>227	29	29
Bacillus subtilis	29	>227	29	29
Staphylococcus epidermidis	15	>227	15	15
MRSA				
CCARM 3089	58	>114	29	29
CCARM 3090	116	>114	29	58
CCARM 3095	58	>114	58	29

3.4. Membrane Depolarization

The examination of peptide-induced membrane permeabilization in intact *S. aureus* cells utilized the membrane-potential-sensitive dye DiSC(3)-5. This dye accumulates in the cytoplasmic membrane under normal membrane potential conditions, leading to fluorescence self-quenching. Membrane potential disruption causes the dye to disperse into the surrounding buffer, resulting in an elevated fluorescence intensity. The antimicrobial peptide melittin, known for membrane disruption, served as a positive control, whereas buforin-2, which does not interact with the membrane, functioned as a negative control.

The initial strong quenching of DiSC(3)-5 fluorescence indicated the dye's accumulation within the membrane. Following a stabilization period of 300 s, peptides were introduced (as indicated by an arrow in Figure 2), introducing a variable to the experiment.

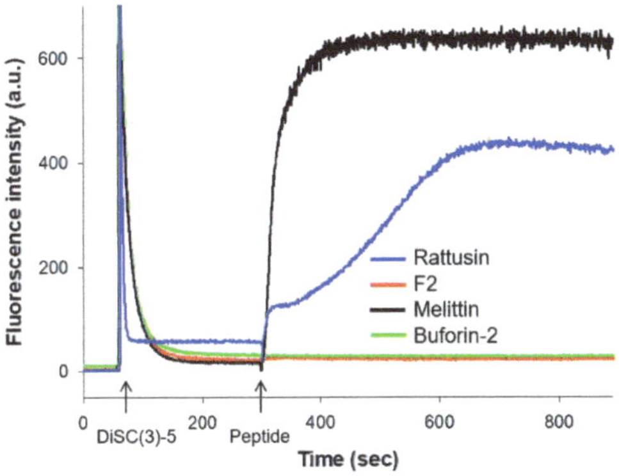

Figure 2. The time course of membrane depolarization in *S. aureus* induced by the antimicrobial peptide rattusin, its derivative fragment F2, and the control peptides melittin and buforin-2. Depolarization was monitored using the fluorescent DiSC(3)-5 dye. The arrows indicate the points of dye and peptide addition.

Rattusin triggered a time-dependent depolarization of the bacterial cytoplasmic membrane, evidenced by a progressive increase in fluorescence intensity, attributable to the collapse of ion gradients that maintain the membrane potential. Melittin rapidly achieved the complete depolarization of *S. aureus* within seconds at a concentration of 4 μM. Conversely, buforin-2 failed to induce any change in membrane potential. Likewise, F2 did not cause any membrane depolarization, implying a distinctive mode of action on the bacterial membrane when compared to the rattusin peptide.

3.5. SYTOX Green Uptake

In the SYTOX Green uptake assay, which serves as an indicator of plasma membrane integrity, melittin demonstrated a significant increase in fluorescence intensity, indicative of its potent membrane-disruptive properties. This effect was rapid and pronounced, with melittin reaching peak fluorescence shortly after treatment application, as seen in Figure 3. Such a response is consistent with melittin's established role in compromising membrane integrity, thereby allowing SYTOX Green to bind to nucleic acids and fluoresce. In stark contrast, the F2 fragment and buforin-2 did not show a similar increase in fluorescence intensity over the course of the assay. The absence of fluorescence enhancement with these peptides suggests that, unlike melittin, they do not cause membrane permeabilization under the conditions tested. Consequently, the data illustrate a clear distinction in the ability of melittin to disrupt cell membranes when compared to F2 and buforin-2.

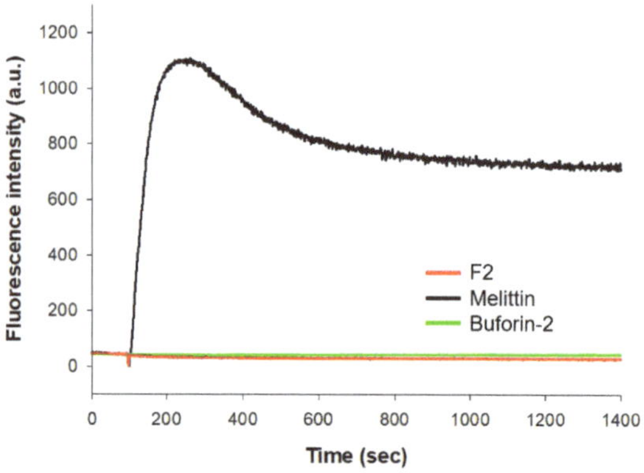

Figure 3. SYTOX Green uptake assay monitoring the permeabilization of *S. aureus* cell membranes by peptides. The concentrations of the peptides used in the experiment were 32 μM for F2, 4 μM for melittin, and 16 μM for buforin-2.

3.6. ONPG Hydrolysis

F2 appears not to interact with the membrane, as evidenced by depolarization and SYTOX experiments. We further investigated whether F2 could affect the inner membrane using an ONPG hydrolysis assay (Figure 4). For this purpose, *E. coli* ML-35 bacteria, from which the outer membrane had been removed, were utilized. Both ONPG and peptides were administered, and the absorbance was monitored at 405 nm. Melittin, known for its membrane-disrupting capabilities, served as the positive control, whereas buforin-2, which can traverse the membrane without causing destruction, acted as the negative control.

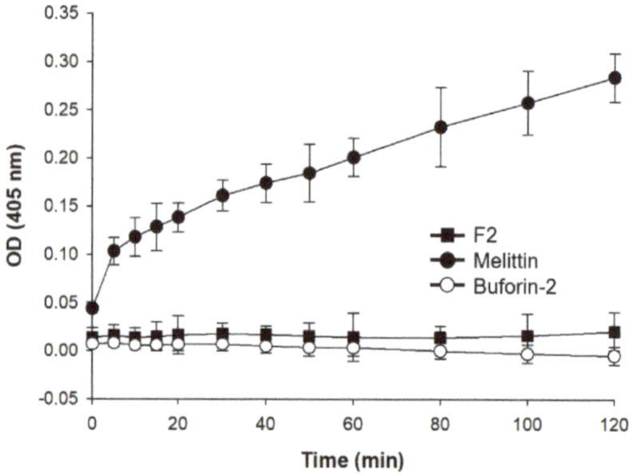

Figure 4. Assay of ONPG hydrolysis by peptides using *E. coli* ML-35. The concentrations of the peptides used in the experiment were 32 μM for F2, 4 μM for melittin, and 16 μM for buforin-2.

Despite the change in absorbance demonstrated by the positive control melittin, F2 did not alter the absorbance, similar to the negative control, buforin-2. This outcome, alongside the results from depolarization and SYTOX experiments, suggests that F2 does not target the inner membrane.

3.7. DNA-Binding Activity

The gel retardation assay elucidated the DNA-binding affinities of peptide variants. As hypothesized, F2 does not target the bacterial membrane, yet it manifests an augmented antimicrobial effect when contrasted with the wild-type rattusin, indicating an alternative mechanism of action. This is likely oriented toward the intracellular milieu, such as interactions with nucleic acids or proteins. To ascertain this, the assay was performed by mixing varying concentrations of the peptide with plasmid DNA.

Buforin-2, with established DNA-binding properties, was employed as a benchmark. At a concentration of 2 μM, buforin-2 successfully demonstrated DNA binding, evidenced by the retardation of the DNA band (Figure 5, left panel). This contrasts with F2, which required a doubled concentration of 4 μM to exhibit similar DNA retardation (Figure 5, middle panel). It is noteworthy that the monomeric variant of F2, specifically the C15S mutant, did not present any DNA retardation up to a concentration of 16 μM (Figure 5, right panel). We analyzed the DNA-binding images using ImageJ (1.54i) to quantify the DNA-binding activity of the peptides (Table S2). This lack of interaction suggests a pivotal role of dimerization in the DNA-binding process of F2.

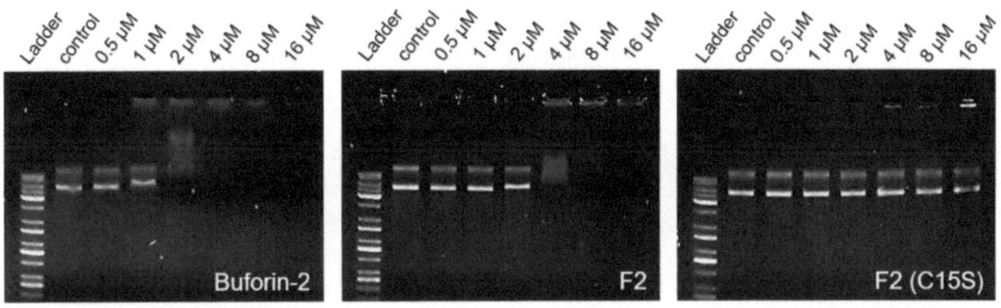

Figure 5. The DNA-binding activity of peptides assessed by the gel retardation assay. Gel electrophoresis illustrating the DNA-binding capability of peptides. The retarded bands signify successful DNA binding, observable for buforin-2 at 2 μM and F2 at 4 μM. No retardation was evident for the monomeric F2 (C15S) up to 16 μM.

3.8. Cytotoxicity

Cytotoxicity assays were conducted using hemolysis and MTT assays for F2, as depicted in Figure 6. In the hemolysis assay, sheep red blood cells (RBCs) were utilized, and F2 was serially diluted from 1 to 512 μg/mL. F2 did not induce hemolysis, even at concentrations up to 512 μg/mL, whereas melittin demonstrated 100% hemolytic activity at concentrations below 10 μg/mL. For the MTT assay, Hs68 cells and HeLa cells were employed. F2 exhibited no cytotoxicity at concentrations up to 512 μg/mL. These results indicate that F2 is highly specific to bacterial cells without affecting mammalian cells.

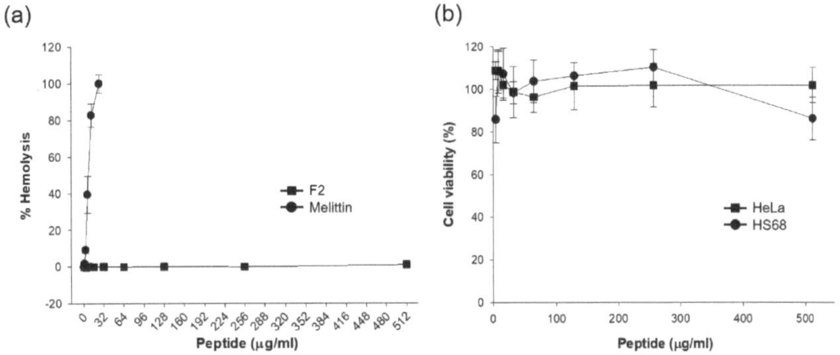

Figure 6. Cytotoxicity analysis of peptide F2. (**a**) Hemolysis assay results displaying the percentage of hemolysis of sheep RBCs after treatment with increasing concentrations of peptide F2 and melittin. (**b**) MTT assay results showing cell viability percentages for Hs68 and HeLa cells upon treatment with varying concentrations of peptide F2.

Further, the MTT assay was implemented to determine the effect of F2 on the viability of mammalian cells. Two cell lines, Hs68 (human fibroblasts) and HeLa (human cervical cancer cells), were treated with F2. The peptide maintained cell viability without notable toxicity up to 512 μg/mL for both cell types (Figure 6b). These findings delineate the specificity of F2's antimicrobial action, highlighting its negligible cytotoxicity to mammalian cells and supporting its potential as a selective antimicrobial agent.

4. Discussion

Finding and improving the functional domains of current antimicrobial peptides (AMPs) is a potential strategy for creating new antibiotics. AMPs like rattusin, known for their antibacterial activities, often have complex structures and high molecular weights, which complicate their synthesis and clinical applications. This study focuses on rattusin, a C2 homodimeric peptide (2 × 33 amino acids) characterized by a robust range of antibacterial activities and significant salt resistance. However, the large size and complexity of rattusin make its synthesis challenging, hence the drive to design shorter, more manageable fragments that retain biological functionality.

We successfully designed and synthesized several short rattusin fragments (F1, F2, F3, and F4), targeting the functional site of the peptide based on its tertiary structure determined through NMR spectroscopy. These fragments were synthesized to explore the peptide's active sequences and investigate the impacts of length and complexity on synthesis yield and antimicrobial activity.

Among the synthesized fragments, F2 exhibited superior antimicrobial properties, significantly outperforming the wild-type peptide. This fragment includes a central cysteine crucial for forming a disulfide-bonded dimer, key to its biological activity. The antimicrobial efficacy of F2 was notably abolished when the cysteine was replaced with serine (F2 (C15S)), highlighting the importance of the dimeric structure facilitated by disulfide bonding.

Interestingly, the monomeric form of F2 (prior to disulfide bonding) showed antimicrobial activity similar to that of the dimeric form. This observation suggests that the monomeric F2 can spontaneously form dimers under physiological conditions, which we confirmed using HPLC analysis after incubation in MIC buffer (Figure 7). This ability to dimerize in situ emphasizes F2's therapeutic potential, allowing for simpler administration and potentially lower manufacturing costs.

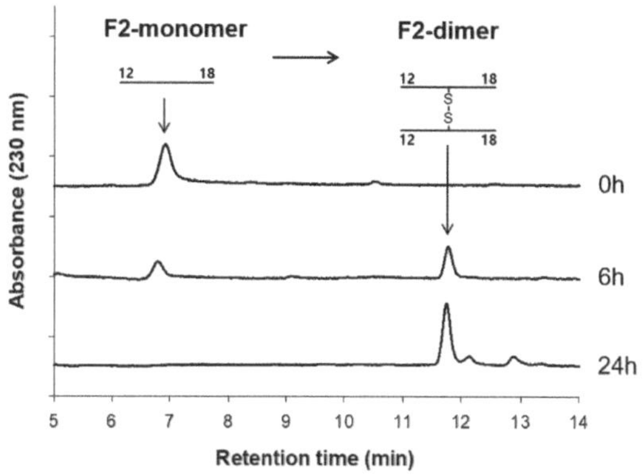

Figure 7. The dimerization of the F2 fragment. The formation of dimers of the F2 peptide monitored by RP-HPLC.

A distinctive feature of F2, compared to the parent rattusin peptide, is its mechanism of action. Unlike rattusin, which disrupts bacterial membranes, F2 targets bacterial DNA directly. This mechanism was elucidated through fluorescence assays and DNA retardation experiments, which demonstrated that the F2 dimer binds to DNA effectively, inhibiting bacterial function at a fundamental level. This mode of action is particularly advantageous, as it reduces the likelihood of bacteria developing resistance, a common drawback of traditional antibiotics, which typically target membrane integrity or protein synthesis.

Moreover, the F2 dimer exhibited remarkably low cytotoxicity toward mammalian cells, as evidenced by hemolysis and MTT assays. It showed negligible hemolytic activity and did not affect cell viability at concentrations significantly higher than its MIC against bacteria. This selective toxicity, combined with its potent antimicrobial activity, positions the F2 dimer as an excellent candidate for further development into a new class of peptide-based antibiotics.

5. Conclusions

The findings from this study underscore the potential of designing shorter AMPs that not only retain but enhance the desirable properties of naturally occurring peptides. The F2 fragment, in particular, emerges as a compelling lead compound for new antibiotic development due to its effective DNA-binding capability and low mammalian cytotoxicity. These characteristics suggest that F2 and peptides like it could serve as foundational structures for the synthesis of new drugs aimed at combating antibiotic-resistant bacteria through mechanisms that differ fundamentally from those of current antibiotics. Future work will focus on optimizing the synthesis of F2 and similar peptides, expanding the range of bacteria against which these peptides are effective, and further delineating their safety profiles in clinical settings. The goal is to develop a new class of AMP-based antibiotics that leverage the unique properties of peptides like F2—targeting bacterial DNA and exhibiting minimal side effects—to provide a potent, safe, and economically viable alternative to traditional antibiotics.

Supplementary Materials: The following supporting information can be downloaded at https://www.mdpi.com/article/10.3390/biom14060659/s1: Figure S1: Analysis of synthesized peptides. The purities and molecular masses of fragment peptides were confirmed using LC-MS. (a) F1, (b) F2, (c) F3, (d) F4, (e) F2 (C15S), (f) F2-AH, and (g) F2-PH. Table S1: Molecular masses of rattusin fragments and its analogs (theoretical and experimental data); Table S2: Quantitative analysis of DNA-binding activity of peptides. Mean values of DNA gel band intensities from the gel retardation assay (Figure 5), assessed using ImageJ (1.54i) software.

Author Contributions: Conceptualization, C.W.L. and H.J.M.; methodology, C.W.L.; investigation, G.P. and H.Y.; writing—original draft preparation, C.W.L. and G.P.; writing—review and editing, C.W.L., H.J.M. and H.Y.; visualization, C.W.L., G.P. and H.Y.; supervision, C.W.L. and H.J.M. All authors have read and agreed to the published version of the manuscript.

Funding: This work was supported by the Basic Science Research Program through the National Research Foundation of Korea (NRF) funded by the Ministry of Education, Science, and Technology of Korea (NRF-2023R1A2C1007203 and RS-2023-00221356 to C.W.L.; RS-2023-00243433 to H.Y.), and Gwangju Women's University (KWU23-049 to H.J.M.).

Institutional Review Board Statement: Not applicable.

Informed Consent Statement: Not applicable.

Data Availability Statement: All relevant data are within the paper and Supplementary Materials.

Conflicts of Interest: The authors declare no conflicts of interest.

References

1. Džidić, S.; Šušković, J.; Kos, B. Antibiotic resistance mechanisms in bacteria: Biochemical and genetic aspects. *Food Technol. Biotechnol.* **2008**, *46*, 11–21.
2. Reynolds, P.E. Structure, biochemistry and mechanism of action of glycopeptide antibiotics. *Eur. J. Clin. Microbiol. Infect. Dis.* **1989**, *8*, 943–950. [CrossRef]
3. Iscla, I.; Wray, R.; Wei, S.; Posner, B.; Blount, P. Streptomycin potency is dependent on MscL channel expression. *Nat. Commun.* **2014**, *5*, 4891. [CrossRef]

4. Kapoor, G.; Saigal, S.; Elongavan, A. Action and resistance mechanisms of antibiotics: A guide for clinicians. *J. Anaesthesiol. Clin. Pharmacol.* **2017**, *33*, 300–305. [CrossRef]
5. Campbell, E.A.; Korzheva, N.; Mustaev, A.; Murakami, K.; Nair, S.; Goldfarb, A.; Darst, S.A. Structural Mechanism for Rifampicin Inhibition of Bacterial RNA Polymerase. *Cell* **2001**, *104*, 901–912. [CrossRef]
6. Ahmed, M.O.; Baptiste, K.E. Vancomycin-Resistant Enterococci: A Review of Antimicrobial Resistance Mechanisms and Perspectives of Human and Animal Health. *Microb. Drug Resist.* **2017**, *24*, 590–606. [CrossRef]
7. Cetinkaya, Y.; Falk, P.; Mayhall, C.G. Vancomycin-resistant enterococci. *Clin. Microbiol. Rev.* **2000**, *13*, 686–707. [CrossRef]
8. Lee, A.S.; de Lencastre, H.; Garau, J.; Kluytmans, J.; Malhotra-Kumar, S.; Peschel, A.; Harbarth, S. Methicillin-resistant *Staphylococcus aureus*. *Nat. Rev. Dis. Primers* **2018**, *4*, 18033. [CrossRef]
9. Turner, N.A.; Sharma-Kuinkel, B.K.; Maskarinec, S.A.; Eichenberger, E.M.; Shah, P.P.; Carugati, M.; Holland, T.L.; Fowler, V.G. Methicillin-resistant *Staphylococcus aureus*: An overview of basic and clinical research. *Nat. Rev. Microbiol.* **2019**, *17*, 203–218. [CrossRef]
10. Gordon, N.C.; Wareham, D.W. A review of clinical and microbiological outcomes following treatment of infections involving multidrug-resistant *Acinetobacter baumannii* with tigecycline. *J. Antimicrob. Chemother.* **2009**, *63*, 775–780. [CrossRef]
11. Dent, L.L.; Marshall, D.R.; Pratap, S.; Hulette, R.B. Multidrug resistant *Acinetobacter baumannii*: A descriptive study in a city hospital. *BMC Infect. Dis.* **2010**, *10*, 196. [CrossRef]
12. Lei, J.; Sun, L.; Huang, S.; Zhu, C.; Li, P.; He, J.; Mackey, V.; Coy, D.H.; He, Q. The antimicrobial peptides and their potential clinical applications. *Am. J. Transl. Res.* **2019**, *11*, 3919–3931.
13. Huan, Y.; Kong, Q.; Mou, H.; Yi, H. Antimicrobial Peptides: Classification, Design, Application and Research Progress in Multiple Fields. *Front. Microbiol.* **2020**, *11*, 582779. [CrossRef]
14. Bahar, A.A.; Ren, D. Antimicrobial peptides. *Pharmaceuticals* **2013**, *6*, 1543–1575. [CrossRef]
15. Zanetti, M. Cathelicidins, multifunctional peptides of the innate immunity. *J. Leukoc. Biol.* **2004**, *75*, 39–48. [CrossRef]
16. Kościuczuk, E.M.; Lisowski, P.; Jarczak, J.; Strzałkowska, N.; Jóźwik, A.; Horbańczuk, J.; Krzyżewski, J.; Zwierzchowski, L.; Bagnicka, E. Cathelicidins: Family of antimicrobial peptides. A review. *Mol. Biol. Rep.* **2012**, *39*, 10957–10970. [CrossRef]
17. Zhang, Q.-Y.; Yan, Z.-B.; Meng, Y.-M.; Hong, X.-Y.; Shao, G.; Ma, J.-J.; Cheng, X.-R.; Liu, J.; Kang, J.; Fu, C.-Y. Antimicrobial peptides: Mechanism of action, activity and clinical potential. *Mil. Med. Res.* **2021**, *8*, 48. [CrossRef]
18. Seyfi, R.; Kahaki, F.A.; Ebrahimi, T.; Montazersaheb, S.; Eyvazi, S.; Babaeipour, V.; Tarhriz, V. Antimicrobial Peptides (AMPs): Roles, Functions and Mechanism of Action. *Int. J. Pept. Res. Ther.* **2020**, *26*, 1451–1463. [CrossRef]
19. Juneyoung, L. Antimicrobial Peptides (AMPs) with Dual Mechanisms: Membrane Disruption and Apoptosis. *J. Microbiol. Biotechnol.* **2015**, *25*, 759–764.
20. Jhong, J.-H.; Chi, Y.-H.; Li, W.-C.; Lin, T.-H.; Huang, K.-Y.; Lee, T.-Y. dbAMP: An integrated resource for exploring antimicrobial peptides with functional activities and physicochemical properties on transcriptome and proteome data. *Nucleic Acids Res.* **2019**, *47*, D285–D297. [CrossRef]
21. Tam, J.P.; Wang, S.; Wong, K.H.; Tan, W.L. Antimicrobial Peptides from Plants. *Pharmaceuticals* **2015**, *8*, 711–757. [CrossRef]
22. Moretta, A.; Salvia, R.; Scieuzo, C.; Di Somma, A.; Vogel, H.; Pucci, P.; Sgambato, A.; Wolff, M.; Falabella, P. A bioinformatic study of antimicrobial peptides identified in the Black Soldier Fly (BSF) *Hermetia illucens* (Diptera: Stratiomyidae). *Sci. Rep.* **2020**, *10*, 16875. [CrossRef]
23. Gan, B.H.; Gaynord, J.; Rowe, S.M.; Deingruber, T.; Spring, D.R. The multifaceted nature of antimicrobial peptides: Current synthetic chemistry approaches and future directions. *Chem. Soc. Rev.* **2021**, *50*, 7820–7880. [CrossRef]
24. Brogden, N.K.; Brogden, K.A. Will new generations of modified antimicrobial peptides improve their potential as pharmaceuticals? *Int. J. Antimicrob. Agents* **2011**, *38*, 217–225. [CrossRef]
25. Yang, S.; Wang, M.; Wang, T.; Sun, M.; Huang, H.; Shi, X.; Duan, S.; Wu, Y.; Zhu, J.; Liu, F. Self-assembled short peptides: Recent advances and strategies for potential pharmaceutical applications. *Mater. Today Bio* **2023**, *20*, 100644. [CrossRef]
26. Wang, L.; Wang, N.; Zhang, W.; Cheng, X.; Yan, Z.; Shao, G.; Wang, X.; Wang, R.; Fu, C. Therapeutic peptides: Current applications and future directions. *Signal Transduct. Target. Ther.* **2022**, *7*, 48. [CrossRef]
27. Drayton, M.; Kizhakkedathu, J.N.; Straus, S.K. Towards Robust Delivery of Antimicrobial Peptides to Combat Bacterial Resistance. *Molecules* **2020**, *25*, 3048. [CrossRef]
28. Patil, A.A.; Ouellette, A.J.; Lu, W.; Zhang, G. Rattusin, an intestinal α-defensin-related peptide in rats with a unique cysteine spacing pattern and salt-insensitive antibacterial activities. *Antimicrob. Agents Chemother.* **2013**, *57*, 1823–1831. [CrossRef]
29. Min, H.J.; Yun, H.; Ji, S.; Rajasekaran, G.; Kim, J.I.; Kim, J.-S.; Shin, S.Y.; Lee, C.W. Rattusin structure reveals a novel defensin scaffold formed by intermolecular disulfide exchanges. *Sci. Rep.* **2017**, *7*, 45282. [CrossRef]
30. Ji, S.; Yun, H.; Park, G.; Min, H.J.; Lee, C.W. Expression and characterization of recombinant rattusin, an α-defensin-related peptide with a homodimeric scaffold formed by intermolecular disulfide exchanges. *Protein Expr. Purif.* **2018**, *147*, 17–21. [CrossRef]

biomolecules

Communication

Preventive Effects of Collagen-Derived Dipeptide Prolyl-Hydroxyproline against Dexamethasone-Induced Muscle Atrophy in Mouse C2C12 Skeletal Myotubes

Yoshifumi Kimira *, Konosuke Osawa, Yoshihiro Osawa and Hiroshi Mano

Department of Clinical Dietetics and Human Nutrition, Faculty of Pharmacy and Pharmaceutical Sciences, Josai University, 1-1 Keyakidai, Sakado-shi 350-0295, Japan
* Correspondence: kimira@josai.ac.jp; Tel.: +81-49-271-7208

Abstract: Glucocorticoids, commonly used to manage inflammatory diseases, can induce muscle atrophy by accelerating the breakdown of muscle proteins. This research delves into the influence of Prolyl-hydroxyproline (Pro-Hyp), a collagen-derived peptide, on muscle atrophy induced with dexamethasone (DEX), a synthetic glucocorticoid, in mouse C2C12 skeletal myotubes. Exposure to DEX (10 μM) for 6 days resulted in a decrease in myotube diameter, along with elevated mRNA and protein levels of two muscle-atrophy-related ubiquitin ligases, muscle atrophy F-box (MAFbx, also known as atrogin-1) and muscle ring finger 1 (MuRF-1). Remarkably, treatment with 0.1 mM of Pro-Hyp mitigated the reduction in myotube thickness caused by DEX, while promoting the phosphorylation of Akt, mammalian target of rapamycin (mTOR), and forkhead box O3a (Foxo3a). This led to the inhibition of the upregulation of the ubiquitin ligases atrogin-1 and MuRF-1. These findings indicate the potential significance of Pro-Hyp as a promising therapeutic target for countering DEX-induced muscle atrophy.

Keywords: collagen-derived peptide; Prolyl-hydroxyproline; muscle atrophy; mouse C2C12 skeletal myotubes; ubiquitin ligases

Citation: Kimira, Y.; Osawa, K.; Osawa, Y.; Mano, H. Preventive Effects of Collagen-Derived Dipeptide Prolyl-Hydroxyproline against Dexamethasone-Induced Muscle Atrophy in Mouse C2C12 Skeletal Myotubes. *Biomolecules* **2023**, *13*, 1617. https://doi.org/10.3390/biom13111617

Academic Editors: Hyung-Sik Won and Ji-Hun Kim

Received: 17 August 2023
Revised: 2 November 2023
Accepted: 3 November 2023
Published: 5 November 2023

1. Introduction

Skeletal muscle atrophy is defined as a reduction in both the size and mass of muscle tissue, which occurs when protein breakdown surpasses protein synthesis [1]. This process leads to exercise intolerance, impeding daily activities due to muscle weakness and fatigue, ultimately compromising the overall quality of life [2].

Synthetic glucocorticoids have demonstrated utility in managing a wide range of inflammatory conditions. Dexamethasone (DEX), a synthetic glucocorticoid, has been used as a therapeutic intervention for various conditions due to its potent anti-inflammatory and protective properties against autoimmune diseases [3]. Nevertheless, despite these benefits, administering high doses and prolonged usage of DEX can result in severe side effects, including the development of muscle atrophy [4]. DEX acts as a catabolic regulator of skeletal muscle by upregulating the transcription of two muscle-specific ubiquitin E3 ligases, muscle atrophy F-box (MAFbx, also known as atrogin-1) and muscle ring finger 1 (MuRF-1), thereby contributing to the increased proteolysis seen during muscle atrophy [5]. Previous studies have indicated the involvement of forkhead box O (Foxo) transcription factors in the regulation of atrogin-1 and MuRF-1 expression during DEX-induced muscle atrophy [6]. Moreover, DEX induces muscle atrophy in mouse myocytes by inhibiting the phosphorylation of muscle protein synthesis factors, including Akt and the mammalian target of rapamycin (mTOR) [7].

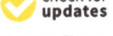

Collagen is a pivotal extracellular matrix protein predominantly found in dense connective tissues such as skin, bone, tendons, or fascia [8–10]. Collagen turnover gives rise to bioactive collagen peptides (CPs) through enzymatic degradation [11,12]. Collagen features

at least one common Glycine (Gly)-X-Y repeat domain, where X and Y are predominantly Proline (Pro) and hydroxyproline (Hyp), respectively. A multitude of bioactive peptides derived from collagen include Hyp in their sequences [13,14]. Certain functional peptides within CPs are absorbed into the bloodstream as oligopeptides [14,15], exerting diverse bioactive effects. Numerous studies have documented the favorable impacts of orally administered CPs on osteoporosis, osteoarthritis, and knee joint discomfort [16–18]. One notable collagen-derived bioactive peptide, Prolyl-hydroxyproline (Pro-Hyp), has been demonstrated to enhance the migration of fibroblasts from mouse skin and facilitate the differentiation of osteoblasts, tendon cells, and chondrocytes [19–23]. Another significant collagen-derived bioactive peptide, hydroxyprolylglycine (Hyp-Gly), has been found to induce muscle hypertrophic effects in C2C12 cells [24].

In addition to its diverse bioactive effects, CP has been recently reported to affect muscle mass positively. In a randomized controlled trial involving premenopausal women (ages 18–50 years), CP supplementation along with resistance training for 12 weeks significantly increased fat-free mass and hand-grip strength [25]. Furthermore, CP supplements also led to increased fat-free mass in middle-aged, untrained men (ages 30–60 years) undergoing resistance training [26].

CP supplementation has also demonstrated an impact on muscle breakdown. Previous research indicated that the intake of 15 g of specific collagen peptides notably increased fat-free mass and leg muscle strength following resistance training in older men with sarcopenia [27]. Recent animal experiments further indicated that CP administration along with treadmill exercise effectively prevented DEX-induced muscle atrophy in mice [28], and CP supplementation also improved age-related sarcopenia in middle-aged mice [29].

Hence, CP may have a significant role in mitigating muscle atrophy. Nonetheless, the influence of specific sequence peptides within CP on suppressing muscle atrophy remains unknown. In this study, we investigated the preventive effects of Pro-Hyp on DEX-induced muscle atrophy in C2C12 myotubular cells.

2. Materials and Methods

2.1. Cell Culture and Treatment

The C2C12 myoblast cell line mouse was obtained from the RIKEN Cell Bank (Tsukuba, Japan). C2C12 myoblast cells were cultured in Dulbecco's Modified Eagle Medium (DMEM, Cat. #11885-084, Gibco, Thermo Fisher Scientific, Waltham, MA, USA) containing 10% fetal bovine serum (FBS, Cat. #7524, Nichirei Biosciences, Tokyo, Japan) and 100 U/mL of penicillin, and maintained in a humidified incubator at 37 °C under a 5% CO_2 atmosphere until they reached 80–90% confluence. Subsequently, to induce differentiation into myotubes, the medium was exchanged for DMEM containing 2% FBS for 6 days, with medium changes every 2 days. For an immunofluorescence analysis, fully differentiated C2C12 cells were treated with 10 μM of DEX (Cat. #D1756, Sigma-Aldrich, St. Louis, MO, USA) for 6 days to induce muscle atrophy. Pro-Hyp (0.01, 0.1 mM, Cat. #4001630, Bachem, Bubendorf, Switzerland) was diluted in the DMEM medium and co-treated with DEX for 6 days. For qRT-PCR and Western blot analyses, fully differentiated C2C12 cells were treated with DEX (10 μM) and Pro-Hyp (0.01, 0.1 mM) for 24 h. DEX was dissolved in dimethyl sulfoxide (DMSO, Cat. #D8418, Sigma-Aldrich, St. Louis, MO, USA), and DMSO (0.01%) was used as the vehicle for DEX. The dose of Pro-Hyp was selected based on the fact that the concentrations used in previous reports of cellular experiments on the physiological effects of Pro-Hyp have also involved 0.1 mM as the upper limit [30].

2.2. Immunofluorescence Analysis

C2C12 myotubes were fixed in 4% paraformaldehyde in phosphate-buffered saline (PBS, Cat. #D163-20145, Wako Pure Chemical Industries, Ltd., Osaka, Japan) for 10 min at room temperature and washed twice with 0.1% Triton X-100 (Cat #160-24751, FUJIFILM Wako Pure Chemical, Osaka, Japan) in PBS. They were subsequently permeabilized with 0.1% Triton X-100 in PBS for 20 min. At room temperature, the cells were blocked with 3% bovine serum albumin in PBS for 1 h. Then, the cells were incubated with the myosin heavy chain (MHC) primary antibody (1:400, Sigma-Aldrich, St. Louis, MO, USA) overnight at 4 °C. After washing three times with 0.1% Tween 20 (Cat #167-11515, FUJIFILM Wako Pure Chemical, Osaka, Japan) in PBS (PBST), the cells were incubated with a secondary antibody conjugated to fluorescein isothiocyanate (FITC, 1:100, Cat. #sc2099, Santa Cruz, TX, USA) for 1 h at room temperature. After washing three times with 0.1% PBST, the nuclei were counterstained with 4′,6-diamidino-2-phenylindole (DAPI, Cat. #S36964, Thermo Fisher Scientific, MA, USA). Fluorescent images were analyzed using a BZ-810 fluorescence microscope (Keyence, Osaka, Japan). Fifty myotubes/group were measured randomly from five different fields. The thickest portion of each myotube was chosen for diameter measurement using BZ-H4M image analysis software (version 1.4.1.1, Keyence, Osaka, Japan).

2.3. RNA Preparation and Quantitative RT-PCR (qPCR)

Total RNA was extracted from the cells using the RNeasy Mini Kit (Qiagen, Hilden, Germany), and cDNA was synthesized from 5 mg of mRNA using the Prime Script Reagent Kit (Takara Bio Japan, Otsu, Japan). qPCR was performed with TB Green® Fast qPCR Mix (Takara Bio Japan, Otsu, Japan). Glyceraldehyde 3-phosphate dehydrogenase (GAPDH) was used as the internal control for normalizing the expression of target genes. The quantitative PCR primers were as follows: 5′-TGTCTGGAGGTCGTTTCCG-3′ (forward) and 5′-CTCGTCTTCGTGTTCCTTGC-3′ (reverse) for MuRF-1; 5′-GAGTGGCATCGCCCAAAAGA-3′ (forward) and 5′-TCTGGAGAAGTTCCCGTATAAGT-3′ (reverse) for atrogin-1; 5′-AGTG AATGAGGCCTTCGAGA-3′ (forward) and 5′-GCA TCTGAGTCGCCACTGTA-3′ (reverse) for MyoD; 5′-ACTCCCTTACGTCCATCGTG-3′ (forward) and 5′-CAGGACAGCCCCACTT AAAA-3′ (reverse) for Myogenin; 5′-ACTGAGCAAGAGAGGCCCTA-3′ (forward) and 5′-TGTGGGTGCAGCGAACTTTA-3′ (reverse) for GAPDH.

2.4. Western Blot Assay

Cells were washed twice with ice-cold PBS and then lysed with a radioimmunoprecipitation assay (RIPA) buffer consisting of 25 mM Tris-HCl (pH 7.6), 150 mM NaCl, 1% NP-40, 1% sodium deoxycholate, and 0.1% sodium dodecyl sulfate (SDS), and containing a protease inhibitor cocktail (Cat. # 87786, Thermo Fisher Scientific, Waltham, MA, USA). Cell lysates were centrifuged at 15,000 rpm for 20 min, and the supernatants were collected as protein samples. The protein concentration of each sample was measured with the bicinchoninic acid (BCA) Protein Assay Reagent (Thermo Fisher Scientific, Waltham, MA, USA). Proteins were separated with sodium dodecyl-sulfate polyacrylamide gel electrophoresis (SDS-PAGE) and transferred to polyvinylidene difluoride (PVDF) membranes using the Trans-Blot Turbo transfer system (Bio-Rad, Hercules, CA, USA). After blocking with 5% skim milk in TBS-T consisting of 10 mM Tris-HCl (pH 7.4), 1.37 M NaCl, and 0.1% Tween 20 for 30 min at room temperature, the membranes were incubated with rabbit anti-atrogin-1 (Cat. #ab168372, abcam, Cambridge, UK), rabbit anti-MuRF-1 (Cat. #ab172479, abcam, Cambridge, UK), rabbit anti-ubiquitin (Cat. #3936; Cell Signaling Technology, Danvers, MA, USA), rabbit anti-Akt (Cat. #2920; Cell Signaling Technology, Danvers, MA, USA), rabbit anti-phospho-Akt (Cat. #4060; Cell Signaling Technology, Danvers, MA, USA), rabbit anti-mTOR (Cat. #2983; Cell Signaling Technology, Danvers, MA, USA), rabbit anti-phospho-mTOR (Cat. #2971; Cell Signaling Technology, Danvers, MA, USA), rabbit anti-Foxo3a (Cat. #12829; Cell Signaling Technology, Danvers, MA, USA), rabbit anti-phospho-Foxo3a (Cat. #9496; Cell Signaling Technology, Danvers, MA, USA), or rabbit anti-β-actin (Cat. #4970; Cell Signaling Technology, Danvers, MA, USA) 1/1000 diluted in a blocking buffer for 1 h at room temperature. The membranes were washed with TBS-T and then incubated for 45 min at room temperature with HRP-conjugated rabbit anti-mouse IgG (Cat. #7074; Cell Signaling Technology, Danvers, MA, USA) 1/2000 diluted in TBS-T. To reprobe with another antibody, blots were incubated in a stripping buffer consisting of 62.5 mM Tris-HCl (pH 6.7), 2% SDS, and 100 mM 2-mercaptoethanol at 50 °C for 30 min and analyzed as described above. Labeled proteins were detected with EZ West Lumi plus (ATTO, Tokyo, Japan). Band intensities were determined using ImageJ software (version 1.54 g, National Institutes of Health, Bethesda, MD, USA).

2.5. Statistical Analysis

Data are expressed as means ± standard deviation (SD). Statistical analyses were performed using SPSS Statistics for Mac, Version 25.0 (IBM Corp., Armonk, NY, USA). Differences among multiple groups were compared using one-way analyses of variance (ANOVA) with Tukey post hoc tests. Values with $p < 0.05$ were considered statistically significant.

3. Results

3.1. Pro-Hyp Suppressed DEX-Induced C2C12 Myotube Atrophy

To evaluate the protective effect of Pro-Hyp on muscle atrophy, the myotube diameters were analyzed with immunofluorescence staining. Figure 1A displays representative photographs of the treated myotubes. Compared to the control group, myotube diameter was reduced by 23.4% after 6 days of treatment with 10 µM of DEX, confirming that DEX effectively induced muscle atrophy. However, in the DEX + 0.01 mM Pro-Hyp treated group, the myotube diameter recovered to 96.3% of the control value. Furthermore, myotube diameter in the DEX + 0.1 mM Pro-Hyp group showed a significant increase compared to the DEX group and was similar to the control group (Figure 1B). These results indicate that Pro-Hyp had protection activity against muscle atrophy in DEX-treated C2C12 myotubes.

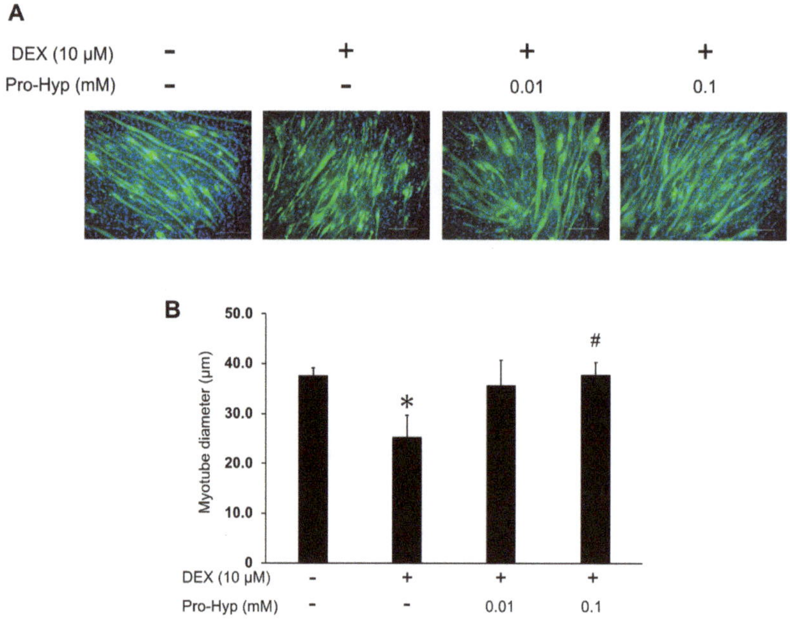

Figure 1. Effects of Pro-Hyp on myotube diameter in DEX-stimulated C2C12 myotubes. (**A**) Representative images of C2C12 myotubes treated with 10 µM of DEX and Pro-Hyp (0.01 mM and 0.1 mM). Fixed cells were reacted with an anti-MHC antibody and a fluorescence-labeled secondary antibody (green). The nuclei were stained with DAPI (blue). The scale bar represents 250 µm. (**B**) Comparison of myotube diameters among the four treatment groups. Data are expressed as means ± SD. * $p < 0.05$ vs. non-treated controls, # $p < 0.05$ vs. DEX-treated groups. $p < 0.05$.

3.2. Pro-Hyp Ameliorates Muscle-Atrophy-Associated Genes in DEX-Induced Myotube Atrophy

To investigate the effect of Pro-Hyp on muscle atrophy in DEX-treated C2C12 myotubes, the mRNA expression levels of atrogin-1 and MuRF-1, muscle-atrophy-related ubiquitin ligases, were assessed through qPCR. Upon exposure to a medium containing DEX, mRNA levels of atrogin-1 and MuRF-1 were significantly higher compared to the control group (Figure 2A,B). However, the DEX + 0.01 mM Pro-Hyp treated group resulted in a 20% reduction in atrogin-1 mRNA expression compared to the DEX group. The DEX + 0.1 mM Pro-Hyp treated group significantly reduced the mRNA expression of atrogin-1 compared to the DEX-treated C2C12 myotubes. Furthermore, Pro-Hyp (0.01 and 0.1 mM) treatment significantly reduced the expression of MuRF-1 compared to the DEX-treated C2C12 myotubes. These findings indicate that Pro-Hyp is associated with downregulating muscle-atrophy-related ubiquitin ligases. We also assessed the mRNA expression levels of MyoD and Myogenin, which are myogenic markers, and observed that exposure to a medium containing DEX significantly decreased the mRNA levels of MyoD and Myogenin in comparison to the control group (Figure 2C,D). However, the simultaneous addition of DEX and Pro-Hyp did not affect the DEX-induced decrease in mRNA expression of these genes. These findings suggest that Pro-Hyp is linked to the downregulation of ubiquitin ligases associated with muscle atrophy without impacting myogenesis in response to DEX-induced muscle atrophy.

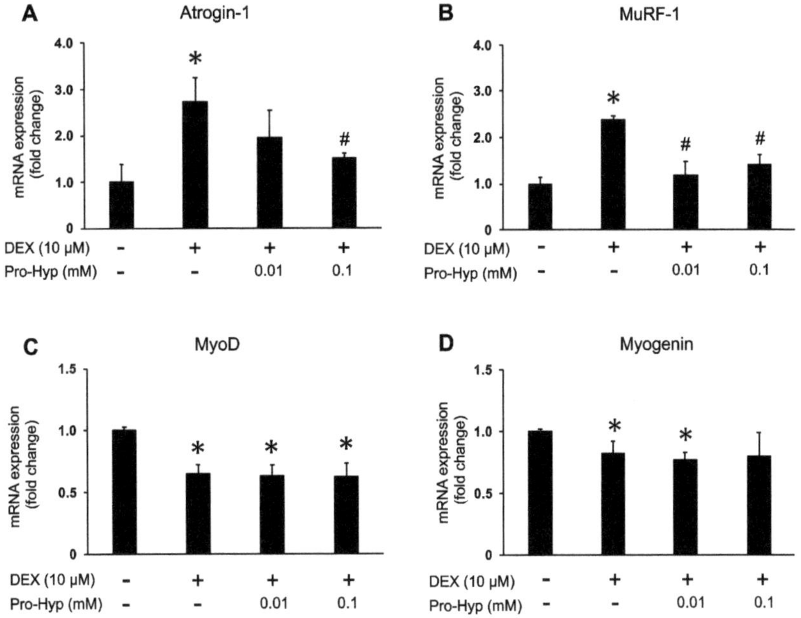

Figure 2. Effects of Pro-Hyp on muscle-atrophy-associated genes and myotube-differentiation-related genes in DEX-stimulated C2C12 myotubes. C2C12 myotubes were treated with 10 μM of DEX and Pro-Hyp (0.01 mM and 0.1 mM) for 24 h. (**A**) Atrogin-1, (**B**) MuRF-1, (**C**) MyoD, and (**D**) Myogenin mRNA levels were examined with qPCR. GAPDH was used as an internal control. Data are expressed as means ± SD. * $p < 0.05$ vs. non-treated controls, # $p < 0.05$ vs. DEX-treated groups. $p < 0.05$.

3.3. Pro-Hyp Attenuates Protein Levels of Muscle-Atrophy-Associated Ubiquitin Ligases and Ubiquitinated Proteins in DEX-Induced Myotube Atrophy

To determine whether Pro-Hyp exerts an inhibitory effect on atrophy in glucocorticoid-induced atrophic conditions, the protein levels of atrogin1 and MuRF-1 were analyzed with a Western blot. DEX treatment increased the protein levels of atrogin-1 and MuRF-1, and they were significantly higher than the control group. In contrast, the DEX + 0.01 mM Pro-Hyp treated group resulted in a 42% reduction in atrogin-1 protein expression compared to the DEX group. The DEX + 0.1 mM Pro-Hyp treated group significantly reduced the protein expression of atrogin-1 compared to the DEX-treated C2C12 myotubes (Figure 3A,B). In addition, the DEX + 0.01 mM Pro-Hyp treated group resulted in a 24% reduction in MuRF-1 protein expression compared to the DEX group. The DEX + 0.1 mM Pro-Hyp treated group significantly reduced the protein expression of MuRF-1 compared to the DEX-treated C2C12 myotubes (Figure 3A,C). To further investigate the inhibition of protein degradation with Pro-Hyp, ubiquitination was analyzed using a Western blot. The results showed that DEX treatment significantly increased the levels of ubiquitinated proteins, while co-treatment with Pro-Hyp and DEX significantly decreased ubiquitinated proteins compared to DEX treatment alone (Figure 3A,D). These results indicate that Pro-Hyp suppresses the expression of ubiquitin ligases atrogin-1 and MuRF-1, consequently inhibiting protein degradation and mitigating DEX-induced muscle atrophy.

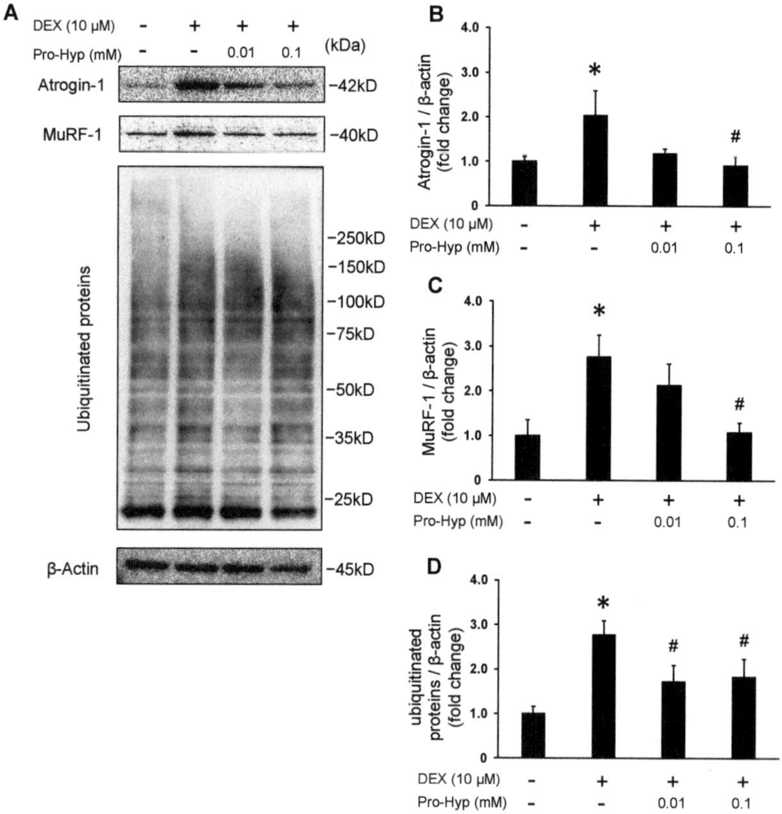

Figure 3. Effects of Pro-Hyp on protein levels of muscle-atrophy-associated ubiquitin ligases and ubiquitinated proteins in DEX-induced myotube atrophy. C2C12 myotubes were treated with 10 μM of DEX and Pro-Hyp (0.01 mM and 0.1 mM) for 24 h. Western blot assay examined atrogin-1, MuRF-1, and ubiquitinated protein level. β-actin was used as an internal control. (**A**) Representative Western blot of total forms of atrogin-1, MuRF-1, ubiquitinated proteins, and β-actin. (**B**) The ratio of total atrogin-1 and β-actin normalized to the control. (**C**) The ratio of total MuRF-1 and β-actin normalized to the control. (**D**) The ratio of ubiquitinated proteins and β-actin normalized to the control. Data are expressed as means ± SD. * $p < 0.05$ vs. non-treated controls, # $p < 0.05$ vs. DEX-treated groups. $p < 0.05$.

3.4. Pro-Hyp Prevented DEX-Induced Muscle Atrophy through Akt/mTOR/Foxo3a Signaling

To explore the mechanism of action of Pro-Hyp in preventing muscle atrophy, we analyzed the Akt, mTOR, and Foxo3a proteins, which are signaling pathway factors associated with protein synthesis and degradation, using a Western blot analysis. DEX treatment resulted in the inhibition of Akt and mTOR phosphorylation. Conversely, both the DEX + 0.01 mM Pro-Hyp and DEX + 0.1 mM Pro-Hyp treatment groups exhibited a significant increase in Akt and mTOR phosphorylation levels compared to C2C12 myotubes treated with DEX alone (Figure 4A–C). Furthermore, DEX treatment led to a significant reduction in the phosphorylation level of Foxo3a when compared to the control group. In contrast, the DEX + 0.01 mM Pro-Hyp treated group showed a significant increase in the phosphorylation level of Foxo3a compared to the DEX-treated group, although it remained significantly lower than the control group. The DEX + 0.1 mM Pro-Hyp treated group displayed a significant increase in the phosphorylation level of Foxo3a compared to the DEX-treated group, with no significant difference when compared to the control group (Figure 4A,D). These results suggest that Pro-Hyp diminishes DEX-induced muscle atrophy by modulating the Akt/mTOR/Foxo3a signaling pathway triggered by DEX.

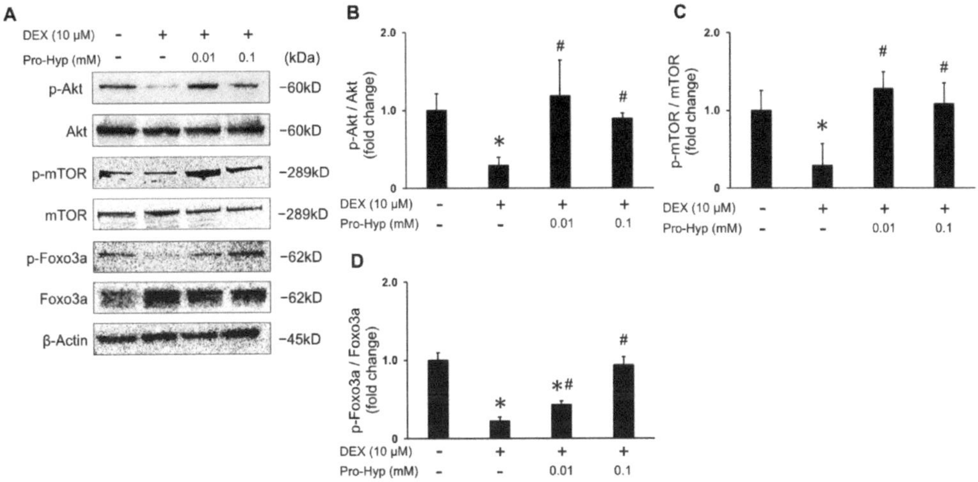

Figure 4. Effects of Pro-Hyp on Akt-mTOR-Foxo3a signaling in DEX-induced myotube atrophy. C2C12 myotubes were treated with 10 μM of DEX and Pro-Hyp (0.01 mM and 0.1 mM) for 24 h. Western blot assay examined Akt, phosphorylated Akt, mTOR, phosphorylated mTOR, Foxo3a, and phosphorylated Foxo3a protein levels. β-actin was used as an internal control. (**A**) Representative Western blot of phosphorylated and total forms of Akt, phosphorylated and total forms of Foxo3a, phosphorylated and total forms of mTOR, and β-actin. (**B**) The ratio of phosphorylated and total Akt normalized to the control. (**C**) The ratio of phosphorylated and total mTOR normalized to the control. (**D**) The ratio of phosphorylated and total Foxo3a normalized to the control. Data are expressed as means ± SD. * $p < 0.05$ vs. non-treated controls, # $p < 0.05$ vs. DEX-treated groups. $p < 0.05$.

4. Discussion

Muscle atrophy not only occurs in various physiological and pathological conditions, such as inactivity, muscle wasting, fasting, sepsis, cachexia, cancer, diabetes, and many chronic diseases, but it also causes increased morbidity and mortality. Therefore, maintaining healthy muscle mass is necessary for a healthy life. Recently, the possible effects of collagen peptide intake on muscle hypertrophy and prevention of muscle atrophy have been reported [25,27]. Still, there are no reports on the impact of specific peptides contained in collagen peptides on muscle atrophy or their molecular mechanisms. In this study, we report the protective activity of Pro-Hyp, a collagen-derived peptide, against DEX-induced C2C12 myotubular atrophy and its mechanism of action.

Many previous studies have shown that DEX reduces the diameter and MHC expression of C2C12 myotubes, which are known to be representative phenotypic modifiers of muscle atrophy [31,32]. In this study, we analyzed the effect of Pro-Hyp on DEX-induced C2C12 myotube atrophy by immunostaining with MHC, a representative marker of myotube differentiation [33]. As shown in Figure 1, the diameter of C2C12 myotubes decreased after DEX treatment but was restored with Pro-Hyp addition (0.01 and 0.1 mM). Thus, Pro-Hyp can prevent muscle atrophy by effectively restoring DEX-induced inhibition of C2C12 myotube differentiation.

Atrogin-1 and MuRF-1 stand out as the two most recognized muscle-specific E3 ubiquitin ligases and serve as crucial markers for muscle atrophy [5,34]. Atrogin-1 becomes evident early in the process, even before the onset of muscle weakness, and plays a role in the degradation of eukaryotic translation initiation factor 3 (eIF3), a key factor in protein translation initiation [35]. On the other hand, MuRF-1 is responsible for degrading MHC protein in DEX-treated skeletal muscle [36]. Several studies have demonstrated that DEX induces muscle atrophy in C2C12 myotubes by increasing the expression of atrogin-1 and MuRF-1 [7,37]. Conversely, myogenic factors like MyoD and Myogenin play a role in activating skeletal muscle formation and differentiation [38]. It has been reported that myoD and Myogenin expression is upregulated during myotube formation [39]. Moreover, DEX administration has been shown to decrease the expression of myoD and Myogenin and hinder myotube formation [7]. In the present study, the mRNA expression of atrogin-1 and MuRF-1 was significantly higher than in the control group. However, when Pro-Hyp and DEX were combined, the mRNA expression of atrogin-1 and MuRF-1 was also reduced (Figure 2A,B). This suppression of the DEX-induced upregulation of atrogin-1 and MuRF-1 mRNA expression with Pro-Hyp was further confirmed at the protein expression level for each respective gene (Figure 3A–C). Pro-Hyp mitigates the DEX-induced upregulation of ubiquitin ligase expression, in line with the observation that the ubiquitinated proteins, previously heightened with DEX administration, were decreased with the addition of Pro-Hyp (Figure 3A,D). Conversely, the mRNA expression levels of MyoD and Myogenin were diminished with DEX treatment compared to the control. However, the addition of Pro-Hyp did not affect the mRNA expression levels of MyoD and Myogenin, which were elevated with DEX treatment. These results suggest that Pro-Hyp effectively suppresses the expression of ubiquitin ligases atrogin-1 and MuRF-1, thereby inhibiting protein degradation with the ubiquitin–proteasome pathway and mitigating DEX-induced muscle atrophy.

Previous reports have indicated that Akt activation elevates mTOR phosphorylation, leading to an upregulation of protein synthesis in muscle tissue [40]. It has also been reported that the inhibition of the Akt/mTOR signaling pathway with DEX results in muscle atrophy [7]. Furthermore, several studies reported that collagen-derived peptides can promote muscle protein synthesis mainly through the Akt/mTOR pathway [24,29]. In the present study, DEX treatment substantially reduced the phosphorylation of Akt and mTOR compared to the control group. However, Pro-Hyp treatment significantly improved the relative phosphorylation levels of Akt and mTOR compared to the DEX-treated group (Figure 4A–C). Consequently, these results indicate that Pro-Hyp promotes the anabolic processes of muscle-specific proteins.

Prior research has indicated the involvement of the Foxo transcription factor in the regulation of atrogin-1 and MuRF-1 expression [41]. In the context of DEX-induced myotube atrophy, there is a reduction in the phosphorylation of Foxo1 and Foxo3a, leading to their translocation to the nucleus, where an upregulation occurs, subsequently increasing the expression of atrogin-1 and MuRF-1. Another relevant factor is the kinase Akt, which has been shown to phosphorylate Foxo during myotube atrophy. This phosphorylation hinders the translocation of Foxo to the nucleus, thereby preventing the upregulation of atrogin-1 and MuRF-1 [42]. Our previous research has identified a mechanism through which Pro-Hyp facilitates the interaction between Foxo1 and Runx2, a master regulator of osteoblast differentiation. This interaction leads to the stimulation of Runx2 promoter activity, ultimately renewing osteoblast differentiation [43]. Notably, Kitakaze et al. demonstrated that Hyp-Gly, a dipeptide derived from collagen, triggers myogenic differentiation by activating the Akt signaling pathway [24]. These reports suggest a potential involvement of collagen-derived dipeptides in intracellular Akt/Foxo signaling. In the present study, the administration of Pro-Hyp prevented the DEX-induced decreases in Akt phosphorylation and Foxo3a phosphorylation (Figure 4A–C). These findings indicate that Pro-Hyp administration inhibits DEX-induced muscle atrophy in C2C12 cells by impeding ubiquitin E3 ligases through the Akt-Foxo3a signaling pathway.

Furthermore, a recent study documented the suppression of DEX-induced muscle atrophy in mice through CP supplementation [28]. In the study, CP effectively curbed muscle atrophy while not impacting the expression of ubiquitin ligases involved in muscle degradation. While these findings contrast with our present study, some investigations employing CP and collagen tripeptide (CTP), which contains elevated collagen tripeptide levels, have indicated that the administration of CP and CTP was regulated in different ways to ameliorate muscle loss caused by aging [29]. These outcomes propose that collagen hydrolysates, comprising peptides of diverse molecular sizes and specific sequences, might offer various mechanisms to counteract muscle atrophy. Subsequent research should also investigate the effects of different molecular sizes and other collagen-derived oligopeptides in inhibiting muscle atrophy. Moreover, several human studies have consistently demonstrated that CP, combined with resistance exercise, leads to amplified muscle strength and diminished muscle weakness [25,27]. It would be beneficial for future research to investigate whether the administration of Pro-Hyp, in combination with resistance exercise, proves effective in mitigating muscle atrophy.

While the current findings support the use of DEX-treated C2C12 myotubes as an in vitro model of muscle atrophy, it is important to acknowledge several potential limitations in this study. First, this study solely investigated and exclusively focused on C2C12 myotubes. We suggest that conducting additional research involving other cell lines, such as L6 myotubes (a rat cell line), or using experimental animals would provide a more comprehensive evaluation of the impact of Pro-Hyp on glucocorticoid-induced muscle wasting and the regulation of myoprotein degradation. Another limitation of the study is its exclusive focus on the ubiquitin–proteasome system as the mechanism of proteolysis. We did not have the opportunity to investigate the impact of Pro-Hyp on muscle proteolysis mediated with catabolic pathways such as the autophagy–lysosome system [44]. Furthermore, our examination was limited to the Akt/mTOR/Foxo3a signaling pathway as the mechanism through which glucocorticoids induce atrophy. It is worth noting that glucocorticoids have been implicated in contributing to muscle atrophy by activating inflammatory signaling pathways [45], although the effects of Pro-Hyp on these pathways has not been explored.

5. Conclusions

In conclusion, the present study provides molecular evidence that Pro-Hyp improves DEX-induced atrophy in C2C12 myotubes through the regulation of the Akt/mTOR/Foxo3a signaling pathway, resulting in the inhibition of the upregulation of the ubiquitin ligases atrogin-1 and MuRF-1. However, further studies are required to investigate other possible anti-atrophy-related mechanisms and in vivo efficacies for Pro-Hyp. Overall, this study highlights the potential importance of Pro-Hyp as an effective therapeutic target for DEX-induced muscle atrophy by decreasing muscle-specific ubiquitin ligase expression.

Supplementary Materials: The following supporting information can be downloaded at: https://www.mdpi.com/article/10.3390/biom13111617/s1.

Author Contributions: Conceptualization, Y.K. and H.M.; methodology, Y.K.; investigation, K.O. and Y.K.; writing—original draft preparation, Y.K.; writing—review and editing, Y.O. and H.M.; visualization, K.O., and Y.K.; supervision, H.M. All authors have read and agreed to the published version of the manuscript.

Funding: This work was supported by JSPS KAKENHI (Grant Number: 23K05095).

Institutional Review Board Statement: Not applicable.

Informed Consent Statement: Not applicable.

Data Availability Statement: All relevant data are within the paper and Supplementary Materials.

Conflicts of Interest: The authors declare no conflict of interest.

References

1. Fanzani, A.; Conraads, V.M.; Penna, F.; Martinet, W. Molecular and Cellular Mechanisms of Skeletal Muscle Atrophy: An Update. *J. Cachexia Sarcopenia Muscle* **2012**, *3*, 163–179. [CrossRef]
2. Mancini, D.M.; Walter, G.; Reichek, N.; Lenkinski, R.; McCully, K.K.; Mullen, J.L.; Wilson, J.R. Contribution of Skeletal Muscle Atrophy to Exercise Intolerance and Altered Muscle Metabolism in Heart Failure. *Circulation* **1992**, *85*, 1364–1373. [CrossRef] [PubMed]
3. Dubashynskaya, N.V.; Bokatyi, A.N.; Skorik, Y.A. Dexamethasone Conjugates: Synthetic Approaches and Medical Prospects. *Biomedicines* **2021**, *9*, 341. [CrossRef]
4. Schakman, O.; Kalista, S.; Barbé, C.; Loumaye, A.; Thissen, J.P. Glucocorticoid-Induced Skeletal Muscle Atrophy. *Int. J. Biochem. Cell Biol.* **2013**, *45*, 2163–2172. [CrossRef]
5. Bodine, S.C.; Baehr, L.M. Skeletal Muscle Atrophy and the E3 Ubiquitin Ligases MuRF1 and MAFbx/Atrogin-1. *Am. J. Physiol. Endocrinol. Metab.* **2014**, *307*, E469–E484. [CrossRef] [PubMed]
6. Stitt, T.N.; Drujan, D.; Clarke, B.A.; Panaro, F.; Timofeyva, Y.; Kline, W.O.; Gonzalez, M.; Yancopoulos, G.D.; Glass, D.J. The IGF-1/PI3K/Akt Pathway Prevents Expression of Muscle Atrophy-Induced Ubiquitin Ligases by Inhibiting FOXO Transcription Factors. *Mol. Cell* **2004**, *14*, 395–403. [CrossRef]
7. Kim, J.; Park, M.Y.; Kim, H.K.; Park, Y.; Whang, K.-Y. Cortisone and Dexamethasone Inhibit Myogenesis by Modulating the AKT/MTOR Signaling Pathway in C2C12. *Biosci. Biotechnol. Biochem.* **2016**, *80*, 2093–2099. [CrossRef]
8. Ricard-Blum, S. The Collagen Family. *Cold Spring Harb. Perspect. Biol.* **2011**, *3*, a004978. [CrossRef] [PubMed]
9. Hulmes, D.J. The Collagen Superfamily—Diverse Structures and Assemblies. *Essays Biochem.* **1992**, *27*, 49–67. [PubMed]
10. Ottani, V.; Raspanti, M.; Ruggeri, A. Collagen Structure and Functional Implications. *Micron* **2001**, *32*, 251–260. [CrossRef]
11. Husek, P.; Svagera, Z.; Vsianský, F.; Franeková, J.; Simek, P. Prolyl-Hydroxyproline Dipeptide in Non-Hydrolyzed Morning Urine and Its Value in Postmenopausal Osteoporosis. *Clin. Chem. Lab. Med.* **2008**, *46*, 1391–1397. [CrossRef]
12. Kusubata, M.; Koyama, Y.-I.; Tometsuka, C.; Shigemura, Y.; Sato, K. Detection of Endogenous and Food-Derived Collagen Dipeptide Prolylhydroxyproline (Pro-Hyp) in Allergic Contact Dermatitis-Affected Mouse Ear. *Biosci. Biotechnol. Biochem.* **2015**, *79*, 1356–1361. [CrossRef] [PubMed]
13. Brodsky, B.; Ramshaw, J.A. The Collagen Triple-Helix Structure. *Matrix Biol.* **1997**, *15*, 545–554. [CrossRef] [PubMed]
14. Iwai, K.; Hasegawa, T.; Taguchi, Y.; Morimatsu, F.; Sato, K.; Nakamura, Y.; Higashi, A.; Kido, Y.; Nakabo, Y.; Ohtsuki, K. Identification of Food-Derived Collagen Peptides in Human Blood after Oral Ingestion of Gelatin Hydrolysates. *J. Agric. Food Chem.* **2005**, *53*, 6531–6536. [CrossRef] [PubMed]
15. Watanabe-Kamiyama, M.; Shimizu, M.; Kamiyama, S.; Taguchi, Y.; Sone, H.; Morimatsu, F.; Shirakawa, H.; Furukawa, Y.; Komai, M. Absorption and Effectiveness of Orally Administered Low Molecular Weight Collagen Hydrolysate in Rats. *J. Agric. Food Chem.* **2010**, *58*, 835–841. [CrossRef] [PubMed]
16. König, D.; Oesser, S.; Scharla, S.; Zdzieblik, D.; Gollhofer, A. Specific Collagen Peptides Improve Bone Mineral Density and Bone Markers in Postmenopausal Women—A Randomized Controlled Study. *Nutrients* **2018**, *10*, 97. [CrossRef]
17. Bello, A.E.; Oesser, S. Collagen Hydrolysate for the Treatment of Osteoarthritis and Other Joint Disorders: A Review of the Literature. *Curr. Med. Res. Opin.* **2006**, *22*, 2221–2232. [CrossRef] [PubMed]
18. Zdzieblik, D.; Oesser, S.; Gollhofer, A.; König, D. Improvement of Activity-Related Knee Joint Discomfort Following Supplementation of Specific Collagen Peptides. *Appl. Physiol. Nutr. Metab.* **2017**, *42*, 588–595. [CrossRef] [PubMed]
19. Shigemura, Y.; Iwai, K.; Morimatsu, F.; Iwamoto, T.; Mori, T.; Oda, C.; Taira, T.; Park, E.Y.; Nakamura, Y.; Sato, K. Effect of Prolyl-Hydroxyproline (Pro-Hyp), a Food-Derived Collagen Peptide in Human Blood, on Growth of Fibroblasts from Mouse Skin. *J. Agric. Food Chem.* **2009**, *57*, 444–449. [CrossRef]
20. Kimira, Y.; Ogura, K.; Taniuchi, Y.; Kataoka, A.; Inoue, N.; Sugihara, F.; Nakatani, S.; Shimizu, J.; Wada, M.; Mano, H. Collagen-Derived Dipeptide Prolyl-Hydroxyproline Promotes Differentiation of MC3T3-E1 Osteoblastic Cells. *Biochem. Biophys. Res. Commun.* **2014**, *453*, 498–501. [CrossRef]

21. Ide, K.; Takahashi, S.; Sakai, K.; Taga, Y.; Ueno, T.; Dickens, D.; Jenkins, R.; Falciani, F.; Sasaki, T.; Ooi, K.; et al. The Dipeptide Prolyl-Hydroxyproline Promotes Cellular Homeostasis and Lamellipodia-Driven Motility via Active B1-Integrin in Adult Tendon Cells. *J. Biol. Chem.* **2021**, *297*, 100819. [CrossRef] [PubMed]
22. Nakatani, S.; Mano, H.; Sampei, C.; Shimizu, J.; Wada, M. Chondroprotective Effect of the Bioactive Peptide Prolyl-Hydroxyproline in Mouse Articular Cartilage in Vitro and in Vivo. *Osteoarthr. Cartil.* **2009**, *17*, 1620–1627. [CrossRef]
23. Kimira, Y.; Sato, T.; Sakamoto, M.; Osawa, Y.; Mano, H. Collagen-Derived Dipeptide Pro-Hyp Enhanced ATDC5 Chondrocyte Differentiation under Hypoxic Conditions. *Molecules* **2023**, *28*, 4664. [CrossRef]
24. Kitakaze, T.; Sakamoto, T.; Kitano, T.; Inoue, N.; Sugihara, F.; Harada, N.; Yamaji, R. The Collagen Derived Dipeptide Hydroxyprolyl-Glycine Promotes C2C12 Myoblast Differentiation and Myotube Hypertrophy. *Biochem. Biophys. Res. Commun.* **2016**, *478*, 1292–1297. [CrossRef] [PubMed]
25. Jendricke, P.; Centner, C.; Zdzieblik, D.; Gollhofer, A.; König, D. Specific Collagen Peptides in Combination with Resistance Training Improve Body Composition and Regional Muscle Strength in Premenopausal Women: A Randomized Controlled Trial. *Nutrients* **2019**, *11*, 892. [CrossRef]
26. Zdzieblik, D.; Jendricke, P.; Oesser, S.; Gollhofer, A.; König, D. The Influence of Specific Bioactive Collagen Peptides on Body Composition and Muscle Strength in Middle-Aged, Untrained Men: A Randomized Controlled Trial. *Int. J. Environ. Res. Public Health* **2021**, *18*, 4837. [CrossRef]
27. Zdzieblik, D.; Oesser, S.; Baumstark, M.W.; Gollhofer, A.; König, D. Collagen Peptide Supplementation in Combination with Resistance Training Improves Body Composition and Increases Muscle Strength in Elderly Sarcopenic Men: A Randomised Controlled Trial. *Br. J. Nutr.* **2015**, *114*, 1237–1245. [CrossRef] [PubMed]
28. Oh, J.; Park, S.H.; Kim, D.S.; Choi, W.; Jang, J.; Rahmawati, L.; Jang, W.Y.; Lim, H.K.; Hwang, J.Y.; Gu, G.R.; et al. The Preventive Effect of Specific Collagen Peptides against Dexamethasone-Induced Muscle Atrophy in Mice. *Molecules* **2023**, *28*, 1950. [CrossRef]
29. Kim, J.E.; Kwon, E.Y.; Han, Y. A Collagen Hydrolysate Containing Tripeptides Ameliorates Sarcopenia in Middle-Aged Mice. *Molecules* **2022**, *27*, 9. [CrossRef]
30. Kimira, Y.; Odaira, H.; Nomura, K.; Taniuchi, Y.; Inoue, N.; Nakatani, S.; Shimizu, J.; Wada, M.; Mano, H. Collagen-Derived Dipeptide Prolyl-Hydroxyproline Promotes Osteogenic Differentiation through Foxg1. *Cell. Mol. Biol. Lett.* **2017**, *22*, 27. [CrossRef]
31. Chen, L.; Chen, L.; Wan, L.; Huo, Y.; Huang, J.; Li, J.; Lu, J.; Xin, B.; Yang, Q.; Guo, C. Matrine Improves Skeletal Muscle Atrophy by Inhibiting E3 Ubiquitin Ligases and Activating the Akt/MTOR/FoxO3α Signaling Pathway in C2C12 Myotubes and Mice. *Oncol. Rep.* **2019**, *42*, 479–494. [CrossRef] [PubMed]
32. Chang, J.S.; Kong, I.D. Irisin Prevents Dexamethasone-Induced Atrophy in C2C12 Myotubes. *Pflug. Arch.* **2020**, *472*, 495–502. [CrossRef] [PubMed]
33. Blau, H.M.; Pavlath, G.K.; Hardeman, E.C.; Chiu, C.P.; Silberstein, L.; Webster, S.G.; Miller, S.C.; Webster, C. Plasticity of the Differentiated State. *Science* **1985**, *230*, 758–766. [CrossRef]
34. Gomes, M.D.; Lecker, S.H.; Jagoe, R.T.; Navon, A.; Goldberg, A.L. Atrogin-1, a Muscle-Specific F-Box Protein Highly Expressed during Muscle Atrophy. *Proc. Natl. Acad. Sci. USA* **2001**, *98*, 14440–14445. [CrossRef] [PubMed]
35. Lagirand-Cantaloube, J.; Offner, N.; Csibi, A.; Leibovitch, M.P.; Batonnet-Pichon, S.; Tintignac, L.A.; Segura, C.T.; Leibovitch, S.A. The Initiation Factor EIF3-f Is a Major Target for Atrogin1/MAFbx Function in Skeletal Muscle Atrophy. *EMBO J.* **2008**, *27*, 1266–1276. [CrossRef]
36. Clarke, B.A.; Drujan, D.; Willis, M.S.; Murphy, L.O.; Corpina, R.A.; Burova, E.; Rakhilin, S.V.; Stitt, T.N.; Patterson, C.; Latres, E.; et al. The E3 Ligase MuRF1 Degrades Myosin Heavy Chain Protein in Dexamethasone-Treated Skeletal Muscle. *Cell Metab.* **2007**, *6*, 376–385. [CrossRef]
37. Castillero, E.; Alamdari, N.; Lecker, S.H.; Hasselgren, P.-O. Suppression of Atrogin-1 and MuRF1 Prevents Dexamethasone-Induced Atrophy of Cultured Myotubes. *Metabolism* **2013**, *62*, 1495–1502. [CrossRef]
38. Dedieu, S.; Mazères, G.; Cottin, P.; Brustis, J.-J. Involvement of Myogenic Regulator Factors during Fusion in the Cell Line C2C12. *Int. J. Dev. Biol.* **2002**, *46*, 235–241.
39. Ferri, P.; Barbieri, E.; Burattini, S.; Guescini, M.; D'Emilio, A.; Biagiotti, L.; Del Grande, P.; De Luca, A.; Stocchi, V.; Falcieri, E. Expression and Subcellular Localization of Myogenic Regulatory Factors during the Differentiation of Skeletal Muscle C2C12 Myoblasts. *J. Cell. Biochem.* **2009**, *108*, 1302–1317. [CrossRef]
40. Hahn-Windgassen, A.; Nogueira, V.; Chen, C.-C.; Skeen, J.E.; Sonenberg, N.; Hay, N. Akt Activates the Mammalian Target of Rapamycin by Regulating Cellular ATP Level and AMPK Activity. *J. Biol. Chem.* **2005**, *280*, 32081–32089. [CrossRef]
41. Milan, G.; Romanello, V.; Pescatore, F.; Armani, A.; Paik, J.-H.; Frasson, L.; Seydel, A.; Zhao, J.; Abraham, R.; Goldberg, A.L.; et al. Regulation of Autophagy and the Ubiquitin–Proteasome System by the FoxO Transcriptional Network during Muscle Atrophy. *Nat. Commun.* **2015**, *6*, 6670. [CrossRef]
42. Sandri, M.; Sandri, C.; Gilbert, A.; Skurk, C.; Calabria, E.; Picard, A.; Walsh, K.; Schiaffino, S.; Lecker, S.H.; Goldberg, A.L. Foxo Transcription Factors Induce the Atrophy-Related Ubiquitin Ligase Atrogin-1 and Cause Skeletal Muscle Atrophy. *Cell* **2004**, *117*, 399–412. [CrossRef] [PubMed]
43. Nomura, K.; Kimira, Y.; Osawa, Y.; Kataoka-Matsushita, A.; Takao, K.; Sugita, Y.; Shimizu, J.; Wada, M.; Mano, H. Stimulation of the Runx2 P1 Promoter by Collagen-Derived Dipeptide Prolyl-Hydroxyproline Bound to Foxg1 and Foxo1 in Osteoblasts. *Biosci. Rep.* **2021**, *41*, BSR20210304. [CrossRef] [PubMed]

44. Sandri, M. Protein Breakdown in Muscle Wasting: Role of Autophagy-Lysosome and Ubiquitin-Proteasome. *Int. J. Biochem. Cell Biol.* **2013**, *45*, 2121–2129. [CrossRef]
45. Sun, H.; Gong, Y.; Qiu, J.; Chen, Y.; Ding, F.; Zhao, Q. TRAF6 Inhibition Rescues Dexamethasone-Induced Muscle Atrophy. *Int. J. Mol. Sci.* **2014**, *15*, 11126–11141. [CrossRef] [PubMed]

biomolecules

MDPI

Article

Synthesis and Antifungal Activity of Fmoc-Protected 1,2,4-Triazolyl-α-Amino Acids and Their Dipeptides Against *Aspergillus* Species

Tatevik Sargsyan [1,2], Lala Stepanyan [1], Henrik Panosyan [3], Heghine Hakobyan [1], Monika Israyelyan [1], Avetis Tsaturyan [1,2], Nelli Hovhannisyan [1,2], Caterina Vicidomini [4], Anna Mkrtchyan [1,2], Ashot Saghyan [1,2,*] and Giovanni N. Roviello [4,*]

1 Scientific and Production Center "Armbiotechnology" NAS RA, 14 Gyurjyan Str., Yerevan 0056, Armenia
2 Institute of Pharmacy, Yerevan State University, 1 Alex Manoogian Str., Yerevan 0025, Armenia
3 Scientific Technological Center of Organic and Pharmaceutical Chemistry, 26, Azatutian Ave., Yerevan 0014, Armenia
4 Institute of Biostructures and Bioimaging, Italian National Council for Research (IBB-CNR), Area di Ricerca Site and Headquarters, Via Pietro Castellino 111, 80131 Naples, Italy
* Correspondence: ashot.saghyan@sci.am (A.S.); giovanni.roviello@cnr.it (G.N.R.); Tel.: +374-43093344 (A.S.); +39-0812203415 (G.N.R.)

Abstract: In recent years, fungal infections have emerged as a significant health concern across veterinary species, especially in livestock such as cattle, where fungal diseases can result in considerable economic losses, as well as in humans. In particular, *Aspergillus* species, notably *Aspergillus flavus* and *Aspergillus versicolor*, are opportunistic pathogens that pose a threat to both animals and humans. This study focuses on the synthesis and antifungal evaluation of novel 9-fluorenylmethoxycarbonyl (Fmoc)-protected 1,2,4-triazolyl-α-amino acids and their dipeptides, designed to combat fungal pathogens. More in detail, we evaluated their antifungal activity against various species, including *Aspergillus versicolor* (ATCC 12134) and *Aspergillus flavus* (ATCC 10567). The results indicated that dipeptide **7a** exhibited promising antifungal activity against *Aspergillus versicolor* with an IC_{50} value of 169.94 μM, demonstrating greater potency than fluconazole, a standard treatment for fungal infections, which showed an IC_{50} of 254.01 μM. Notably, dipeptide **7a** showed slightly enhanced antifungal efficacy compared to fluconazole also in *Aspergillus flavus* (IC_{50} 176.69 μM vs. 184.64 μM), suggesting that this dipeptide might be more potent even against this strain. Remarkably, **3a** and **7a** are also more potent than fluconazole against *A. candidus* 10711. On the other hand, the protected amino acid **3a** demonstrated consistent inhibition across all tested *Aspergillus* strains, but with an IC_{50} value of 267.86 μM for *Aspergillus flavus*, it was less potent than fluconazole (IC_{50} 184.64 μM), still showing some potential as a good antifungal molecule. Overall, our findings indicate that the synthesized 1,2,4-triazolyl derivatives **3a** and **7a** hold significant promise as potential antifungal agents in treating *Aspergillus*-induced diseases in cattle, as well as for broader applications in human health. Our mechanistic studies based on molecular docking revealed that compounds **3a** and **7a** bind to the same region of the sterol 14-α demethylase as fluconazole. Given the rising concerns about antifungal resistance, these amino acid derivatives, with their unique bioactive structures, could serve as a novel class of therapeutic agents. Further research into their in vivo efficacy and safety profiles is warranted to fully realize their potential as antifungal drugs in clinical and agricultural settings.

check for updates

Academic Editors: Hyung-Sik Won and Ji-Hun Kim

Received: 21 November 2024
Revised: 15 December 2024
Accepted: 24 December 2024
Published: 4 January 2025

Citation: Sargsyan, T.; Stepanyan, L.; Panosyan, H.; Hakobyan, H.; Israyelyan, M.; Tsaturyan, A.; Hovhannisyan, N.; Vicidomini, C.; Mkrtchyan, A.; Saghyan, A.; et al. Synthesis and Antifungal Activity of Fmoc-Protected 1,2,4-Triazolyl-α-Amino Acids and Their Dipeptides Against *Aspergillus* Species. *Biomolecules* **2025**, *15*, 61. https://doi.org/10.3390/biom15010061

Keywords: 1,2,4-triazoles; antifungal peptides; synthesis; dipeptides; fluconazole; non-protein amino acids; *Aspergillus candidus; Aspergillus versicolor; Aspergillus flavus; Alternaria alternate; Ulocladium botrytis; Aureobasidium pullulans*

1. Introduction

In recent years, fungi have been recognized as integral components of commensal microbiota in various parts of the body, including the intestines, oral cavity, skin, lungs, and vagina [1,2]. They have served as a food source and played a significant role in food processing for thousands of years. Additionally, fungi may be utilized in numerous industrial processes, contributing to the production of peptides, enzymes, vitamins, organic acids, and antibiotics [3,4]. However, alongside their beneficial properties [5], fungi can act as pathogens for plants, humans, and animals. Zoonotic infections have been acknowledged for centuries and represent a significant portion of emerging and reemerging infectious diseases globally. Notably, there has been an increasing number of recalcitrant fungal diseases in animals over the last two decades, primarily stemming from opportunistic and pathogenic fungi [6,7], which can also be transmitted to humans. Opportunistic fungi have a preferred habitat independent from the living host and cause infection after accidental penetration of intact skin barriers or in the case of immunologic defects or other debilitating conditions that exist in the host [8]. In contrast, several other pathogens are characterized by their dependence on vertebrate hosts; obligate pathogens, in particular, require a host to complete their life cycle and essential functions such as nutrient acquisition, growth, habitat establishment, and reproduction [9,10].

1.1. Fungal Strains Affecting Animal Species

Some of the more relevant fungal strains include *Aspergillus, Alternaria alternata, Cladobotryum botrytis*, and *Aureobasidium pullulans*. Aspergillosis is an airborne fungal infection caused by molds in the genus *Aspergillus*. It primarily spreads through the inhalation of conidia, although infection can also occur via ingestion or contaminated wounds [11]. The clinical spectrum of *Aspergillus*-associated diseases in humans ranges from chronic localized aspergillomas to acute invasive aspergillosis, with severity often linked to the patient's underlying health conditions [12,13]. In animals, the clinical manifestations of aspergillosis vary widely depending on the species and environmental factors. Here is a concise table (Table 1) summarizing how *Aspergillus* infections affect different animal species [14,15].

Fungal infections, particularly those caused by *Aspergillus* species, are a growing concern in veterinary medicine, especially in livestock such as cattle. *Aspergillus flavus* and *Aspergillus* versicolor are known opportunistic pathogens that can lead to significant health issues in animals, including mycotic abortion, respiratory infections, and gastrointestinal diseases. In cattle, *Aspergillus* infections often occur in late pregnancy, where they can cause abortion, a serious condition with major implications for both animal health and farm productivity [16]. Furthermore, these infections can lead to chronic respiratory conditions, reduced fertility, and diminished milk production, all of which contribute to considerable economic losses in the agricultural sector. In addition to direct impacts on cattle health, *Aspergillus* species are also of concern due to their ability to develop resistance to commonly used antifungal treatments. With the increasing prevalence of such infections in immunocompromised animals and the limited number of effective antifungal agents available, there is an urgent need for novel, more effective therapeutic approaches. This situation underscores the critical importance of developing targeted antifungal therapies that not only address the immediate health risks posed by *Aspergillus* species but also reduce the likelihood of resistance development, a growing challenge in both veterinary and human medicine [14,17].

Table 1. *Aspergillus* infections and their clinical manifestations in different animal species.

Species	*Aspergillus*-Related Conditions	Clinical Manifestations	Affected Systems/Organs
Birds	Aspergillosis	Respiratory distress, weight loss, lethargy	Primarily lungs (respiratory system)
Cattle	Mycotic abortion	Abortion or stillbirth, particularly in late pregnancy	Uterus, placenta
Horses	Laryngeal pouch mycosis	Respiratory issues, coughing, nasal discharge	Laryngeal pouch, respiratory system
	Mycotic keratitis	Eye infections, corneal ulcers, vision impairment	Eyes (cornea)
Dogs	Nasal/paranasal aspergillosis	Nasal discharge, facial pain, sinus issues	Nasal and paranasal tissues
	Intervertebral space infection	Neurological symptoms (e.g., ataxia, paralysis)	Spine (intervertebral spaces)
	Renal aspergillosis	Kidney dysfunction, potential kidney failure	Kidneys
Cats	Sinonasal, sino-orbital aspergillosis	Respiratory distress, nasal discharge, eye problems (e.g., conjunctivitis, exophthalmos)	Sinuses, orbital region, lungs (pulmonary system)

Aureobasidium pullulans is a dematiaceous, yeast-like fungus that is ubiquitous in nature and can colonize human hair and skin. It has been implicated clinically as causing skin and soft tissue infections, meningitis, splenic abscesses, and peritonitis [18,19]. Like other saprophytic fungi, *A. pullulans* can cause disease in the setting of immunocompromised conditions [20]. *Ulocladium*, viewed as a harmless fungus, is now recognized for its potential to cause mycotoxicoses linked to contaminated crops like wheat. Its pathogenic capabilities have come to light, with reported cases of keratitis and onychomycosis in immunocompetent patients, along with skin infections in immunocompromised individuals [21–23]. *Alternaria species* are ubiquitous fungi known for their dark pigmentation due to melanin. They are significant plant pathogens, causing considerable economic losses in various food crops. In addition to affecting plants, Alternaria spp. can also infect animals, including warm-blooded species and humans, with increasing clinical relevance, particularly among immunocompromised patients. Their role as potent airborne allergens is noteworthy, as they contribute to allergic respiratory conditions, including severe asthma [24,25].

1.2. Antifungal Drugs

Four major classes of antifungal agents dominate the market: azoles, which inhibit the synthesis of ergosterol; polyenes, which interact with fungal membrane sterols physicochemically; echinocandins, which inhibit glucan synthesis; and fluorinated pyrimidines, which interfere with pyrimidine metabolism, leading to the inhibition of DNA and RNA biosynthesis [26]. 1,2,4-Triazoles are a class of heterocyclic compounds that play an important role in medicine and chemistry due to their biological and pharmacological properties; they have a wide range of biological activities such as antibacterial, antifungal, antiviral, insecticidal, and herbicidal [27,28].. This group of biologically active compounds acts by inhibiting the activity of the cytochrome P450-dependent enzyme lanosterol-14α-demethylase

(CYP51), which is an important enzyme in the ergosterol biosynthesis of fungi [29]. Some azoles bind to the heme within CYP51, causing a blockade of the ergosterol biosynthesis pathway of fungi, which leads to agglomeration of 14-demethylated sterols [30]. Recently, new 1,2,4-triazole derivatives have been obtained and evaluated for fungicidal activity, and some have shown potential activity against certain fungi. In previous years, many research papers have highlighted the importance of 1,2,4-triazoles having powerful antifungal and antibacterial properties [25,31]. However, the high mortality of invasive fungal infections, the long course of treatments required, narrow spectrum activity, and cross-resistance due to similar mechanisms of action across drugs has triggered the search for safer alternatives with reduced toxicity or other enhanced features. Drug resistance development, the increasing number of immunodeficiency- and/or immunosuppression-related diseases, and limited therapeutic options available are triggering the search for novel alternatives. Recent advancements in the study of oxidative processes and xenobiotic metabolism in plants [32]., computational drug discovery methods [33], and marine-derived therapeutic innovations [34,35] highlight the growing intersection of natural substance research with modern medicine [36,37]., offering promising avenues for novel treatments. As for new antifungals, these should be less toxic for the host, with targeted or broader antimicrobial spectra (for diseases of known and unknown etiology, respectively) and modes of actions that limit the potential for the emergence of resistance among pathogenic fungi. Given these criteria, antimicrobial peptides with antifungal properties, i.e., antifungal peptides (AFPs), have emerged as powerful candidates due to their efficacy and high selectivity. These peptides have a broad spectrum of activity against bacteria, fungi, and viruses and are less likely to develop resistance compared to conventional antibiotics [38–41]. Antifungal peptides (AFPs) are typically classified based on origin: natural, semisynthetic, or synthetic [42,43]. Semisynthetic and synthetic amino acids [44] and peptides are designed to improve pharmacological properties, reduce side effects, and lower immunogenicity compared to natural peptides and proteins [45,46]. These modifications also enhance stability and bioavailability for clinical use. For example, replacing the linoleoyl side chain of echinocandin B with octyloxybenzoyl (cilofungin) or pentyloxyterphenyl (anidulafungin) reduces hemolytic activity [47]. Structure–activity relationships (SAR) help guide the design of these peptides, with key factors such as net charge, hydrophobicity, amphipathicity, and peptide length influencing antifungal activity. Hydrophobicity and amphipathicity are crucial for membrane disruption, though higher levels may increase toxicity. Short antimicrobial peptides (SAMPs) (2–10 amino acids) are gaining attention due to their lower toxicity, greater stability, and simpler synthesis [48]. Combinatorial libraries and de novo design strategies, along with targeting fungal virulence traits and multiligand molecules like dendrimers, are employed to develop more effective peptides [49].

1.3. *Aim of This Work*

In summary, synthetic and semisynthetic peptides offer significant potential for improving antifungal therapies, with better targeting, stability, and reduced toxicity compared to natural peptides [50]. When designing and synthesizing highly bioactive compounds, it is possible to synthesize hybrid molecules containing two active fragments: triazoles and peptide moieties—a new and useful strategy [51]. The combination of these two groups yields new peptides that may have the following properties:

(i) Membrane disruption: the triazole ring can insert into fungal membranes, disrupting their integrity, causing leakage of cellular contents, and leading to cell death;
(ii) Inhibition of ergosterol biosynthesis: similar to other triazole drugs, these peptides may inhibit ergosterol synthesis, a key component of fungal cell membranes, impairing membrane function;

(iii) Cell wall disruption: triazole peptides may interfere with the synthesis of fungal cell wall components (e.g., chitin, β-glucan), weakening the cell wall and causing osmotic lysis;
(iv) DNA and protein synthesis inhibition: the triazole ring can bind to metal ions involved in DNA replication and interfere with enzymes crucial for protein synthesis;
(v) Increased stability and bioavailability: the incorporation of triazole increases the peptide's stability, bioavailability, and resistance to enzymatic degradation;
(vi) Immune modulation: some peptides may enhance immune recognition and responses, aiding in fungal clearance.

Overall, triazole-containing peptides work by disrupting fungal cell structures and interfering with essential biosynthetic pathways, making them effective in combating fungal infections [52,53].. Thus, to develop new and effective fungicidal agents based on 1,2,4-triazole derivatives linked to amino acid residues, we synthesized novel dipeptides incorporating 1,2,4-triazole along with alanine and glycine. Additionally, we employed the protective group 9-fluorenylmethoxycarbonyl (Fmoc), which also possesses inherent antimicrobial activity due to its lipophilic nature [54]. In our design, the Fmoc group provides lipophilicity, enhancing interaction with the fungal membrane. The triazole moiety inhibits the fungal enzyme lanosterol 14α-demethylase, disrupting ergosterol synthesis and compromising membrane integrity. The glycine at the C-terminus imparts flexibility, minimizes steric hindrance, and potentially improves solubility and stability, supporting the compound's overall antifungal activity (Scheme 1).

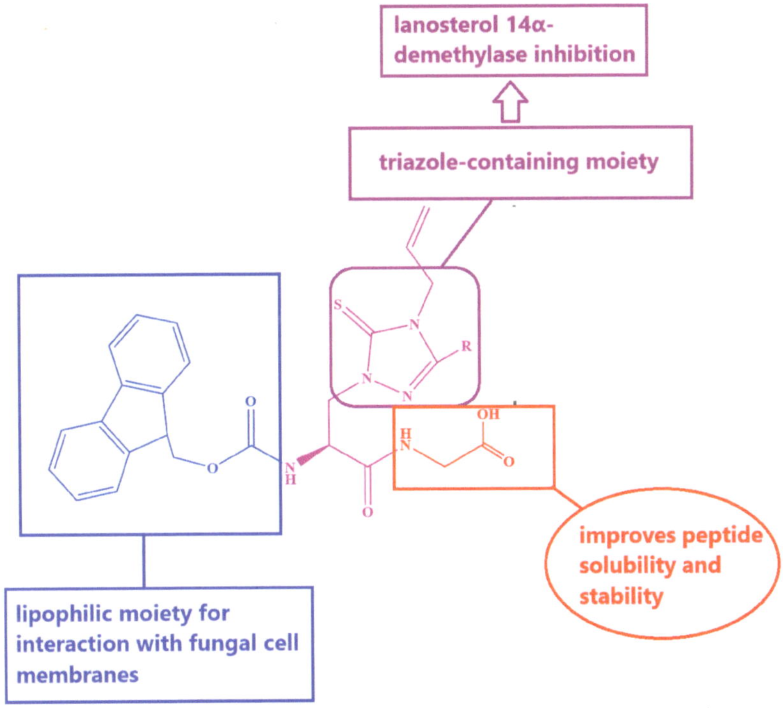

Scheme 1. Schematic representation of the rationale for the structural moieties in our Fmoc dipeptide for antifungal properties.

This dual functionality of Fmoc—acting both as a protective group and as an active antimicrobial component—provides a valuable strategy for developing more effective drugs [55,56], which we aimed to investigate in the context of antifungal applications, as described in the sections below.

2. Materials and Methods

2.1. Materials

The materials used in this study included dimethylsulfoxide (DMSO), DCC, N-hydroxysuccinimide, Fmoc-OSu, Gly, C_6H_{14}, $C_4H_8O_2$, $CH_3COOC_2H_5$, CH_2Cl_2, $NaHCO_3$, Na_2CO_3, and NaOH, which were purchased from Sigma Aldrich (St. Louis, MA, USA). The non-proteinogenic amino acids (S)-β-4-allyl-3-(2-methoxyphenyl)-5-thioxo-1,2,4-triazol-1-yl]alanine and (S)-β-[4-allyl-3-(furan-2-yl)-5-thioxo-1,2,4-triazol-1-yl]alanine were synthesized at the "Armbiotechnology" Scientific and Production Center (SPC) of National Academy of Sciences of the Republic of Armenia (NAS RA). All physicochemical properties of the non-proteinogenic amino acids are described in the catalog of the "Armbiotechnology" SPC of NAS RA, available at (http://www.armbiotech.am/, accessed on 13 December 2024). All chemicals were obtained from commercial suppliers and used without further purification. All solvents were freshly distilled before use. Thin-layer chromatography (TLC) was performed on Merck aluminum foil-backed sheets precoated with 0.2 mm Kieselgel 60 F254 (Darmstadt, Germany). The proton (^1H) and carbon-13 (^{13}C) nuclear magnetic resonance (NMR) spectra were recorded on a Varian Mercury 300 MHz spectrometer, using tetramethylsilane (TMS) as the internal standard (Palo Alto, CA, USA). Melting points were determined using an electrothermal apparatus (Bibby Scientific, Stone, UK). Mass Spectrometry Analysis. Sample preparation: 0.1 mg of test substance was dissolved in 1 mL of methanol. The sample solution was filtered through a 0.45 μm syringe filter PTFE 100. Sample analysis utilized a Prominence I LC-2030C 3D Plus instrument from Shimadzu, Kyoto, Japan. The mobile phase comprised a mixture of 0.1% formic acid aqueous solution (20%) and methanol (80%). A flow rate of 0.2 mL/min was maintained, with the column temperature set at 30 °C. The injection volume stood at 0.1 μL. Detection of the sample employed a basic quadrupole MS system (LC-MS-2020, Shimadzu, Kyoto, Japan) operating in positive ionization mode via electrospray ionization (ESI). Nitrogen gas served as both the nebulizing and drying agent, with the interface temperature, heat block, and DL temperature set at 350 °C, 200 °C, and 250 °C, respectively. Data acquisition and processing were performed using Shimadzu's LabSolutions software (version 5.99 SP2, Shimadzu, Kyoto, Japan). The m/z values of the target ions were monitored under the specified experimental conditions. IR characterization: the infrared analysis made use of an ATR (Attenuated Total Reflection) accessory, which allowed us to conduct a direct examination of the powder samples using a IRTracer-100 instrument (Shimadzu, Kyoto, Japan) using a KBr prism (4000–350 cm^{-1}) with single reflection, at resolution 4 cm^{-1}.

2.2. Synthesis of Derivatives of 9-Fluorenylmethoxycarbonyl Protected α-Amino Acids

Briefly, 0.0043 mol of the α-amino acid was dissolved in 0.0043 mol of 15% Na_2CO_3 and stirred at room temperature until a transparent solution formed, after which 0.0058 mol of 9-fluorenyl-methoxycarbonyl-N-oxysuccinimide ester, dissolved in 1 mL of 1,4-dioxane and 1 mL of acetone, was added to the reaction mixture. After the completion of the reaction, the reaction mixture was diluted twice with distilled water and the pH was adjusted to 6.5 with hydrochloric acid, during which the crystals of the protected amino acid precipitated at the bottom of the flask. The reaction was monitored by TLC.

As a result of the synthesis of 9-fluorenylmethoxycarbonyl-(S)-β-4-allyl-3-(2-methoxyphenyl)-5-thioxo-1,2,4-triazol-1-yl]-alanine, a white crystalline solid was obtained (75% yield) and exhibited a melting point of 104–106 °C. Found (%) C, 64.34; H, 4.67; N, 9.87; Calc for $C_{30}H_{28}N_4O_5S$ (%) C, 64.73; H, 5.07; N, 10.07. ESI MS (m/z): 556.64 (found) 557.10 (expected for $[C_{30}H_{28}N_4O_5S]+H^+$). ATR-IR, ν, cm^{-1}: ATR-IR, ν, cm^{-1}: 3869.20 (N-H); 3587.60 (O-H); 2924.09 (C–H allyl); 1693.50 (C=O, ester), 1681.93 (C=O acid); 1608.63 (C=O carbamate); 1519.91 (C=N carbamate); 1485.19 (C=C aromtic); 1442.75 (C=S), 1330.88 ($-OCH_3$); 1284.59 (C-N); 1219.01 (C-N); 1037.70 (C–N heterocyclic).

^{1}H NMR spectra (DMSO/CCl_4 1/3, δ, p.p.m, Hz): 10.9 (1H, COOH); 7.75–7.71 m (2H, Ar); 7.68–7.61 m (2H, Ar); 7.50–7.43 m (1H, Ar); 7.41 b.d (1H, J = 8,2, NH); 7.37–7.19 m (5H, Ar); 7.03–6.99 m (1H, Ar); 6.96–6.90 m (1H, Ar); 5.64 ddt (1H, J = 17.1, 10.5, 5.5, =CH); 4.94 br.d (1H, J = 10.5, CH_2); 4,80 br.d (1H, J = 17.1, =CH_2); 4.75–4.68 m (2H); 4.55–4.46 m (3H); 4.29–4.11 m (3H, OCH_2CH); 3.75 s (3H, CH_3): ^{13}C: 170.5; 166.9; 156.8; 155.2; 147.8; 143.6; 143.4; 140.5; 140.4; 132.1; 131.4; 130.7; 127.0; 126.9; 126.5; 125.1; 125.0; 120.1; 119.3; 119.2; 117.0; 114.4; 110.9; 65.9 (OCH_2); 55.1 (OCH_3); 52.1 (NCH); 48.9 (CH_2); 46.7 (CH_2); 46.5 (CH).

As a result of the synthesis of 9-fluorenylmethoxycarbonyl-(*S*)-β-[4-allyl-3-(furan-2-yl)-5-thioxo-1,2,4-triazol-1-yl]-alanine, a white crystalline solid was obtained (73% yield) and exhibited a melting point of 140–142 °C. Found (%) C, 62.81; H, 4.82; N, 10.38; Calc for $C_{27}H_{24}N_4O_5S$ (%) C, 62.78; H, 4.68; N, 10.85. ESI MS (*m*/*z*): 516.57 (found) 517.00 (expected for $[C_{27}H_{24}N_4O_5S]+H+$). ATR-IR, ν, cm^{-1}: 3734.19 (NH); 3491.16 (OH); 3066.82 (C-H aromatic); 2924.09 (C–H allyl); 1712.79 (C=O, acid), 1624.06 (C=O carbamate); 1523.76 (C=N carbamate); 1354.03 (C=S), 1334.74 (C–H); 1172.72 (C–O ether), 1103.28 (C–N); 1076.28 (C–N heterocyclic); 1049.28 (C–N).

^{1}H NMR spectra (DMSO/CCl_4 1/3; δ, p.p.m, Hz): 7.44 br.d (J = 7.9, NH); 6.92 dd (J = 3.5, 0.8); 6.51 dd (J = 3.5, 1.8); 5.89 ddt (J = 17.1, 10.6, 5.1); 5.14 br.t (J = 10.6); 5.11 br.d (J = 17.1); 4.97–4.83 m; 4.78–4.55 m (2H); 4.46 m (3H); 4.21–4.10 m (3H, OCH_2CH): ^{13}C: 170.4; 167.4; 155.3; 144.3; 143.6; 143.4; 141.4; 140.5; 140.4; 139.7; 130.6; 126.9; 126.5; 125.1; 125.0; 119.2; 117.2 (=CH_2); 112.4 (C-4 fur); 111.4 (C-4 fur); 65.9 (OCH_2); 51.8 (NCH); 49.3 (NCH_2); 47.0 (NCH_2); 46.5 (CH); 40.3 (NCH_2).

2.3. Synthesis of N-Oxysuccinimide Esters

Briefly, 1.75 g (8.5 mmol) of DCC previously dissolved in 3 mL of dioxane was added to a solution of (7.9 mmol) of derivatives of 9-fluorenylmethoxycarbonyl protected α-amino acid and 0.95 g (8.2 mmol) of N-hydroxysuccinimide in a mixture of 1.0 mL of dioxane and 2.7 mL of methylene chloride at 0 °C. The reaction mixture was stirred for 2 h at 0 °C and left overnight in the refrigerator. The reaction progress was monitored by TLC (chloroform/ethyl acetate/methanol, 2:4:1). The resulting precipitate of dicyclohexylurea (DCU) was filtered, and the filtrate containing the intermediate product succinimide ester of the amino acid was concentrated under vacuum to form an oily mass. As a result, stable intermediate compound **3a** was synthesized in 70% yield and **3b** in 75% yield, which were immediately used in the synthesis of peptides.

2.4. Synthesis of Dipeptides

Briefly, 0.085 g (1 mmol) of $NaHCO_3$ was introduced into a solution of 0.08 g (1.5 mmol) of glycine in 2 mL of 0.5 M NaOH, and then 1.6 mmol of N-hydroxysuccinimide ester of 9-fluorenylmethoxycarbonyl protected α-amino acids in 4 mL of dioxane was added. The reaction mixture was stirred for 3 h at room temperature, then transferred to a separatory funnel and 6 mL of ethyl acetate, 3 mL of 10% citric acid solution, and 0.2 g of NaCl were added. After intense stirring, the organic layer was separated and dried with magnesium sulfate and the solvent was distilled off under vacuum at 50 °C. The residual matter was crystallized from a mixture of ethyl acetate and petroleum ether in a ratio of 1/3. As a result, **4a** (yield 65%) and **4b** (yield 60%) dipeptides were synthesized. The dipeptide 9-fluorenylmethoxycarbonyl-(S)-β-[4-allyl-3-(2-methoxyphenyl)-5-thioxo-

1,2,4–triazol-1-yl]-α-alanylglycine is a white crystalline substance with a melting point of 182–183 °C. Found (%) C, 62.29; H, 5.39; N, 11.61; Calc for $C_{32}H_{31}N_5O_6S$ (%) C, 62.63; H, 5.09; N, 11.41. ESI MS (*m/z*): 613.69 (found) 614.01 (expected for $[C_{32}H_{31}N_5O_6S]$+H^+). ATR-IR, ν, cm^{-1}: 3869.20 (NH); 3649.32 (NH); 3587.6 (OH); 3066.82 (C-H arom); 1716.65 (C=O, acid), 1693.50 (C=O eter); 1616.35 (C=O carbamate); 1581.63 (C=N carbamate); 1535.34 (C=C, aromatic); 1431.18 (C=S), 1365.6 (-OCH_3); 1334.74 (C–O); 1296.16 (C–N); 1234.44 (C–N); 1118.71 (C–N heterocyclic); 1083.9 (C–N heterocyclic).

^{1}H NMR spectra (DMSO/CCl_4 1/3, δ, p.p.m, Hz): 12.0 v.b. (1H, COOH); 8.16 br.t (1H, J = 5.4, $NHCH_2$); 7.75–7.70 m (2H, Ar-H and NH); 7.68–7.61 m (2H); 7.48–7.19 m (7H); 7.50–7.40 m (2H); 7.01–6.88 m (2H); 5.69–5.54 m (1H, =CH Ally); 4.93–4.73 m (3H); 4.65–4.45 m (4H); 4.28–4.06 m (3H, OCH_2CH); 3.82 b.d. (2H, J = 5.4, CH_2NH); 3.71 s (3H, CH_3): 170.3; 168.5; 166.9; 156.8; 155.2; 147.9; 143.6; 143.4; 140.5; 140.4; 132.1; 131.4; 130.7; 127.0; 126.9; 126.5; 125.2; 125.0; 120.1; 119.23; 119.19; 116.9; 114.4; 110.9; 66.1 (OCH_2); 55.0; 53.4 (OCH_3); 49.6; 46.7 (NCH_2); 46.5 (CH); 40.7 (NCH_2).

The dipeptide 9-fluorenylmethoxycarbonyl-(*S*)-β-[4-allyl-3-(furan-2-yl)-5-thioxo-1,2,4-triazol-1-yl]-α–alanylglycine is a white crystalline substance with a melting point of 169–170 °C. Found (%) C, 60.85; H, 5.1; N, 12.36; Calc for $C_{29}H_{27}N_5O_6S$ (%) C, 60.72; H, 4.74; N, 12.21. ESI MS (*m/z*): 573.62 (found) 574.05 (expected for $[C_{29}H_{27}N_5O_6S]$+H^+). ATR-IR, ν, cm^{-1}: 3649.32 (NH); 3630.03 (NH); 3471.87 (OH); 2927.94 (C–H allyl); 1701.22 (C=O, acid), 1581.63 (C=O carbamate); 1519.91 (C=N carbamate); 1446.61 (C=C, aromatic); 1354.03 (C=S), 1172.72 (C–O, ether), 1122.57 (C–O, acid); 1103.28 (C–N); 1045.42 (C–N).

^{1}H NMR spectra (DMSO/CCl_4 1/3, δ, p.p.m, Hz): 8.17 br.t (1H, J = 5.6, CH_2NH); 7.74–7.70 m (2H, Ar.); 7.68–7.58 m (3H, Ar + H-5 fur.); 7.74–7.70 m (2H, Ar.); 7.39 br.d. (1H, J = 9.1, NHCH); 7.36–7.30 m (2H, Ar.); 7.28–7.21 m (2H, Ar.); 6.90 br.d. (1H, J = 3.3, H-3 fur.); 6.48 dd (1H, J = 3.3, 1.8, H-4 fur.); 5.87 ddt (1H, J = 16.6, 11.1, 5.0, =CH); 5.15–5.05 m (2H, =CH_2); 4.95–4.81 m (2H, CH_2, All); 4.77 td (1H, J = 9.1, 4.1); 4.63 dd (1H, J = 13.7, 4.1); 4.47 dd (1H, J = 13.7, 9.4); 4.29–4.03 m (3H); 3.83 dd (1H, J = 18.0, 5.6, CH_2NH); 3.81 dd (1H, J = 18.0, 5.6, CH_2NH).

^{13}C: 170.4; 168.5; 167.5; 155.3; 144.3; 143.6; 143.4; 141.5; 140.5; 140.4; 139.7; 130.6; 127.0; 126.5; 125.2; 125.0; 119.3; 117.1 (=CH_2); 112.5 (C-3 fur.); 111.4 (C-4 fur.); 66.1 (OCH_2); 53.2 (NCH); 50.0 (NCH_2); 47.0 (NCH_2); 46.5 (CH); 40.7 (NCH_2).

2.5. Antifungal Activity Assessment

In our work, the antifungal activity of the synthesized compounds was evaluated against various fungal strains: *Aspergillus versicolor* 12134, *Aspergillus flavus* 10567, *Aspergillus candidus* 10711, *Alternaria alternata* 8126, *Ulocladium botrytis* 12027, and *Aureobasidium pullulans* 8269. The compounds were dissolved in DMSO to prepare 0.05 M solutions and tested at three different concentrations (89 μM, 183 μM, 278 μM) in 90 mL Czapek medium. Each sample was tested in triplicate across Petri dishes, with three strains per dish. The Petri dishes were incubated at 28 °C for 5–7 days. Fungal growth was assessed visually and with the aid of a magnifying glass. The intensity of fungal growth was compared to control plates to evaluate the antifungal effect of the compounds. To obtain comparative data during the research, the obtained data were compared with those obtained using a fluconazole solution of the same molarity. The data are presented in the Supporting Information and Results and Discussion sections. The histograms related to fungal growth inhibition were obtained by analyzing colony intensities using ImageJ (Rasband, W.S., U.S. National Institutes of Health, Bethesda, MD, USA, https://imagej.nih.gov/ij/, accessed on 13 November 2024). ImageJ is an open-source image analysis software widely used in scientific research for digital image processing and intensity quantification. For data collection, the plates with fungal colonies were compared before and after treatment with the compounds isolated and described in our manuscript. The procedure was performed three times in different areas of the analyzed images to ensure adequate representation of the results. The intensity values were provided as the mean ± standard deviation (SD = ±2–10%). This methodology was chosen as a modification of a standard method (CLSI M38-A2, reference protocol for antifungal testing).

2.6. Molecular Docking

The fungal sterol 14-α demethylase model used in our simulations corresponds to the structure with PDB ID: 5F3B, which was visualized using Discovery Studio (DS) 2021 software (Accelrys, San Diego, CA, USA) [57], with the ligand removed manually. The complex predictions were obtained by docking the ligands fluconazole, **3a**, and **7a** with the target protein using the HDOCK software (http://hdock.phys.hust.edu.cn/, accessed on 1 November 2024), [58], with default parameters. The ligand structures were generated using the MolView program (https://molview.org/, accessed on 1 November 2024, The Netherlands, v2.4), which, after energy minimization, allowed us to create three-dimensional models saved as pdb files and visualized in DS. HDOCK, which is suitable for both macromolecule–macromolecule and small molecule–macromolecule docking [54–59], was used for the blind docking described in this study. The software employs the iterative knowledge-based scoring function ITScore-PP to rank the top 10 poses obtained after the docking simulations. The HDOCK score, which is an energy score represented as a dimensionless value, indicates the binding strength between the molecules, with larger negative values reflecting stronger interactions. This scoring method has been shown to correlate well with experimental binding affinities [60]. The top-ranked pose (top 1) and the top 1 to top 3 poses for the complexes predicted by HDOCK are considered in our analysis.

3. Results

3.1. Synthesis of Dipeptides

The synthesis of dipeptides **7a** and **7b** containing non-protein amino acids **2a** and **2b** was carried out according to Scheme 2. In the first stage, the protected amino acids 9-fluorenylmethoxycarbonyl (Fmoc)-protected alanine (**3a**, **3b**) were synthesized. The reaction was carried out in a slightly alkaline medium at room temperature (Scheme 2) according to a previously published procedure [61], the experimental conditions of which were optimized by us in the present work. After testing the solvents acetone, isopropanol, and dioxane, we came to the conclusion that the best option for protecting the triazole-containing amino acids was a solvent mixture in an equal ratio of 1,4-dioxane/acetone.

When working up the reaction mixture, it was not possible to get rid of the excess Fmoc-N-hydroxysuccinimide ester and the resulting N-hydroxysuccinimide using the standard method, since they are almost equally soluble in both diethyl ether and ethyl acetate. An accessible and effective method was developed for processing the reaction mixture. By adding water and adjusting the pH to 5.5 with 0.1 N HCl, excess Fmoc-N-hydroxysuccinimide ester was removed, causing the protected amino acid to precipitate immediately at the first stage. This is explained by the fact that the solubility of 9-fluorenylmethoxycarbonyl-N-hydroxysuccinimide ester in water is higher than the solubility of the protected amino acids. Subsequently, a small amount of residual **1** was removed using diethyl ether, since this ester was more soluble in diethyl ether than the protected amino acids. During the neutralization of the reaction mixture, the molarity of hydrochloric acid was adjusted, since concentrated hydrochloric acid could cause unwanted transformations or reactions of the synthesized compounds. The optimal concentration was 0.1 N, at which the protected amino acids remained stable. The subsequent step was the transformation of the Fmoc-amino acids into succinimide esters. This was achieved by activating the carboxyl groups of the Fmoc-amino acids with N-hydroxysuccinimide (HOSu) (**4**) in the presence of dicyclohexylcarbodiimide (DCC) as a coupling reagent. The reaction was carried out in a solvent mixture of dioxane and methylene chloride, resulting in N-hydroxysuccinimide esters **5a** and **5b** [62]. In the next step, glycine (6) was condensed with N-hydroxysuccinimide esters of the Fmoc-amino acids **5a** and **5b**. The condensation reactions were carried out in different media using different molar ratios of sodium hydroxide and sodium carbonate. Optimal results were achieved with a $NaOH/Na_2CO_3$ molar ratio of 2:1. Reactions carried out with NaOH alone, in the absence of Na_2CO_3, resulted in increased formation of by-products. Thus, the dipeptides **7a** and **7b** were successfully synthesized, as shown in Scheme 2.

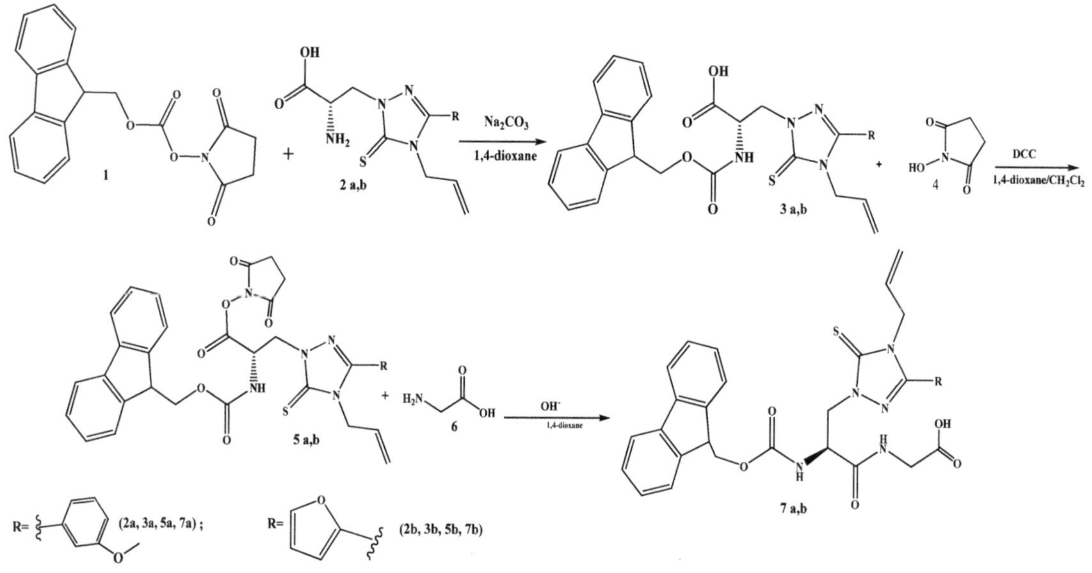

Scheme 2. Schematic representation of the synthesis pathway for the dipeptides **7a** and **7b**.

3.2. Antifungal Activity

An in vitro study was conducted to evaluate the antifungal effects of fluconazole, the synthesized amino acids, and their corresponding dipeptide derivatives, with the aim of obtaining comparative data. The following fungal strains were selected as study subjects: *Aspergillus versicolor* 12134, *Aspergillus flavus* 10567, *Aspergillus candidus* 10711, *Alternaria altenata* 8126, *Ulocladium botrytis* 12027, *Aureobasidium pullulans* 8269. The influence of different concentrations of all samples (89 μM, 183 μM, and 278 μM) on the activity of the aforementioned fungi was studied.

The results are depicted in Figure S1, which illustrates the observed antifungal activities based on visual appearance, and in Table 2, which lists the antifungal activities of the three different concentrations of the compounds and the reference fluconazole against the selected fungal strains. Taking into account the above data, the percentage of inhibition of strains *Aspergillus versicolor* 12134, *A. flavus* 10567, and *A. candidus* 10711 by the two most active compounds (**3a** and **7a**) was calculated and compared to fluconazole (Figure 1A–C). Table 2 presents the antifungal activity of fluconazole and the test compounds (**2a**, **2b**, **3a**, **3b**, **7a**, **7b**) at varying concentrations against the six fungal strains. These strains are identified by their corresponding strain numbers, as registered in the Microbial Depository Center and include *Aspergillus versicolor* 12134, *A. flavus* 10567, *A. candidus* 10711, *Alternaria alternata* 8126, *Ulocladium botrytis* 12027, and *Aureobasidium pullulans* 8269. The data are shown for the above-mentioned three different concentrations (89 μM, 183 μM, and 278 μM), with the antifungal response indicated as follows.

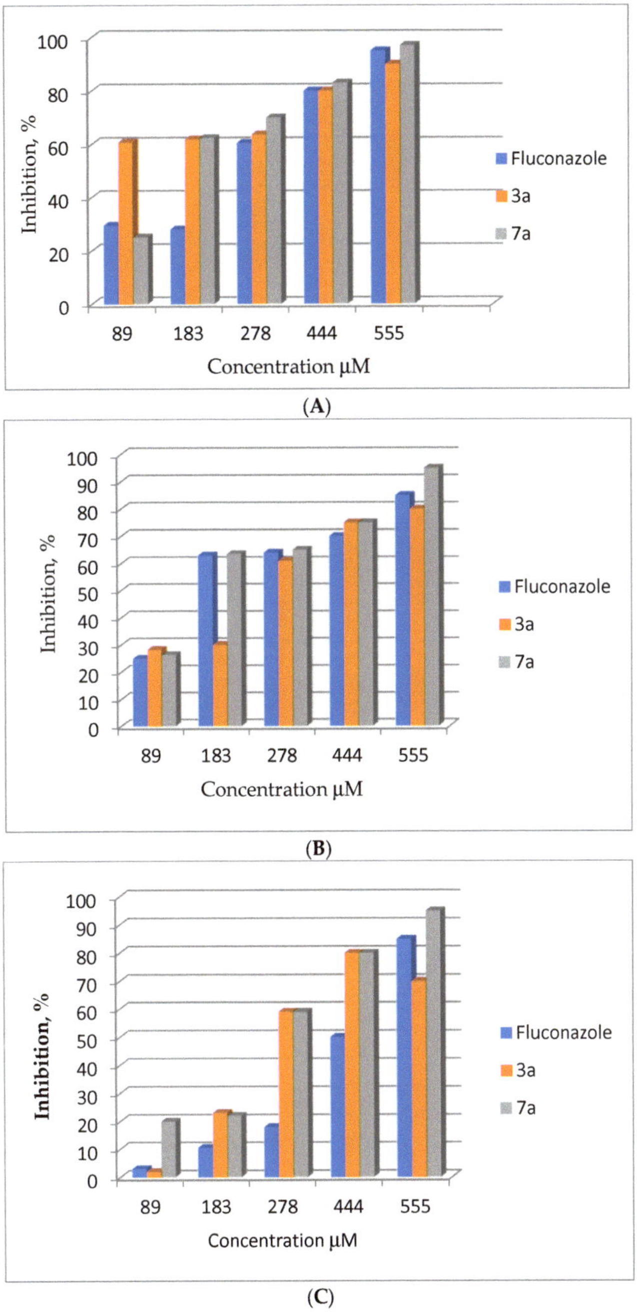

Figure 1. Histograms showing the antifungal effects of compounds **3a**, **7a**, and fluconazole on *A. versicolor* 12134 (**A**), *A. flavus* 10567 (**B**), and *A. candidus* 10711 (**C**). For photographs of the fungal plates treated with the different compounds, please refer to Figure S1 in the Supporting Information. The X-axis indicates the concentrations of fluconazole and compounds **3a** and **7a** in the cultures.

Table 2. Antifungal activity of test compounds against various fungal strains.

Concentration of Test Compounds		Names and Numbers of Strains According to the Microbial Depository Center					
		Aspergillus versicolor 12134	*A.flavus* 10567	*A.candidus* 10711	*Alternaria alternata* 8126	*Ulocladium botrytis* 12027	*Aureobasidium pullulans* 8269
Fluconazole	89 µM	+	+	-	++	++	+++
	183 µM	+	++	+	++	+++	+++
	278 µM	++	++	+	+++	+++	+++
2a	89 µM	-	-	-	-	-	-
	183 µM	+	-	-	+	-	+
	278 µM	+	+	-	+	+	+
3a	89 µM	++	+	-	-	+	-
	183 µM	++	+	+	+	+	+
	278 µM	++	++	++	++	++	++
7a	89 µM	+	+	+	+	+	-
	183 µM	++	++	+	++	++	-
	278 µM	++	++	++	++	++	-
2b	89 µM	-	-	-	-	-	-
	183 µM	+	+	-	-	-	-
	278 µM	+	+	+	+	+	-
3b	89 µM	+	+	-	+	+	-
	183 µM	+	+	+	+	+	+
	278 µM	-	++	+	++	++	++
7b	89 µM	-	+	-	-	-	-
	183 µM	-	+	+	-	-	-
	278 µM	+	++	+	+	+	-

"-": No activity (inhibition % 0–10%); "+": Low activity (inhibition % 10–30%); "++": Moderate activity (inhibition % 40–70%); "+++": High activity (inhibition % 70–90%).

For each concentration, the presence or absence of antifungal activity was recorded for each strain, with higher concentrations generally leading to more pronounced antifungal effects. The experiments revealed that several samples had an effect on the selected strains. When comparing the numerical data to fluconazole, dipeptide **7a** at a dose of 89 µM was found to suppress the growth of *Aspergillus versicolor* 12134 and *A. flavus* 10567 strains with the same effectiveness as fluconazole (Figure 1A,B). An increase in the amount of fluconazole to 183 µM does not change the suppressive action on *Aspergillus versicolor*, while in the case of the dipeptide, the suppressive action increases significantly. In the case of 278 µM, the suppressive action of fluconazole practically coincides with the suppression of dipeptide in the case of 183 µM, and the noteworthy suppressive effects caused by the protected amino acid **3a** at concentrations of 89, 183, and 278 µM on *Aspergillus versicolor* are not significantly different from each other and are of the same order of magnitude as the suppression observed with 278 µM of fluconazole. In the case of *A. candidus* 10711, fluconazole is generally a weaker inhibitor compared to compounds **3a** and **7a** (Figure 1C).

Additionally, 278 µM of compound **3a** shows the same activity as 278 µM of compound **7a**. This suggests that compounds **3a** and **7a** exhibit similar effects at this concentration and are more effective than fluconazole *A. candidus* 10711 (Figures 1C and S1). In the case of the strains different from *Aspergillus*, the effect of fluconazole is more pronounced than that of the test compounds, but a certain inhibitory effect is still present. To obtain more quantitative and comparative data, additional experiments were conducted with *Aspergillus* species using fluconazole, as well as compounds **3a** and **7a**. While initial assays were performed at 89 μM, 183 μM, and 278 μM, these were subsequently extended to higher concentrations of 444 μM and 555 μM. The inhibition percentages observed at 555 μM and the corresponding apparent IC_{50} (Figure S2) values for each substance are summarized in Table 3. Although complete (100%) inhibition was not achieved, significant partial inhibition was observed, further demonstrating the compounds' strong antifungal activity, as shown in Figure S1. The findings revealed that dipeptide **7a** exhibited notable antifungal activity against *Aspergillus versicolor*, with an IC_{50} of 169.94 μM, indicating higher potency than fluconazole, a widely used antifungal agent, which had an IC_{50} of 254.01 μM. Interestingly, dipeptide **7a** demonstrated slightly improved antifungal effectiveness compared to fluconazole in *Aspergillus flavus* too (IC_{50} 176.69 μM vs. 184.64 μM), highlighting its potential efficacy against this strain. Moreover, the protected amino acid **3a** showed consistent inhibitory activity across all tested strains. However, with an IC_{50} of 267.86 μM for *Aspergillus flavus*, it was less potent than fluconazole (IC_{50} 184.64 μM), though it still holds promise as a viable antifungal compound. Remarkably, **3a** and **7a** are also more potent than fluconazole against *A. candidus* 10711 (Table 3).

Table 3. IC_{50} values and inhibition percentages of fluconazole, compound **3a**, and compound **7a** at a concentration of 555 μM against *Aspergillus* species.

***Aspergillus* Species**	**Compound**	**Inhibition at 555 μM (%)**	**IC_{50} (μM)**	**SD**
Aspergillus versicolor 12134	fluconazole	95	254.01	0.05
	3a	90	-	0.09
	7a	97	169.94	0.09
Aspergillus flavus 10567	fluconazole	85	184.64	0.09
	3a	80	267.86	0.06
	7a	95	176.69	0.1
Aspergillus candidus 10711	fluconazole	85	476.20	0.08
	3a	70	240.35	0.04
	7a	95	248.94	0.04

3.3. In Silico Exploration of the Mechanism Behind the Activity of Compounds 3a and 7a Against Aspergillus Species: Molecular Docking of the Antifungal Molecules with Sterol 14- α Demethylase

Given the particularly interesting antifungal properties of compounds **3a** and **7a**, especially their pronounced effects on *Aspergillus* species, we sought to investigate the underlying mechanism of action responsible for this observed activity. To explore this, we selected one of the key proteins involved in fungal activity whose inhibition is linked to the action of triazole-containing antifungal drugs. Specifically, we focused on the sterol 14-α demethylase from *Aspergillus* species [63], a well-known target for azole-based antifungals like fluconazole [64].

To study the interaction of fluconazole and our test compounds (**3a** and **7a**) with this target protein, we performed molecular docking simulations using the HDOCK docking software [54,65]. Blind docking simulations were carried out on the protein target (PDB ID 5FRB [61]), which represents the sterol 14-alpha demethylase from an *Aspergillus* species, using fluconazole as a reference ligand, alongside the .pdb files for compounds **3a** and **7a**. As shown in Figure 2, our docking results revealed that both compound **3a** and compound **7a**, but especially compound **3a**, bind to a similar region of the protein as fluconazole. This similarity is visually confirmed by the overlap in the binding locations of the ligands, which are depicted in yellow for clarity (Figure 2). A more detailed analysis, shown in Table 4, compares the receptor interface residues common between the fluconazole–protein complex and those formed with compounds **3a** and **7a**. While the fluconazole and compound **7a** complexes share four common interface residues (TYR 122, ILE 373, LEU 503, PHE 504), compound **3a** interacts with a larger number of common residues: TYR 122, LEU 125, THR 126, TYR 136, ALA 307, GLY 308, SER 311, ILE 373, LEU 503, PHE 504, and HEM 580. The interaction diagrams for the complexes of **3a**, **7a**, and fluconazole with the protein are also shown in the Supporting Information (Figure S3). In terms of binding affinity, both compounds **3a** and **7a** demonstrate comparable, or slightly stronger, binding than fluconazole.

Table 4. HDOCK scores for the top 1 pose and average scores for poses 1–3 (± standard deviation) of fluconazole and compounds **3a** and **7a** are presented. The receptor interface residues for the top 1 poses are listed with their respective ligand—residue distances in Angstroms (Å). Common residues across all complexes are also indicated.

Compound	HDOCK Score (Top 1 Pose)	HDOCK Score (Avg. Top 1–3 ± SD)	Receptor Interface Residues for the Top 1 Poses (Residue—Ligand Distance/Å)	Common Residues
Fluconazole	−193.30	−183.27 ± 11.13	TYR 122 (3.460 Å), LEU 125 (4.013 Å), THR 126 (3.484 Å), PHE 130 (3.176 Å), VAL 135 (3.295 Å), TYR 136 (3.261 Å), ALA 307 (2.987 Å), GLY 308 (4.884 Å), SER 311 (3.536 Å), ILE 373 (3.680 Å), LEU 503 (4.080 Å), PHE 504 (2.951 Å), HEM 580 (2.982 Å)	TYR 122, LEU 125, THR 126, TYR 136, ALA 307, GLY 308, SER 311, ILE 373, LEU 503, PHE 504, HEM 580
3a	−207.97	−192.63 ± 11.86	TYR 68 (2.876 Å), LEU 91 (3.496 Å), VAL 121 (3.717 Å), TYR 122 (1.493 Å), LEU 125 (2.678 Å), THR 126 (1.979 Å), TYR 136 (4.045 Å), PHE 229 (4.538 Å), PHE 234 (2.725 Å), ALA 307 (2.652 Å), GLY 308 (4.381 Å), SER 311 (3.302 Å), ILE 373 (2.803 Å), HIS 374 (3.010 Å), SER 375 (3.111 Å), ILE 376 (3.278 Å), ILE 377 (3.117 Å), ARG 378 (4.992 Å), ASN 398 (4.823 Å), TYR 500 (4.472 Å), SER 502 (4.805 Å), LEU 503 (2.285 Å), PHE 504 (3.955 Å), HEM 580 (3.095 Å)	TYR 122, LEU 125, THR 126, TYR 136, ALA 307, GLY 308, SER 311, ILE 373, LEU 503, PHE 504, HEM 580
7a	−206.62	−190.42 ± 11.51	THR 65 (3.017 Å), ILE 66 (3.865 Å), TYR 68 (3.957 Å), GLY 69 (2.937 Å), ILE 70 (3.821 Å), LEU 91 (2.091 Å), LEU 92 (3.069 Å), GLY 93 (3.464 Å), LYS 94 (2.725 Å), THR 96 (4.979 Å), TYR 122 (4.669 Å), PRO 231 (3.321 Å), ILE 232 (3.429 Å), PHE 234 (2.594 Å), MET 235 (2.112 Å), ILE 373 (4.311 Å), HIS 374 (3.240 Å), SER 375 (2.883 Å), ILE 377 (3.910 Å), TYR 500 (2.672 Å), SER 501 (3.521 Å), SER 502 (2.803 Å), LEU 503 (3.029 Å), PHE 504 (4.955 Å)	TYR 122, ILE 373, LEU 503, PHE 504

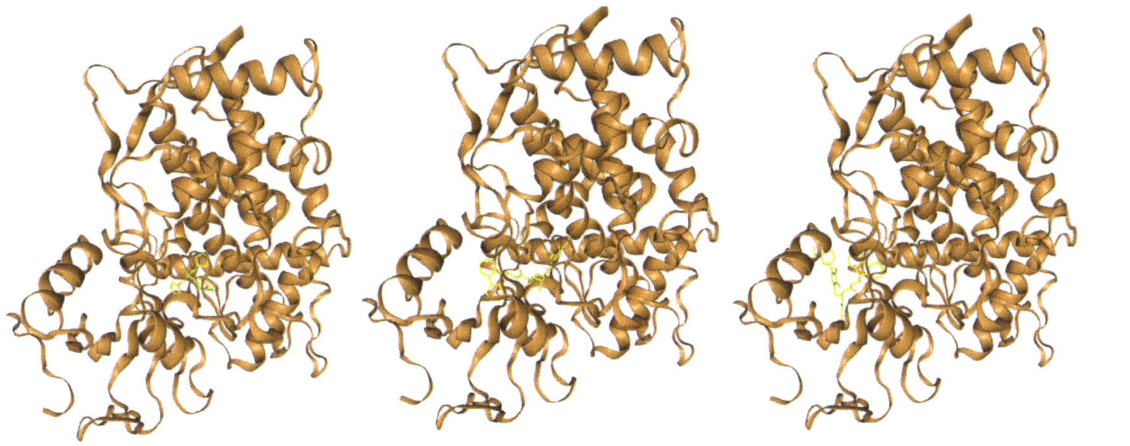

(a) (b) (c)

Figure 2. Molecular docking complex views (top 1 pose) of PDB ID 5FRB, sterol 14-α demethylase (unliganded) in complex with fluconazole (**a**), compound **3a** (**b**), and compound **7a** (**c**) visualized using the HDOCK software. The ligand is highlighted in yellow color.

The HDOCK scores (both top 1 poses and the averages across poses 1–3) indicate that fluconazole binds with slightly lower affinity to the sterol 14-α demethylase than either of the test compounds, **3a** and **7a** (−193.30, 183.27 ± 11.13 vs. −207.97, 192.63 ± 11.86 and −206.62, −190.42 ± 11.51, respectively. Table 4).

This finding supports the hypothesis that compounds **3a** and **7a** may exert their antifungal effects through a mechanism similar to fluconazole, leading to similar or slightly enhanced binding to the target protein, which contributes to its antifungal activity, particularly against *Aspergillus* species as experimentally found.

4. Discussion

The synthesis of Fmoc-amino acids and their conversion into peptides [66,67], including dipeptides, highlights the effective use of optimized methods in peptide chemistry. The careful selection of solvent systems is essential for achieving high chemical yields during the reaction process. Selecting a solvent mixture of 1,4-dioxane and acetone in a 1:1 ratio for the protection of triazole-containing amino acids proved effective. This solvent system not only facilitated the protection of the amino acids but also contributed to the overall chemical yield.

The difficulty in separating excess 9-fluorenylmethoxycarbonyl-N-oxysuccinimide ester highlighted the common challenges encountered in solution-phase synthesis of peptides [68]. The development of a new purification strategy by adjusting the water content to exploit solubility differences was an innovative solution, emphasizing the importance of process optimization in synthetic peptide chemistry. Additionally, regulating the concentration of hydrochloric acid during neutralization was crucial. The observed degradation of synthesized compounds in the presence of concentrated acid underscores the sensitivity of these reactions to pH. Since the use of concentrated acid led to the decomposition of final products and the formation of side compounds, experimental results identified 0.1N hydrochloric acid as the optimal condition. The transition from Fmoc-amino acids to dipeptides involved activating the carboxyl groups with N-hydroxysuccinimide and dicyclohexylcarbodiimide, enabling efficient coupling with glycine. The variation in molar ratios of sodium hydroxide and sodium carbonate significantly influenced the reaction outcome. An optimal 2:1 (NaOH/Na_2CO_3) ratio minimized by-product formation, underscoring the importance of selecting appropriate base conditions in peptide coupling reactions. The successful synthesis of dipeptides **7a** and **7b** using this approach highlights the robustness of the employed methods and their scalability potential. The herein presented antifungal study revealed that synthesized compounds, especially dipeptides **3a** and **7a**, comparable to fluconazole, exhibited significant antifungal activity against various strains, particularly against *Aspergillus versicolor* and *A. flavus* (Table 2, Figures S1 and 1). The concentration-dependent effects highlighted the importance of dosage, with dipeptide 8 showing increased efficacy at higher concentrations. Given the pronounced antifungal effects of compounds **3a** and **7a**, particularly against *Aspergillus* species, we investigated their underlying mechanism of action. We focused on the sterol 14-α demethylase [69] from *Aspergillus*, a well-known target of azole-based antifungals like fluconazole. To study the interaction of fluconazole, compound **3a**, and compound **7a** with this target, we conducted molecular docking simulations using HDOCK software, targeting the protein structure (PDB ID 5FRB) from an *Aspergillus* species. More in detail, we removed the ligand VT-1598 [70] from the structure of sterol 14 α-demethylase (CYP51B) of *Aspergillus fumigatus* [71], which was then used in the docking studies. Our docking results revealed that compounds **3a** and **7a** bind to a similar region of the sterol 14-α demethylase as fluconazole. Notably, compound **3a** displayed a broader interaction profile, engaging more receptor interface residues than fluconazole or compound **7a**. Binding affinity analysis showed that compounds **3a** and **7a** exhibited slightly stronger or comparable binding to the sterol 14-α demethylase than fluconazole, with HDOCK scores of −207.97 (± 11.86) and −206.62 (± 11.51) for compounds **3a** and **7a**, respectively, compared to fluconazole's score of −193.30 (± 11.13). These results suggest that compounds **3a** and **7a** may exert their antifungal activity through a similar, if not enhanced, mechanism to fluconazole, contributing to their efficacy against *Aspergillus* species. Interestingly, compounds **3a** and **7a** share several interface residues within their complex structures with the antifungal drug VT-1598 [61]. Specifically, compound **3a** shares the following residues with VT-1598: TYR 68, TYR 122, LEU 125, THR 126, TYR 136, PHE 234, ALA 307, GLY 308, SER 311, ILE 373, HIS 374, SER 375, LEU 503, and PHE 504. On the other hand, compound **7a** shares the following residues with VT-1598: TYR 68, TYR 122, PHE 234, ILE 373, HIS 374, SER 375, LEU 503, and PHE 504. Remarkably, these residues have been shown to play important roles in the antifungal activity of VT-1598. Notably, HIS 374 (acting as a proton donor) stands out as a critical residue for antifungal–protein binding, further corroborating its importance in the interaction between the compound and the protein target [61]. While fluconazole generally demonstrated superior effectiveness across *Alternaria alternata* 8126, *Ulocladium botrytis* 12027, and *Aureobasidium pullulans* 8269, which are notable for their roles in various research studies on fungal diseases [72,73], the presence of inhibitory effects from the synthesized compounds suggests for *Aspergillus* species potential for their use in combination therapies or as adjuncts to other drugs. These findings encourage further investigation into the mechanisms of action and structure–activity relationships of the synthesized compounds, aimed at optimization of their antifungal properties and development of new therapeutic strategies against fungal infections.

5. Conclusions

This study demonstrates the successful synthesis of novel Fmoc-protected 1,2,4-triazolyl-α-amino acids and their corresponding dipeptides, targeting antifungal activity against *Aspergillus* species, which are notorious pathogens in both human and veterinary medicine. The synthesized compounds were tested for their ability to inhibit the growth of multiple fungal strains, including *Aspergillus versicolor* and *Aspergillus flavus*. The solution-phase synthesis of the Fmoc-protected 1,2,4-triazolyl-α-amino acids **3a** and **3b**, followed by their conversion into the dipeptides **7a** and **7b**, involved an optimized strategy that included solvent selection, protection strategies, and the careful tuning of reaction conditions. Notably, a solvent system comprising 1,4-dioxane and acetone proved to be the most effective for protecting the triazole-containing amino acids, ensuring high yields and minimal side reactions. The development of a novel purification method to separate excess reagents, such as 9-fluorenylmethoxycarbonyl-N-oxysuccinimide ester, was an innovative contribution from a synthetic perspective. On the other hand, our antifungal activity studies revealed that the dipeptide **7a** exhibited superior antifungal effects to the antifungal drug fluconazole against *Aspergillus versicolor* and *Aspergillus flavus*. Our mechanistic studies based on molecular docking revealed that compounds **3a** and **7a** bind to a similar region of the sterol 14-α demethylase as fluconazole. The dose-dependent enhancement of the antifungal effect in the dipeptide **7a** suggests its potential as a more effective therapeutic agent. Although fluconazole was more effective against strains different from *Aspergillus*, some of the tested compounds still demonstrated detectable inhibitory effects, supporting the hypothesis that these new derivatives could serve as adjunctive or alternative therapies to conventional antifungals. The promising activity of the synthesized dipeptide **7a**, particularly against *Aspergillus* species, suggests that these structures could be valuable candidates for further development into treatments for fungal infections. Moreover, given the rising concern about antifungal resistance [74], these compounds could also serve as a platform for the design of next-generation antifungal agents that are both potent and less prone to resistance. In conclusion, the synthesis and characterization of Fmoc-protected 1,2,4-triazolyl-α-amino acids and dipeptides represents a significant step toward the development of new antifungal agents. The results of this study underscore the potential of these compounds in treating fungal infections, and their use could be an important strategy to mitigate the impact of *Aspergillus* infections in both humans and animals. Further research, including in vivo studies, is essential to fully assess the clinical applicability, toxicity profiles, and broader spectrum of activity of these compounds.

Supplementary Materials: The following supporting information can be downloaded at: https://www.mdpi.com/article/10.3390/biom15010061/s1, including NMR, ESI MS, and IR characterization spectra, biological data related to antifungal assays, and in silico data. Figure S1. Photographs from the antifungal test (visual inspection) showing the antifungal activities of the compounds developed in the present work, alongside fluconazole as the reference antifungal drug, against the following fungal strains: *A. versicolor* 12134 (I), *A. flavus* 10567 (II), *A. candidus* 10711 (III), *Aureobasidium pullulans* 8269 (IV), *Alternaria altenata* 8126 (V), *Ulocladium botrytis* 12027 (VI); Figure S2. Plots of inhibition rates versus concentration for the determination of IC50 values (Table 3) for the following fungal strains: (a, b, c) *A. versicolor* 12134; (d, e, f) *A. flavus* 10567; and (g, h, i) *A. candidus* 10711; Figure S3. 3D interaction diagrams for the complexes of Comp 3a, Comp 7a, and fluconazole with the protein as obtained using PLIP (Protein-Ligand Interaction Profiler).

Author Contributions: The individual contributions of the authors are as follows: Conceptualization, T.S.; Methodology, N.H., M.I., L.S. and A.S.; Investigation, A.T., H.P., C.V. and H.H.; Validation, A.T., H.P. and A.S.; Formal Analysis, T.S., A.M. and A.S.; Resources, T.S., A.S. and G.N.R.; Data Curation, C.V. and T.S.; Writing—Original Draft Preparation, T.S. and G.N.R.; Supervision, G.N.R.; Project Administration, T.S. and G.N.R.; Funding Acquisition, T.S. and G.N.R. All authors have read and agreed to the published version of the manuscript.

Funding: This research was supported by the Higher Education and Science Committee of MESCs RA (Republic of Armenia), under research project No. 24WS-1D012.

Institutional Review Board Statement: Not applicable.

Informed Consent Statement: Not applicable.

Data Availability Statement: The original contributions presented in the study are included in the article; further inquiries can be directed to the corresponding authors.

Acknowledgments: G.N. Roviello and T. Sargsyan would like to express their sincere gratitude to the Higher Education and Science Committee of the RA Ministry of Education, Science, Culture, and Sports of Armenia for their support through the Adjunct Research Professorship Program 2024. This opportunity has significantly contributed to the advancement of this research.

Conflicts of Interest: The authors declare no conflicts of interest.

References

1. Enaud, R.; Vandenborght, L.E.; Coron, N.; Bazin, T.; Prevel, R.; Schaeverbeke, T.; Berger, P.; Fayon, M.; Lamireau, T.; Delhaes, L. The Mycobiome: A Neglected Component in the Microbiota-Gut-Brain Axis. *Microorganisms* **2018**, *6*, 22. [CrossRef]
2. Kapitan, M.; Niemiec, M.J.; Steimle, A.; Frick, J.S.; Jacobsen, I.D. Fungi as Part of the Microbiota and Interactions with Intestinal Bacteria. In *Fungal Physiology and Immunopathogenesis. Current Topics in Microbiology and Immunology*; Rodrigues, M., Ed.; Springer: Cham, Switzerland, 2019; Volume 422, pp. 265–301. [CrossRef]
3. Money, N.P. Fungi and biotechnology. In *The Fungi*, 3rd ed.; Watkinson, S.C., Boddy, L., Money, N.P., Eds.; Academic Press: Cambridge, MA, USA, 2016; pp. 401–424.
4. Mukherjee, D.; Singh, S.; Kumar, M.; Kumar, V.; Datta, S.; Dhanjal, D.S. Fungal Biotechnology: Role and Aspects. In *Fungi and their Role in Sustainable Development: Current Perspectives*; Gehlot, P., Singh, J., Eds.; Springer: Singapore, 2018; pp. 91–103.
5. Elmastaş, M.; Işıldak, Ö.; Türkekul, İ.; Temur, N. Determination of antioxidant activity and antioxidant compounds in wild edible mushrooms. *J. Food Compos. Anal.* **2007**, *20*, 337–345. [CrossRef]
6. Fisher, M.C.; Henk, D.A.; Briggs, C.J.; Brownstein, J.S.; Madoff, L.C.; McCraw, S.L.; Gurr, S.J. Emerging fungal threats to animal, plant and ecosystem health. *Nature* **2012**, *484*, 186–194. [CrossRef]
7. Seyedmousavi, S.; Bosco, S.M.G.; de Hoog, S.; Ebel, F.; Elad, D.; Gomes, R.R.; Jacobsen, I.D.; Jensen, H.E.; Martel, A.; Mignon, B.; et al. Fungal infections in animals: A patchwork of different situations. *Med. Mycol.* **2018**, *56*, 165–187. [CrossRef]
8. Casadevall, A.; Pirofski, L.A. Host-pathogen interactions: Basic concepts of microbial commensalism, colonization, infection, and disease. *Infect. Immun.* **2000**, *68*, 6511–6518. [CrossRef] [PubMed]
9. Guarro, J.; Gené, J.; Stchigel, A.M. Developments in fungal taxonomy. *Clin. Microbiol. Rev.* **1999**, *12*, 454–500. [CrossRef] [PubMed] [PubMed Central]
10. Seyedmousavi, S.; Guillot, J.; Tolooe, A.; Verweij, P.E.; de Hoog, G.S. Neglected fungal zoonoses: Hidden threats to man and animals. *Clin. Microbiol. Infect.* **2015**, *21*, 416–425. [CrossRef] [PubMed]
11. Desoubeaux, G.; Bailly, É.; Chandenier, J. Diagnosis of invasive pulmonary aspergillosis: Updates and recommendations. *Med. Mal. Infect.* **2014**, *44*, 89–101. [CrossRef] [PubMed]
12. Latgé, J.P. Aspergillus fumigatus and aspergillosis. *Clin. Microbiol. Rev.* **1999**, *12*, 310–350. [CrossRef]
13. Paulussen, C.; Hallsworth, J.E.; Álvarez-Pérez, S.; Nierman, W.C.; Hamill, P.G.; Blain, D.; Rediers, H.; Lievens, B. Ecology of aspergillosis: Insights into the pathogenic potency of Aspergillus fumigatus and some other Aspergillus species. *Microb. Biotechnol.* **2017**, *10*, 296–322. [CrossRef] [PubMed]
14. Seyedmousavi, S.; Guillot, J.; Arné, P.; de Hoog, G.S.; Mouton, J.W.; Melchers, W.J.; Verweij, P.E. Aspergillus and aspergilloses in wild and domestic animals: A global health concern with parallels to human disease. *Med. Mycol.* **2015**, *53*, 765–797. [CrossRef] [PubMed]
15. Desoubeaux, G.; Cray, C. Animal Models of Aspergillosis. *Comp. Med.* **2018**, *68*, 109–123. [PubMed]
16. Henker, L.C.; Lorenzett, M.P.; Lopes, B.C.; Dos Santos, I.R.; Bandinelli, M.B.; Bassuino, D.M.; Juffo, G.D.; Antoniassi, N.A.B.; Pescador, C.A.; Sonne, L.; et al. Pathological and etiological characterization of cases of bovine abortion due to sporadic bacterial and mycotic infections. *Braz. J. Microbiol.* **2022**, *53*, 2251–2262. [CrossRef] [PubMed]
17. Elad, D.; Segal, E. Diagnostic Aspects of Veterinary and Human Aspergillosis. *Front. Microbiol.* **2018**, *9*, 1303. [CrossRef]
18. Mittal, J.; Szymczak, W.A.; Pirofski, L.A.; Galen, B.T. Fungemia caused by *Aureobasidium pullulans* in a patient with advanced AIDS: A case report and review of the medical literature. *JMM Case Rep.* **2018**, *5*, e005144. [CrossRef] [PubMed]
19. Verdecia, J.; Jankowski, C.A.; Reynolds, M.L.; McCarter, Y.; Ravi, M. Fungemia due to *Aureobasidium pullulans*. *Med. Mycol. Case Rep.* **2022**, *37*, 26–28. [CrossRef] [PubMed]
20. Mehta, S.R.; Johns, S.; Stark, P.; Fierer, J. Successful treatment of *Aureobasidium pullulans* central catheter-related fungemia and septic pulmonary emboli. *IDCases* **2017**, *10*, 65–67. [CrossRef] [PubMed]
21. Kaur, R.; Wadhwa, A.; Gulati, A.; Agrawal, A. An unusual phaeoid fungi: Ulocladium, as a cause of chronic allergic fungal sinusitis. *Iran. J. Microbiol.* **2010**, *2*, 95–97.
22. Badenoch, P.R.; Halliday, C.L.; Ellis, D.H.; Billing, K.J.; Mills, R.A. Ulocladium atrum keratitis. *J. Clin. Microbiol.* **2006**, *44*, 1190–1193. [CrossRef]

23. Durán, M.T.; Del Pozo, J.; Yebra, M.T.; Crespo, M.G.; Paniagua, M.J.; Cabezón, M.A.; Guarro, J. Cutaneous infection caused by Ulocladium chartarum in a heart transplant recipient: Case report and review. *Acta Derm. Venereol.* **2003**, *83*, 218–221. [CrossRef] [PubMed]
24. Martins, L.M.L. Allergy to Fungi in Veterinary Medicine: *Alternaria*, Dermatophytes and *Malassezia* Pay the Bill! *J. Fungi* **2022**, *8*, 235. [CrossRef] [PubMed]
25. Fernandes, C.; Casadevall, A.; Gonçalves, T. Mechanisms of *Alternaria* pathogenesis in animals and plants. *FEMS Microbiol. Rev.* **2023**, *47*, fuad061. [CrossRef]
26. Roemer, T.; Krysan, D.J. Antifungal drug development: Challenges, unmet clinical needs, and new approaches. *Cold Spring Harb. Perspect. Med.* **2014**, *4*, a019703. [CrossRef] [PubMed]
27. Jin, R.; Liu, J.; Zhang, G.; Li, J.; Zhang, S.; Guo, H. Design, Synthesis, and Antifungal Activities of Novel 1,2,4-Triazole Schiff Base Derivatives. *Chem. Biodivers.* **2018**, *15*, e1800263. [CrossRef] [PubMed]
28. Wu, W.-N.; Jiang, Y.-M.; Du, H.-T.; Yang, M.-F. Synthesis and antifungal activity of novel 1,2,4-triazole derivatives containing an amide moiety. *J. Heterocycl. Chem.* **2019**, *57*, 1379–1386. [CrossRef]
29. Campoy, S.; Adrio, J.L. Antifungals. *Biochem. Pharmacol.* **2017**, *133*, 86–96. [CrossRef]
30. Dawson, J.H.; Sono, M. Cytochrome P-450 and chloroperoxidase: Thiolate-ligated heme enzymes. Spectroscopic determination of their active-site structures and mechanistic implications of thiolate ligation. *Chem. Rev.* **1987**, *87*, 1255–1276. [CrossRef]
31. Kazeminejad, Z.; Marzi, M.; Shiroudi, A.; Kouhpayeh, S.A.; Farjam, M.; Zarenezhad, E. Novel 1, 2, 4-Triazoles as Antifungal Agents. *Biomed Res. Int.* **2022**, *22*, 4584846. [CrossRef] [PubMed]
32. Vicidomini, C.; Palumbo, R.; Moccia, M.; Roviello, G.N. Oxidative Processes and Xenobiotic Metabolism in Plants: Mechanisms of Defense and Potential Therapeutic Implications. *J. Xenobiotics* **2024**, *14*, 1541–1569. [CrossRef]
33. Vicidomini, C.; Fontanella, F.; D'Alessandro, T.; Roviello, G.N. A Survey on Computational Methods in Drug Discovery for Neurodegenerative Diseases. *Biomolecules* **2024**, *14*, 1330. [CrossRef] [PubMed]
34. Costanzo, M.; De Giglio, M.A.R.; Gilhen-Baker, M.; Roviello, G.N. The Chemical Basis of Seawater Therapies: A Review. *Environ. Chem. Lett.* **2024**, *22*, 2133–2149. [CrossRef]
35. Gamberi, C.; Leverette, C.L.; Davis, A.C.; Ismail, M.; Piccialli, I.; Borbone, N.; Oliviero, G.; Vicidomini, C.; Palumbo, R.; Roviello, G.N. Oceanic Breakthroughs: Marine-Derived Innovations in Vaccination, Therapy, and Immune Health. *Vaccines* **2024**, *12*, 1263. [CrossRef] [PubMed]
36. Marasco, D.; Vicidomini, C.; Krupa, P.; Cioffi, F.; Huy, P.D.Q.; Li, M.S.; Florio, D.; Broersen, K.; De Pandis, M.F.; Roviello, G.N. Plant isoquinoline alkaloids as potential neurodrugs: A comparative study of the effects of benzo[c]phenanthridine and berberine-based compounds on β-amyloid aggregation. *Chem. Biol. Interact.* **2020**, *330*, 109300. [CrossRef] [PubMed]
37. Mittova, V.; Pirtskhalava, M.; Bidzinashvili, R.; Vakhania, M.; Mindiashvili, T.; Kobiashvili, M. Effects of different drying, extraction methods, and solvent polarity on the antioxidant properties of Paeonia daurica subsp. mlokosewitschii leaves. *Mod. Issues Med. Manag.* **2023**, *26*, 66–77. [CrossRef]
38. Sharma, K.K.; Ravi, R.; Maurya, I.K.; Kapadia, A.; Khan, S.I.; Kumar, V.; Tikoo, K.; Jain, R. Modified histidine containing amphipathic ultrashort antifungal peptide, His[2-p-(n-butyl)phenyl]-Trp-Arg-OMe exhibits potent anticryptococcal activity. *Eur. J. Med. Chem.* **2021**, *223*, 113635. [CrossRef] [PubMed]
39. Sharma, K.K.; Maurya, I.K.; Khan, S.I.; Jacob, M.R.; Kumar, V.; Tikoo, K.; Jain, R. Discovery of a Membrane-Active, Ring-Modified Histidine Containing Ultrashort Amphiphilic Peptide That Exhibits Potent Inhibition of Cryptococcus neoformans. *J. Med. Chem.* **2017**, *60*, 6607–6621. [CrossRef] [PubMed]
40. Tivari, S.R.; Kokate, S.V.; Sobhia, E.M.; Kumar, S.G.; Shelar, U.B.; Jadeja, Y.S. A Series of Novel Bioactive Cyclic Peptides: Synthesis by Head-to-Tail Cyclization Approach, Antimicrobial Activity and Molecular Docking Studies. *ChemistrySelect* **2022**, *7*, e202201481. [CrossRef]
41. Tivari, S.R.; Kokate, S.V.; Belmonte-Vázquez, J.L.; Pawar, T.J.; Patel, H.; Ahmad, I.; Gayke, M.S.; Bhosale, R.S.; Jain, V.D.; Muteeb, G.; et al. Synthesis and Evaluation of Biological Activities for a Novel 1,2,3,4-Tetrahydroisoquinoline Conjugate with Dipeptide Derivatives: Insights from Molecular Docking and Molecular Dynamics Simulations. *ACS Omega* **2023**, *8*, 48843–48854. [CrossRef] [PubMed]
42. De Lucca, A.J. Antifungal Peptides: Potential Candidates for the Treatment of Fungal Infections. *Expert Opin. Investig. Drugs* **2000**, *9*, 273–299. [CrossRef]
43. Skwarecki, A.S.; Schielmann, M.; Martynow, D.; Kawczyński, M.; Wiśniewska, A.; Milewska, M.J.; Milewski, S. Antifungal dipeptides incorporating an inhibitor of homoserine dehydrogenase. *J. Pept. Sci.* **2018**, *24*, e3060. [CrossRef]
44. Saghyan, A.S.; Simonyan, H.M.; Petrosyan, S.G.; Geolchanyan, A.V.; Roviello, G.N.; Musumeci, D.; Roviello, V. Thiophenyl-substituted triazolyl-thione L-alanine: Asymmetric synthesis, aggregation, and biological properties. *Amino Acids* **2014**, *46*, 695–702. [CrossRef] [PubMed]
45. Pirtskhalava, M.; Vakhania, M.; Mindiashvili, T.; Kobiashvili, M.; Velijanashvili, M. Use of monoclonal antibodies (mAbs) and their future prospects. *Mod. Issues Med. Manag.* **2022**, *23*, 4–25. [CrossRef]

46. Pirtskhalava, M.; Vakhania, M.; Tavkhelidze, T.; Gogodze, M.; Mindiashvili, T.; Kobiashvili, M.; Mittova, V. Hepatoprotective effect of protein extract of Potamogeton perfoliatus L. against carbon-tetrachloride (CCl_4)-induced hepatic injury in mice. *Mod. Issues Med. Manag.* **2023**, *26*, 30–39. [CrossRef]
47. Emri, T.; Majoros, L.; Tóth, V.; Pócsi, I. Echinocandins: Production and applications. *Appl. Microbiol. Biotechnol.* **2013**, *97*, 3267–3284. [CrossRef] [PubMed]
48. Duncan, V.M.S.; O'Neil, D.A. Commercialization of Antifungal Peptides. *Fungal Biol. Rev.* **2013**, *26*, 156–165. [CrossRef]
49. Agrawal, P.; Bhalla, S.; Chaudhary, K.; Kumar, R.; Sharma, M.K.; Gajendra, P.S. Raghava In Silico Approach for Prediction of Antifungal Peptides. *Front. Microbiol.* **2018**, *9*, 323. [CrossRef] [PubMed]
50. Fernández de Ullivarri, M.; Arbulu, S.; Garcia-Gutierrez, E.; Cotter, P.D. Antifungal Peptides as Therapeutic Agents. *Front. Cell. Infect. Microbiol.* **2020**, *10*, 105. [CrossRef] [PubMed]
51. El-Bahnsawye, M.; Hussein, M.K.A.; Elmongy, E.I.; Awad, H.M.; Tolan, A.A.E.; Moemen, Y.S.; El-Shaarawy, A.; El-Sayed, I.E. Design, Synthesis, and Antiproliferative Activity of Novel Neocryptolepine-Rhodanine Hybrids. *Molecules* **2022**, *27*, 7599. [CrossRef] [PubMed]
52. Grabeck, J.; Mayer, J.; Miltz, A.; Casoria, M.; Quagliata, M.; Meinberger, D.; Klatt, A.R.; Wielert, I.; Maier, B.; Papini, A.M.; et al. Triazole-Bridged Peptides with Enhanced Antimicrobial Activity and Potency against Pathogenic Bacteria. *ACS Infect. Dis.* **2024**, *10*, 2717–2727. [CrossRef] [PubMed]
53. Staśkiewicz, A.; Ledwoń, P.; Rovero, P.; Papini, A.M.; Latajka, R. Triazole-Modified Peptidomimetics: An Opportunity for Drug Discovery and Development. *Front. Chem.* **2021**, *9*, 674705. [CrossRef] [PubMed]
54. Righetto, G.M.; Lopes, J.L.d.S.; Bispo, P.J.M.; André, C.; Souza, J.M.; Andricopulo, A.D.; Beltramini, L.M.; Camargo, I.L.B.d.C. Antimicrobial Activity of an Fmoc-Plantaricin 149 Derivative Peptide against Multidrug-Resistant Bacteria. *Antibiotics* **2023**, *12*, 391. [CrossRef] [PubMed]
55. Apostolidou, C.P.; Kokotidou, C.; Platania, V.; Nikolaou, V.; Landrou, G.; Nikoloudakis, E.; Charalambidis, G.; Chatzinikolaidou, M.; Coutsolelos, A.G.; Mitraki, A. Antimicrobial Potency of Fmoc-Phe-Phe Dipeptide Hydrogels with Encapsulated Porphyrin Chromophores Is a Promising Alternative in Antimicrobial Resistance. *Biomolecules* **2024**, *14*, 226. [CrossRef]
56. Misra, S.; Mukherjee, S.; Ghosh, A.; Singh, P.; Mondal, S.; Ray, D.; Bhattacharya, G.; Ganguly, D.; Ghosh, A.; Aswal, V.K.; et al. Single Amino-Acid Based Self-Assembled Biomaterials with Potent Antimicrobial Activity. *Chem. A Eur. J.* **2021**, *27*, 16744–16753. [CrossRef] [PubMed]
57. Pawar, S.S.; Rohane, S.H. Review on Discovery Studio: An Important Tool for Molecular Docking. *Asian J. Res. Chem.* **2021**, *14*, 1–3. [CrossRef]
58. Yan, Y.; Zhang, D.; Zhou, P.; Li, B.; Huang, S.-Y. HDOCK: A web server for protein–protein and protein–DNA/RNA docking based on a hybrid strategy. *Nucleic Acids Res.* **2017**, *45*, W365–W373. [CrossRef] [PubMed]
59. Scognamiglio, P.L.; Riccardi, C.; Palumbo, R.; Gale, T.F.; Musumeci, D.; Roviello, G.N. Self-Assembly of Thyminyl L-Tryptophanamide (TrpT) Building Blocks for the Potential Development of Drug Delivery Nanosystems. *J. Nanostruct. Chem.* **2023**, *14*, 335–353. [CrossRef]
60. Huang, S.-Y.; Zou, X. An Iterative Knowledge-Based Scoring Function for Protein-Protein Recognition. *Proteins Struct. Funct. Bioinform.* **2008**, *72*, 557–579. [CrossRef] [PubMed]
61. Sargsyan, T.H.; Stepanyan, L.A.; Israyelyan, M.H.; Gasparyan, A.A.; Saghyan, A.S. The Synthesis and in vitro Study of 9-fluorenylmethoxycarbonyl Protected Non-Protein Amino Acids Antimicrobial Activity. *Eurasian Chem. Technol. J.* **2023**, *25*, 235–240. [CrossRef]
62. Sargsyan, A.; Hakobyan, H.; Mardiyan, Z.; Jamharyan, S.; Dadayan, A.; Sargsyan, T.; Hovhannisyan, N. Modeling, Synthesis, and In Vitro Screening of Unusual Amino Acids and Peptides as Protease Inhibitors. *J. Chem. Technol. Metall.* **2023**, *58*, 615–620. [CrossRef]
63. Hargrove, T.Y.; Garvey, E.P.; Hoekstra, W.J.; Yates, C.M.; Wawrzak, Z.; Rachakonda, G.; Villalta, F.; Lepesheva, G.I. Crystal Structure of the New Investigational Drug Candidate VT-1598 in Complex with Aspergillus Fumigatus Sterol 14α-Demethylase Provides Insights into Its Broad-Spectrum Antifungal Activity. *Antimicrob. Agents Chemother.* **2017**, *61*, e00570-17. [CrossRef] [PubMed]
64. Sagatova, A.A.; Keniya, M.V.; Wilson, R.K.; Monk, B.C.; Tyndall, J.D.A. Structural Insights into Binding of the Antifungal Drug Fluconazole to Saccharomyces Cerevisiae Lanosterol 14α-Demethylase. *Antimicrob. Agents Chemother.* **2015**, *59*, 4982–4989. [CrossRef] [PubMed]
65. Li, H.; Huang, E.; Zhang, Y.; Huang, S.-Y.; Xiao, Y. HDOCK Update for Modeling Protein—RNA/DNA Complex Structures. *Protein Sci.* **2022**, *31*, e4441. [CrossRef] [PubMed]
66. Roviello, V.; Musumeci, D.; Mokhir, A.; Roviello, G.N. Evidence of Protein Binding by a Nucleopeptide Based on a Thymine-Decorated L-Diaminopropanoic Acid through CD and In Silico Studies. *Curr. Med. Chem.* **2021**, *28*, 5004–5015. [CrossRef]
67. Roviello, G.N.; Ricci, A.; Bucci, E.M.; Pedone, C. Synthesis, Biological Evaluation, and Supramolecular Assembly of Novel Analogues of Peptidyl Nucleosides. *Mol. Biosyst.* **2011**, *7*, 1773–1778. [CrossRef]

68. Hughes, A.B. (Ed.) *Amino Acids, Peptides and Proteins in Organic Chemistry: Building Blocks, Catalysis and Coupling Chemistry*; Wiley-VCH Verlag GmbH & Co. KGaA: Weinheim, Germany, 2011; ISBN 9783527321025/9783527631803. [CrossRef]
69. Warrilow, A.G.S.; Melo, N.; Martel, C.M.; Parker, J.E.; Nes, W.D.; Kelly, S.L.; Kelly, D.E. Expression, Purification, and Characterization of *Aspergillus fumigatus* Sterol 14-Alpha Demethylase (CYP51) Isoenzymes A and B. *Antimicrob. Agents Chemother.* **2010**, *54*, 4225–4234. [CrossRef] [PubMed]
70. Wiederhold, N.P.; Lockhart, S.R.; Najvar, L.K.; Berkow, E.L.; Jaramillo, R.; Olivo, M.; Garvey, E.P.; Yates, C.M.; Schotzinger, R.J.; Catano, G.; et al. The Fungal Cyp51-Specific Inhibitor VT-1598 Demonstrates In Vitro and In Vivo Activity against *Candida auris*. *Antimicrob. Agents Chemother.* **2019**, *63*, e02233-18. [CrossRef] [PubMed]
71. Van de Veerdonk, F.L.; Gresnigt, M.S.; Romani, L.; Netea, M.G.; Latgé, J.-P. *Aspergillus fumigatus* Morphology and Dynamic Host Interactions. *Nat. Rev. Microbiol.* **2017**, *15*, 661–674. [CrossRef]
72. De Hoog, G.S.; Horré, R. Molecular Taxonomy of the *Alternaria* and *Ulocladium* Species from Humans and Their Identification in the Routine Laboratory. *Mycoses* **2002**, *45*, 259–276. [CrossRef] [PubMed]
73. Zalar, P.; Gostincar, C.; de Hoog, G.S.; Ursic, V.; Sudhadham, M.; Gunde-Cimerman, N. Redefinition of *Aureobasidium pullulans* and Its Varieties. *Stud. Mycol.* **2008**, *61*, 21–38. [CrossRef] [PubMed]
74. Hendrickson, J.A.; Hu, C.; Aitken, S.L.; Beyda, N. Antifungal Resistance: A Concerning Trend for the Present and Future. *Curr. Infect. Dis. Rep.* **2019**, *21*, 47. [CrossRef] [PubMed]

biomolecules

Article

Enhancing Selective Antimicrobial and Antibiofilm Activities of Melittin through 6-Aminohexanoic Acid Substitution

Naveenkumar Radhakrishnan [1], Sukumar Dinesh Kumar [1], Song-Yub Shin [2] and Sungtae Yang [3,*]

[1] Department of Biomedical Sciences, School of Medicine, Chosun University, Gwangju 61452, Republic of Korea; naveens4596@gmail.com (N.R.); sdkumarphd@gmail.com (S.D.K.)
[2] Department of Cellular and Molecular Medicine, School of Medicine, Chosun University, Gwangju 61452, Republic of Korea; syshin@chosun.ac.kr
[3] Department of Microbiology, School of Medicine, Chosun University, Gwangju 61452, Republic of Korea
* Correspondence: styang@chosun.ac.kr

Abstract: Leucine residues are commonly found in the hydrophobic face of antimicrobial peptides (AMPs) and are crucial for membrane permeabilization, leading to the cell death of invading pathogens. Melittin, which contains four leucine residues, demonstrates broad-spectrum antimicrobial properties but also significant cytotoxicity against mammalian cells. To enhance the cell selectivity of melittin, this study synthesized five analogs by replacing leucine with its structural isomer, 6-aminohexanoic acid. Among these analogs, Mel-LX3 exhibited potent antibacterial activity against both Gram-positive and Gram-negative bacteria. Importantly, Mel-LX3 displayed significantly reduced hemolytic and cytotoxic effects compared to melittin. Mechanistic studies, including membrane depolarization, SYTOX green uptake, FACScan analysis, and inner/outer membrane permeation assays, demonstrated that Mel-LX3 effectively permeabilized bacterial membranes similar to melittin. Notably, Mel-LX3 showed robust antibacterial activity against methicillin-resistant *Staphylococcus aureus* (MRSA) and multidrug-resistant *Pseudomonas aeruginosa* (MDRPA). Furthermore, Mel-LX3 effectively inhibited biofilm formation and eradicated existing biofilms of MDRPA. With its improved selective antimicrobial and antibiofilm activities, Mel-LX3 emerges as a promising candidate for the development of novel antimicrobial agents. We propose that the substitution of leucine with 6-aminohexanoic acid in AMPs represents a significant strategy for combating resistant bacteria.

Keywords: antimicrobial peptide; melittin; 6-aminohexanoic acid; leucine; drug-resistant bacteria

Citation: Radhakrishnan, N.; Kumar, S.D.; Shin, S.-Y.; Yang, S. Enhancing Selective Antimicrobial and Antibiofilm Activities of Melittin through 6-Aminohexanoic Acid Substitution. *Biomolecules* **2024**, *14*, 699. https://doi.org/10.3390/biom14060699

Academic Editors: Hyung-Sik Won and Ji-Hun Kim

Received: 22 May 2024
Revised: 10 June 2024
Accepted: 11 June 2024
Published: 14 June 2024

1. Introduction

Antimicrobial peptides (AMPs) are derived from a wide range of living organisms and assist in combating invading pathogens [1,2]. These peptides demonstrate broad-spectrum antimicrobial activity, effectively targeting bacteria, viruses, and fungi [3,4]. Unlike conventional antibiotics, which often target specific cellular components or processes, AMPs exert their antimicrobial effects through various mechanisms, including membrane disruption, inhibition of intracellular targets, and modulation of immune responses [5,6]. With the rise of antibiotic-resistant pathogens and given that bacteria are known to have difficulty developing resistance to AMPs, there is a growing interest in AMPs as alternative strategies for combating infectious diseases [7–9]. Research efforts are focused on understanding the structure–function relationships of AMPs, identifying new sources, and exploring their therapeutic potential in various medical and biotechnological applications [10–12].

Melittin (GIGAVLKVLTTGLPALISWIKRKRQQ), derived from the venom of the European honeybee (*Apis melifera*), is a compelling AMP that has attracted significant attention in scientific research and medical applications [13–15]. Recent studies have assessed melittin for its therapeutic potential in various diseases, including rheumatoid arthritis [16,17], chronic pain [18], anti-nociceptive effects [19,20], anti-mutagenic properties [21], anticancer activity [22,23], and radioprotective effects [24]. However, its clinical translation is hindered by its inherent cytotoxicity towards mammalian cells. Melittin contains the leucine zipper motif, and its structure is marked by an amphipathic bent helix due to the presence of proline in the central region [25]. These structural features contribute to its ability to disrupt lipid membranes, leading to cell lysis and death. This mechanism of action makes melittin effective against a broad spectrum of microorganisms and mammalian cells alike [26–28]. For example, the leucine zipper can contribute to the ability of melittin to form oligomers or aggregates, which can enhance its cytolytic activity by facilitating membrane disruption and pore formation [29,30]. Therefore, understanding this structural feature is crucial for elucidating the mechanism of action of melittin and its pivotal role in membrane disruption, which underpins its antimicrobial and cytolytic activities.

6-Aminohexanoic acid is an unnatural amino acid characterized by a six-carbon aliphatic chain, comprising an amino group at one end and a carboxylic acid group at the other. Despite sharing the same molecular weight as leucine, 6-aminohexanoic acid offers flexibility and mobility due to its central aliphatic chain (Figure S1). This structural divergence confers unique properties and biological activities on 6-aminohexanoic acid [31,32]. In this study, to modify the leucine zipper motif and to enhance the structural flexibility of melittin, each or all leucine residues at four positions (L6, L9, L13, and L16) of melittin were substituted with 6-aminohexanoic acids (Table 1). To assess the cell selectivity of the peptides, we examined their antibacterial activities against Gram-positive and Gram-negative bacteria, as well as their cytotoxicity against mammalian cells. The secondary structures of melittin and its analogs were analyzed in various environments using circular dichroism, while the interactions of the peptides with biological and/or artificial membranes were investigated using fluorescence spectroscopy. Furthermore, we evaluated the antimicrobial and antibiofilm activities of the peptides against drug-resistant bacteria. We discovered that Mel-LX3, wherein leucine at position 13 was replaced by 6-Aminohexanoic acid, exhibited improved cell selectivity and antibiofilm activity against drug-resistant bacteria.

Table 1. Amino acid sequences and physicochemical properties of melittin and its analogs.

Peptides	Sequences	Rt [a] (min)	Net Charge	Mass (g/mol)	Mass Analysis [b] m/z Calculated	m/z Observed
Melittin	GIGAVLKVLTTGLPALISWIKRKRQQ	30.64	6	2847.49	949.83	949.8
Mel-LX1	GIGAV**X**KVLTTGLPALISWIKRKRQQ	24.93	6	2847.49	949.83	949.8
Mel-LX2	GIGAVLKV**X**TTGLPALISWIKRKRQQ	24.76	6	2847.49	949.83	949.7
Mel-LX3	GIGAVLKVLTTG**X**PALISWIKRKRQQ	26.80	6	2847.49	949.83	949.7
Mel-LX4	GIGAVLKVLTTGLPA**X**ISWIKRKRQQ	24.75	6	2847.49	949.83	949.7
Mel-LX5	GIGAV**X**KV**X**TTG**X**PA**X**ISWIKRKRQQ	18.76	6	2847.49	949.83	949.7

[a] Retention time (Rt) was evaluated by RP-HPLC with C_{18} reversed-phase column. [b] Molecular masses were analyzed by ESI-MS. m/z: mass-to-charge ratio of $[M+3H]^{3+}$. The X shown in bold indicates 6-aminohexanoic acid.

2. Materials and Methods

2.1. Materials

Resins of amide-methyl benzhydrylamine (MBHA) and amino acids pre-treated with 9-fluorenyl-methoxycarbonyl (Fmoc) protective groups were acquired from Novabiochem (La Jolla, CA, USA) for peptide synthesis. Several reagents were sourced from Sigma-Aldrich (St. Louis, MO, USA), including 2,2,2-trifluoroethanol, N-phenyl-1-napthylamine (NPN), sodium dodecyl sulfate (SDS), *o*-nitrophenyl-β-galactosidase (ONPG), 3,3′-Dipropylthiadicarbocyanine iodide (diSC$_3$-5), and calcein. SYTOX green dye was supplied from Thermo Fisher Scientific, South Korea. All the buffers were made by using Milli-Q ultrapure water (Merck Millipore, USA). The bacterial strains utilized in this study comprised *Staphylococcus aureus* (KCTC 1621), *Staphylococcus epidermitis* (KCTC 1917), *Bacillus subtilis* (KCTC 3068), *Escherichia coli* (KCTC 1682), *Salmonella typhimurium* (KCTC 1926), and *Pseudomonas aeruginosa* (KCTC 1637). These strains were acquired from the Research Institute of Bioscience and Biotechnology (KRIBB)'s Korean Collection for Type Cultures

(KCTC) of South Korea. Additionally, multidrug-resistant *Pseudomonas aeruginosa* (CCARM 2095) and methicillin-resistant strains of *Staphylococcus aureus* (CCARM 3090) were obtained from Seoul Women's University in South Korea.

2.2. Peptide Synthesis

The Fmoc-based solid-phase method was employed to synthesize all peptides with MBHA resin [33]. Peptide purity was assessed using an RP-HPLC C_{18} column (Vydac, 250 × 20 mm, 15 µm, 300 Å). The molecular masses of the peptides were determined using a triple-quadrupole mass spectrometer equipped with an electrospray ionization liquid chromatography–mass spectrometry (ESI-LC-MS) system (API2000, AB SCIEX).

2.3. Circular Dichroism (CD) Spectroscopy

CD spectroscopy was employed to analyze the secondary structure of the peptides under various environmental conditions, as described previously [34,35]. CD spectra were recorded between 190 and 250 nm at a scan speed of 10 nm/min at 25 °C in 10 mM sodium phosphate buffer (pH 7.4), 30 mM SDS micelles, and 50% trifluoroethanol (TFE) using a spectropolarimeter J-715 (Jasco-Tokyo, Japan) equipped with a 0.1 cm long rectangular quartz cell. Three scans were performed for each peptide, and the results were compiled and averaged. Peptides were concentrated to a final concentration of 100 µg/µL. The mean residue ellipticity ([θ]M) was calculated using the formula $[\theta]M = (\theta_{obs} \times 1000)/(c \times l \times n)$, where θ_{obs} represents the observed ellipticity corrected for the buffer at a given wavelength (mdeg), c is the peptide concentration (µM), l is the path length (mm), and n is the number of amino acids in the peptide sequence.

2.4. Antimicrobial Activity

Peptides were assessed for their antibacterial activity against four Gram-positive and four Gram-negative bacteria, including drug-resistant strains, in accordance with Clinical and Laboratory Standards Institute (CLSI) guidelines [36]. The minimum inhibitory concentration (MIC) was determined using a microtiter broth dilution method. All bacterial strains were incubated overnight at 37 °C. Cultured bacteria were then diluted 10-fold in Muller–Hinton Broth (MHB) medium (Difco, Detroit, MI, USA) and incubated for 3 h to reach mid-log phase. Following the establishment of mid-log phase cultures, bacteria were inoculated into sterile 96-well plates containing serially diluted peptides. The MIC was defined as the lowest concentration of peptides that prevented observable turbidity after incubation of the plates at 37 °C for 18 to 24 h.

2.5. Hemolytic Activity

The hemolytic activity of peptides was assessed by measuring the release of hemoglobin from sheep red blood cells (sRBCs), as described previously [37]. To create a 4% *v*/*v* erythrocyte dilution, fresh sRBCs were washed with phosphate-buffered saline (PBS), centrifuged, and then resuspended in PBS. Next, 100 µL of serially diluted peptides was added to a sterile 96-well plate, followed by the addition of 100 µL of sRBCs. The plate was then incubated at 37 °C for one hour. After incubation, the plate was centrifuged at 1000 relative centrifugal force (RCF), and the supernatant was transferred to a new 96-well plate. Hemoglobin release was measured at 405 nm using a microplate ELISA reader. A total of 0.1% Triton X-100 treatment was utilized to induce 100% hemolysis, while PBS was employed as the reference for 0% hemolysis. The percentage of hemolytic activity was determined using the formula % Hemolysis = [(Abs in peptide solution − Abs in PBS)/(Abs of 0.1% Triton X-100 − Abs of PBS)] × 100.

2.6. Cytotoxicity against RAW 264.7 Cells

We conducted the MTT assay (3-(4,5-dimethylthiazol-2-yl)-2,5-diphenyltetrazolium bromide) dye reduction experiment against RAW 264.7 macrophage cells to evaluate the cytotoxicity of the peptides, following previously published methods [38,39]. RAW 264.7 cells were cultured for 24 h in the presence of 5% CO_2 at 37 °C after seeding them in 96-well plates (2 × 10^4 cells/well). Subsequently, the peptides were treated at increasing concentrations and allowed to interact with the cells for 48 h. Following the incubation period, 20 μL of MTT solution (5 mg/mL in PBS) was added to each well, and the plate was further incubated at 37 °C for 4 h. The absorbance was then measured at 550 nm using a microplate ELISA reader after dissolving the formazan crystals in dimethyl sulfoxide (DMSO). Treatment with 0.1% Triton X-100 served as a positive control for 100% cytotoxicity. Each experiment was performed in triplicate.

2.7. Membrane Depolarization

The evaluation of membrane potential was conducted by employing the voltage-sensitive fluorescent dye diSC_3-5, as described previously [40]. Gram-positive *S. aureus* cells were centrifuged after reaching the mid-log point at 37 °C, corresponding to an OD600 of 0.5. Subsequently, the bacteria were resuspended in a washing buffer at OD600 nm = 0.05, following two washes with the same buffer solution containing 20 mM glucose and 5 mM HEPES at pH 7.4. Upon adding 20 nM diSC_3-5 to the cell suspension, the dye was allowed to fully absorb into the bacterial membrane until a stable fluorescence value was achieved. The intensity of fluorescence emitted from diSC_3-5 (excitation = 622 nm, emission = 670 nm) increased following the addition of peptides, serving as an indicator of membrane depolarization. The addition of 0.1% Triton X-100 completely abolished the membrane potential.

2.8. SYTOX Green Uptake Assay

The SYTOX green experiment was utilized to assess the impact of peptides on bacterial membrane permeabilization [41]. *S. aureus* cells in the mid-log phase (OD600 = 0.5) were washed three times in a buffer containing 20 mM glucose and 5 mM HEPES (pH 7.4). Subsequently, the bacterial cell suspensions were diluted in a buffer consisting of 5 mM HEPES, 100 mM KCl, and 20 mM glucose, at pH 7.4, to a concentration of 1 × 10^6 CFU/mL. After incubating for fifteen minutes in complete darkness, 0.5 μM SYTOX green was added to the bacterial suspensions. The Shimadzu fluorescence spectrophotometer RF-5300PC (Shimadzu Scientific Instruments, Kyoto, Japan) was employed to monitor SYTOX green fluorescence following the addition of peptides at a concentration of 2 × MIC. In the Shimadzu fluorescence spectrophotometer, the excitation and emission wavelengths were set at 485 nm and 520 nm, respectively.

2.9. Membrane Permeability Assay

The fluorescent probe NPN (1-N-phenylnaphthylamine) was utilized to measure the outer membrane permeability of Gram-negative *E. coli* [38]. Mid-log phase *E. coli* cells were diluted to an OD600 of 0.05 after being washed three times in a buffer containing 5 mM HEPES, 20 mM glucose, and 5 mM KCN at pH 7.4. A 1 mM stock solution of NPN was prepared by dissolving NPN in acetone. To achieve a final concentration of 10 μM, 30 μL of the stock solution was added to the bacterial suspension. The fluorescence was observed with an emission wavelength (λ) of 420 nm and an excitation wavelength (λ) of 350 nm until stable fluorescence was reached. Fluorescence was then measured over time after the peptides were added, with the concentration increasing until it reached a steady state. ONPG (o-nitrophenyl-β-galactosidase), a non-chromogenic substrate used for cytoplasmic membrane β-galactosidase enzyme, was employed to assess the release of β-galactosidase from *E. coli* ML-35, aiming to determine the inner membrane permeability of peptides [42]. A 1.5 mM solution of ONPG was added to a sample buffer consisting of 10 mM sodium phosphate and 100 mM NaCl at pH 7.4, which was used to suspend mid-log phase *E. coli* ML-35 bacteria to an OD600 of 0.5. Spectrophotometry at 405 nm was used to assess peptide-induced membrane permeabilization. The fluorescence of ONPG increases when it is hydrolyzed to form o-nitrophenol. The permeability of the inner membrane of *E. coli* ML-35 bacteria was assessed by the influx of ONPG, a substance that was then broken down into o-nitrophenol, forming a yellow product, by the presence of β-galactosidase in the cytoplasm.

2.10. Antibiofilm Activity

We assessed the antibiofilm activity of the peptides by determining their minimum biofilm eradication concentration (MBEC) and minimum biofilm inhibition concentration (MBIC) against drug-resistant bacteria, including MDRPA and MRSA, as previously described [43,44]. A 96-well plate containing a subculture of 1×10^6 CFU/200 μL of bacteria was incubated overnight at 37 °C with or without peptides to test for biofilm inhibition and eradication. The untreated culture served as the negative control, and LL-37 was used as the control peptide.

2.11. Confocal Laser Scanning Microscopy

Drug-resistant bacteria, including MDRPA and MRSA, were cultured to a concentration of 1×10^6 CFU/mL in 24-well plates, and discs were submerged in MHB supplemented with glucose for a full day to facilitate biofilm formation [37]. Subsequently, discs containing planktonic cells were transferred to new 24-well plates containing peptides, following three washes with PBS. The plates were then incubated for 6 h. Afterward, the discs were removed, washed twice with PBS, and stained simultaneously with 40 μM propidium iodide (PI) and 6.7 μM SYTO 9. The biofilm mass was visualized as a planar image using confocal laser scanning microscopy (ZEISS Microscopy LSM 710 Meta, Jena, Germany) and analyzed using the ZEN 2009 Light Edition software, version 4.2.0.121, following a 30 min dark incubation period at 37 °C.

2.12. FACScan Analysis

A flow cytometer was utilized to assess bacterial membrane integrity by quantifying the uptake of PI by the cells [37]. In brief, bacterial cells in the mid-log phase of MRSA and MDRPA were diluted to achieve an OD600 of 0.5. An equal volume of PBS and cell suspension was added to the mixture, which was then centrifuged at 8000 RPM for 5 min. The resulting cell pellets were resuspended in PBS. Subsequently, 10 μL of PI was added, and the mixture was incubated for 15 min. Peptides at a concentration of 2 × MIC were then added to the mixture, followed by an additional fifteen-minute incubation. A FACScan device (Agilent, Santa Clara, CA, USA) was used to quantify PI fluorescence.

3. Results and Discussion

3.1. Peptide Design and Characterization

Melittin contains four leucine residues at positions 6, 9, 13, and 16. In this study, we systematically substituted four leucine residues (L6, L9, L13, and L16) in melittin with 6-aminohexanoic acids, aiming to alter the leucine zipper motif and enhance the structural flexibility of melittin. Specifically, Mel-LX1, Mel-LX2, Mel-LX3, and Mel-LX4 represent individual substitutions of leucine residues at positions 6, 9, 13, and 16 with 6-aminohexanoic acid, respectively. Meanwhile, Mel-LX5 serves as an analog with simultaneous substitution of all four leucine residues.

The synthesized melittin and its analogs underwent mass spectroscopic examination, precisely determining the molecular weight of the peptides (Figure S2). Despite the identical molecular weights of the peptides, analysis by RP-HPLC revealed distinct changes in retention times (Figure S3). The results obtained from RP-HPLC and mass spectroscopy for melittin and its analogs indicated that the peptides were synthesized with adequate purity and precision. Table 1 provides the sequences, HPLC retention times, net charges, and mass analyses of melittin and its analogs.

3.2. CD Spectroscopy

CD spectroscopy was used to analyze the secondary structure of melittin and its analogs in an aqueous solution and in membrane-mimicking environments (30 mM SDS and 50% TFE), as shown in Figure 1. In an aqueous solution, melittin molecules are known to be monomeric and have a random coil structure at low concentrations, whereas at high concentrations, melittin folds into α-helical tetramers. The CD spectra of melittin at 100 μg/μL concentration in a 10 mM sodium phosphate buffer showed characteristic α-helical patterns, with molar lower mean residue ellipticity at 208 nm and 222 nm, whereas all its analogs (Mel-LX1, Mel-LX2, Mel-LX3, Mel-LX4, and Mel-LX5) exhibited a characteristic disordered structure, with the lowest point occurring at about 198 nm. In our conditions, melittin appears to be a tetramer in aqueous buffer, and the analogs are monomers. When exposed to a solution containing 30 mM SDS and 50% TFE, all peptides displayed two distinct negative bands at 208 and 222 nm, indicating that the peptides mostly adopted stable α-helical conformations in the membrane-mimicking environment. Compared to melittin, Mel-LX1, Mel-LX2, and Mel-LX4 showed relatively lower intensity, and Mel-LX5 had the lowest, suggesting that the incorporation of 6-aminohexanoic acid provides structural flexibility in the lipid bilayers. Mel-LX3 displayed comparable levels of α-helical structure to melittin, suggesting that both Mel-LX3 and melittin are likely to interact with membranes in a similar manner. It is noteworthy that the proline at position 14 of melittin introduces a kink of an α-helix. The substitution of leucine at position 13 for 6-aminohexanoic acid appears to have less effect on structural changes compared to other positions.

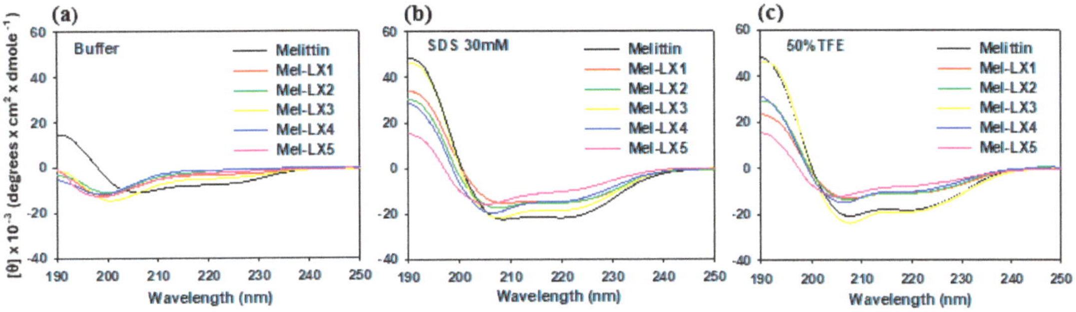

Figure 1. CD spectra of melittin and its analogs in (**a**) 10 mM sodium phosphate buffer, (**b**) 30 mM SDS, and (**c**) 50% TFE.

3.3. Antibacterial Activity of Melittin and Its Analogs

The antibacterial activity of melittin and its analogs was assessed against four Gram-positive bacteria, including MRSA, and four Gram-negative bacteria, including MDRPA. Melittin demonstrated antibacterial activity, with MIC values ranging from 4 to 16 μM against all tested strains. In comparison to melittin, Mel-LX1, Mel-LX2, and Mel-LX4 displayed 4- to 16-fold lower activity, while Mel-LX5 was almost inactive. However, Mel-LX3 was similarly active as melittin against both Gram-positive and Gram-negative bacteria. Importantly, Mel-LX3 effectively inhibited the growth of drug-resistant bacteria, including MRSA and MDRPA. The potent antibacterial activity of Mel-LX3 suggests that the leucine at position 13 contributes less significantly to its effectiveness against bacterial strains.

3.4. Hemolytic and Cytotoxic Activities of Melittin and Its Analogs

We then examined the hemolytic impact of the peptides on sRBCs, as depicted in Figure 2a. At a concentration of 2 μM, melittin induced nearly 100% hemolysis, whereas all melittin analogs exhibited minimal hemolytic activity of less than 5%. Even at a concentration of 64 μM, hemolysis by Mel-LX1, Mel-LX2, Mel-LX3, Mel-LX4, and Mel-LX5 was 11%, 6%, 27%, 3%, and 2%, respectively. We further assessed the cytotoxicity of the peptides against RAW 264.7 macrophage cells, as depicted in Figure 2b. Melittin resulted in less than 10% cell survival rate at 4 μM, whereas all analogs displayed over 80% cell survival at the same concentration. These findings suggest that regardless of the leucine position in melittin, substitution of the leucine residue with 6-aminohexanoic acid significantly diminishes its hemolytic and cytotoxic effects. These results align with prior research indicating the crucial role of leucine residues in the hemolytic activity and cytotoxicity of melittin [30,45]. The hemolytic activity of melittin is closely related to its hydrophobicity, and its oligomerization in aqueous buffer is likely driven by these hydrophobic interactions.

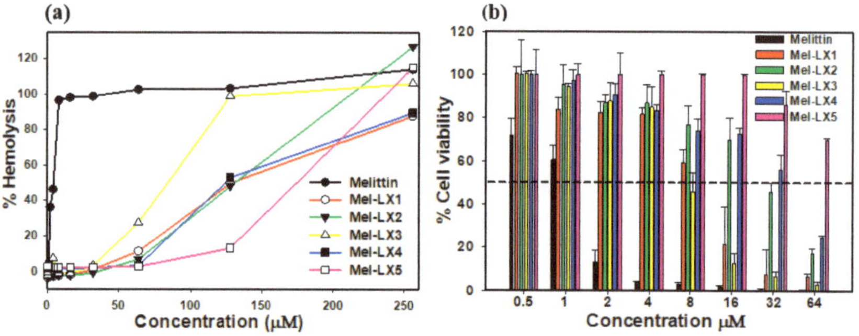

Figure 2. Hemolytic and cytotoxic activities of melittin and Mel-LX3. (**a**) Percentage of hemolysis of sRBCs induced by the peptides. (**b**) Percentage of cell viability in RAW264.7 mouse macrophages. Cell viability was assessed using an MTT dye reduction assay.

To evaluate cell selectivity towards bacterial and mammalian cells, the therapeutic index (TI) was calculated based on antibacterial and hemolytic activities (Table 2). The TI was determined as the ratio of the 10% hemolysis (HC_{10}) to the geometric mean (GM) of the MIC. A higher TI indicates better cell selectivity. Among the melittin analogs, Mel-LX3 exhibited the highest TI value of 5.12, significantly higher than melittin's TI of 0.19. Other analogs, such as Mel-LX1, Mel-LX2, Mel-LX4, and Mel-LX5, showed TI values of 0.65, 2.28, 2.13, and 0.66, respectively. Notably, Mel-LX3 demonstrated the most enhanced selectivity for bacteria over mammalian cells.

Table 2. Antibacterial activities of melittin and its analogs against Gram-positive and Gram-negative bacteria.

Microorganism	MIC (μM)					
	Melittin	Mel-LX1	Mel-LX2	Mel-LX3	Mel-LX4	Mel-LX5
Gram-positive organisms						
S. aureus (KCTC 1621)	8	64	32	8	32	>128
S. epidermidis (KCTC 1917)	8	32	32	16	32	>64
B. subtilis (KCTC 3068)	16	16	16	16	32	>64
MRSA (CCARM 3090)	4	>128	128	4	128	>128
Gram-negative organisms						
E. coli (KCTC 1682)	8	64	32	16	32	>128
P. aeruginosa (KCTC 1637)	16	64	64	16	64	>64
S. typhimurium (KCTC 1926)	16	32	16	16	32	>64
MDRPA (CCARM 2095)	8	>128	128	8	128	>128
GM (μM) [a]	10.5	98	56	12.5	60	192
HC_{10} (μM) [b]	2	64	128	64	128	128
TI (HC_{10}/GM) [c]	0.19	0.65	2.28	5.12	2.13	0.66

[a] Geometric mean (GM) of the minimum inhibitory concentration (MIC). [b] HC_{10} is the minimum inhibitory concentration that causes 10% hemolysis of sRBC. [c] Therapeutic index (TI) is the ratio of HC_{10}/GM.

3.5. Membrane Permeabilization of Gram-Positive Bacteria

Many AMPs with an amphipathic α-helical structure permeabilize the cytoplasmic membrane of Gram-positive bacteria, causing a breakdown in transmembrane potential, resulting in cell death [46]. We assessed the effects of melittin and Mel-LX3 on the membrane depolarization of Gram-positive *S. aureus* by monitoring the fluorescence intensity of diSC$_3$-5, a dye that is sensitive to potential (Figure 3a). Buforin-2, known to be an intracellular target without membrane permeabilization, was used as a negative control. Both melittin and Mel-LX3 at two times the MIC induced rapid depolarization of the membrane against *S. aureus*. Both peptides caused depolarization of the cytoplasmic membrane, which increased fluorescence within 2 min. We then evaluated the membrane permeability of *S. aureus* using SYTOX green, which is a cationic dye that can only pass through compromised membranes (Figure 3b). Buforin-2 as a negative control did not affect fluorescence intensity, but both melittin and Mel-LX3 at 2 × MIC resulted in a rapid increase in fluorescence, reaching the highest levels within 2 min. These results imply that the primary antimicrobial mechanism of Mel-LX3 is related to membrane permeabilization of Gram-positive *S. aureus*.

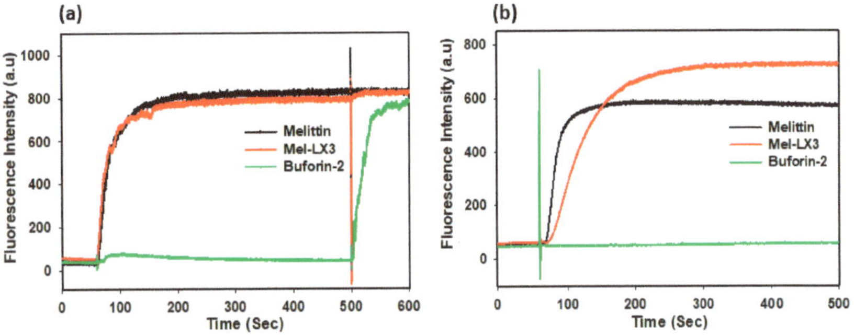

Figure 3. Membrane permeabilization of Gram-positive bacteria induced by melittin and Mel-LX3. (**a**) Membrane depolarization of *S. aureus*. Cytoplasmic membrane depolarization was measured using the fluorescent intensity of the membrane potential-sensitive dye DiSC$_3$-5 when treated with melittin and Mel-LX3 at 2 × MIC. (**b**) SYTOX green entry due to membrane alterations. Increased fluorescence when treading the peptides at 2 × MIC indicates the entry of the SYTOX green probe into *S. aureus* cells.

3.6. Membrane Permeabilization of Gram-Negative Bacteria

Given the presence of both outer and inner membranes in Gram-negative bacteria, we examined the permeability of these membranes in *E. coli* induced by melittin and Mel-LX3. The outer membrane permeability of *E. coli* was evaluated using N-phenyl-1-naphthylamine (NPN) fluorescence, which exhibits weak fluorescence in the intact outer membrane but becomes more pronounced when the outer membrane is compromised (Figure 4a). The outer membrane permeability of *E. coli* increased in a dose-dependent manner in response to melittin and Mel-LX3. Notably, Mel-LX3 at a concentration below the MIC (2 μM) significantly permeabilized the outer membranes of *E. coli*, similar to melittin. No appreciable outer membrane permeability was observed when buforin-2 was applied. To analyze the inner membrane permeability of Gram-negative bacteria induced by the peptides, we measured the hydrolysis of ortho-nitrophenyl-β-D-galactosidase (ONPG) due to the release of cytoplasmic β-galactosidase from *E. coli* ML-35 (Figure 4b). We observed that fluorescence intensity increased with the concentration of melittin and Mel-LX3, indicating that the peptides induce inner membrane permeability in a dose-dependent manner. These results indicate that Mel-LX3 is capable of permeabilizing both the outer and inner membranes of Gram-negative bacteria, similar to melittin.

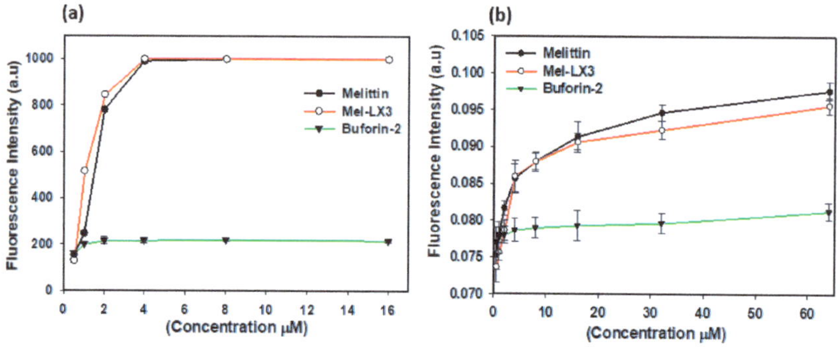

Figure 4. Membrane permeabilization of Gram-negative bacteria. (**a**) Permeabilization of outer membranes. NPN uptake in *E. coli* (KCTC 1682) was monitored in the presence of varying peptide concentrations. (**b**) Permeabilization of inner membranes. Hydrolysis of ONPG occurs due to the release of cytoplasmic β-galactosidase from *E. coli* ML-35 bacterial cells treated with peptides at different concentrations.

3.7. Flow Cytometric Analysis

A flow cytometric analysis was conducted to evaluate the membrane integrity of drug-resistant bacteria (MRSA and MDRPA) following treatment with melittin and Mel-LX3 (Figure 5). Propidium iodide (PI), a DNA intercalating dye, was used as an indicator to assess membrane integrity and cell death via flow cytometry. In the absence of peptides, minimal PI staining was observed in the bacteria, indicating intact cell membranes. As expected, the negative control, buforin-2, resulted in less than 10% PI staining of the bacteria, suggesting that buforin-2 does not disrupt the bacterial membrane. In contrast, both melittin and Mel-LX3 led to significant PI staining, with melittin resulting in 98% and 97% PI staining of MRSA and MDRPA, respectively, and Mel-LX3 inducing 94% PI staining of both MRSA and MDRPA. These findings suggest that both peptides are capable of damaging the bacterial cell membrane. This analysis supports the hypothesis that Mel-LX3 damages bacterial cell membrane integrity, potentially contributing to its antimicrobial properties against these resistant bacteria.

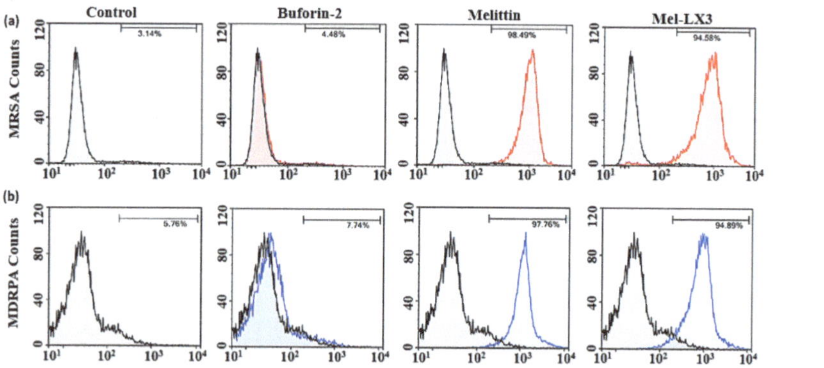

Figure 5. Membrane integrity of drug-resistant bacteria. Flow cytometry was used to monitor membrane integrity of (**a**) MRSA and (**b**) MDRPA in the absence and presence of peptides.

3.8. Antibiofilm Activity

Biofilms represent a significant threat to environmental health as they enable bacteria to form resilient communities, leading to various diseases and fostering antibiotic resistance [47,48]. We investigated whether melittin and Mel-LX3 can inhibit the growth of biofilms of MRSA and MDRPA, as well as eradicate preformed biofilms. LL-37, known for its antibiofilm properties, was used as a control. Figure 6 illustrates the antibiofilm activity of melittin and Mel-LX3 against drug-resistant bacteria, including MRSA and MDRPA. When exposed to the peptides, LL-37 inhibited biofilm formation by approximately 50% at concentrations ranging from 8 to 16 μM. In contrast, melittin and Mel-LX3 effectively inhibited nearly 90% of biofilm formation at concentrations of 4 μM for MRSA and 8 μM for MDRPA (Figure 6a,b). Moreover, both melittin and Mel-LX3 demonstrated nearly 90% MBEC at 64 μM for MRSA and 8 μM for MDRPA (Figure 6c,d). Particularly noteworthy is their significantly stronger biofilm eradication activity against MDRPA compared to LL37. We then employed confocal laser scanning microscopy to visualize the impact on live/dead biofilm bacteria (Figure 6e,f). Live cells were stained with a green fluorescence dye (SYTO-9), while dead cells were stained with a red fluorescence dye (PI). The treatment of biofilm-formed MRSA and MDRPA with melittin or Mel-LX3 resulted in a notable decrease in the number of live cells and a significant increase in the number of dead cells. This suggests that both melittin and Mel-LX3 are effective in killing biofilm-formed MDRPA and MRSA.

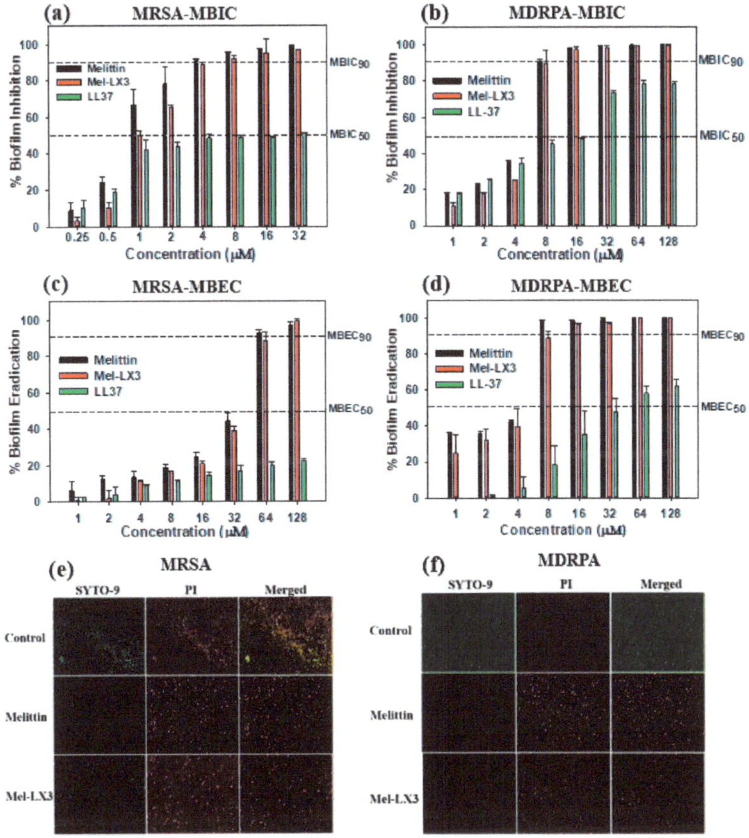

Figure 6. Antibiofilm activity of melittin and Mel-LX3 against drug-resistant bacteria. (**a**) Biofilm inhibition by peptides against MRSA. (**b**) Biofilm inhibition by peptides against MDRPA. (**c**) Biofilm eradication by peptides against MRSA. (**d**) Biofilm eradication by peptides against MDRPA. The dashed lines represent the 50% and 90% inhibition and eradication concentrations. Visualization of antibiofilm properties of the peptides against (**e**) MRSA and (**f**) MDRPA. Live and dead cells are illustrated in green (SYTO 9) and red (PI) fluorescence, respectively.

4. Conclusions

This study synthesized five analogs of melittin by substituting leucine residues with the structural isomer 6-aminohexanoic acid with the aim of enhancing cell selectivity. Among the analogs, Mel-LX3 exhibited potent antibacterial activity against both Gram-positive and Gram-negative bacteria, comparable to melittin, while demonstrating significantly reduced hemolytic and cytotoxic effects. Mechanistic studies revealed that Mel-LX3 effectively permeabilized bacterial membranes, leading to its enhanced antibacterial efficacy. Particularly noteworthy is the ability of Mel-LX3 to combat MRSA and MDRPA, as well as its effectiveness in inhibiting and eradicating biofilms, especially in MDRPA strains. With its improved bacterial selectivity and anti-biofilm activity, Mel-LX3 emerges as a promising candidate for the development of new antimicrobial agents. The substitution of leucine with 6-aminohexanoic acid in AMPs represents a promising strategy for addressing resistant bacteria by reducing toxicity and maintaining antibacterial efficacy, offering potential solutions to combat infectious diseases in the future.

Supplementary Materials: The following supporting information can be downloaded at https://www.mdpi.com/article/10.3390/biom14060699/s1: Figure S1: Chemical structures of leucine and 6-aminohexanoic acid; Figure S2: ESI-MS spectra of peptides; Figure S3: Analytical RP-HPLC profiles of peptides.

Author Contributions: Conceptualization, N.R. and S.Y.; methodology, N.R. and S.-Y.S.; validation, S.-Y.S. and S.Y.; investigation, N.R. and S.D.K.; writing—original draft preparation, N.R.; writing—review and editing, S.Y. and N.R.; supervision, S.Y. All authors have read and agreed to the published version of the manuscript.

Funding: This study was supported by a research fund from Chosun University (2022).

Institutional Review Board Statement: Not applicable.

Informed Consent Statement: Not applicable.

Data Availability Statement: Data are contained within this article and the Supplementary Materials.

Conflicts of Interest: The authors declare no conflicts of interest.

References

1. Mookherjee, N.; Anderson, M.A.; Haagsman, H.P.; Davidson, D.J. Antimicrobial host defence peptides: Functions and clinical potential. *Nat. Rev. Drug Discov.* **2020**, *19*, 311–332. [CrossRef] [PubMed]
2. Huan, Y.; Kong, Q.; Mou, H.; Yi, H. Antimicrobial peptides: Classification, design, application and research progress in multiple fields. *Front. Microbiol.* **2020**, *11*, 582779. [CrossRef] [PubMed]
3. Reddy, K.; Yedery, R.; Aranha, C. Antimicrobial peptides: Premises and promises. *Int. J. Antimicrob. Agents* **2004**, *24*, 536–547. [CrossRef] [PubMed]
4. Gan, B.H.; Gaynord, J.; Rowe, S.M.; Deingruber, T.; Spring, D.R. The multifaceted nature of antimicrobial peptides: Current synthetic chemistry approaches and future directions. *Chem. Soc. Rev.* **2021**, *50*, 7820–7880. [CrossRef] [PubMed]
5. Moravej, H.; Moravej, Z.; Yazdanparast, M.; Heiat, M.; Mirhosseini, A.; Moosazadeh Moghaddam, M.; Mirnejad, R. Antimicrobial peptides: Features, action, and their resistance mechanisms in bacteria. *Microb. Drug Resist.* **2018**, *24*, 747–767. [CrossRef]
6. Zhang, Q.-Y.; Yan, Z.-B.; Meng, Y.-M.; Hong, X.-Y.; Shao, G.; Ma, J.-J.; Cheng, X.R.; Liu, J.; Kang, J.; Fu, C.Y. Antimicrobial peptides: Mechanism of action, activity and clinical potential. *Mil. Med. Res.* **2021**, *8*, 48. [CrossRef] [PubMed]
7. Mba, I.E.; Nweze, E.I. Focus: Antimicrobial resistance: Antimicrobial peptides therapy: An emerging alternative for treating drug-resistant bacteria. *Yale J. Biol. Med.* **2022**, *95*, 445.
8. Moretta, A.; Scieuzo, C.; Petrone, A.M.; Salvia, R.; Manniello, M.D.; Franco, A.; Lucchetti, D.; Vassallo, A.; Vogel, H.; Sgambato, A.; et al. Antimicrobial peptides: A new hope in biomedical and pharmaceutical fields. *Front. Cell. Infect. Microbiol.* **2021**, *11*, 668632. [CrossRef]
9. Li, W.; Separovic, F.; O'Brien-Simpson, N.M.; Wade, J.D. Chemically modified and conjugated antimicrobial peptides against superbugs. *Chem. Soc. Rev.* **2021**, *50*, 4932–4973. [CrossRef]
10. Silva, O.N.; Mulder, K.C.; Barbosa, A.E.; Otero-Gonzalez, A.J.; Lopez-Abarrategui, C.; Rezende, T.M.; Dias, S.C. Exploring the pharmacological potential of promiscuous host-defense peptides: From natural screenings to biotechnological applications. *Front. Microbiol.* **2011**, *2*, 232.
11. Nayab, S.; Aslam, M.A.; Rahman, S.U.; Sindhu, Z.U.D.; Sajid, S.; Zafar, N.; Razaq, M.; Kanwar, R.; Amanullah. A review of antimicrobial peptides: Its function, mode of action and therapeutic potential. *Int. J. Pept. Res. Ther.* **2022**, *28*, 46. [CrossRef]

12. Erdem Büyükkiraz, M.; Kesmen, Z. Antimicrobial peptides (AMPs): A promising class of antimicrobial compounds. *J. Appl. Microbiol.* **2022**, *132*, 1573–1596. [CrossRef] [PubMed]
13. Guha, S.; Ferrie, R.P.; Ghimire, J.; Ventura, C.R.; Wu, E.; Sun, L.; Kim, S.Y.; Wiedman, G.R.; Hristova, K.; Wimley, W.C. Applications and evolution of melittin, the quintessential membrane active peptide. *Biochem. Pharmacol.* **2021**, *193*, 114769. [CrossRef]
14. Lee, M.-T.; Sun, T.-L.; Hung, W.-C.; Huang, H.W. Process of inducing pores in membranes by melittin. *Proc. Natl. Acad. Sci. USA* **2013**, *110*, 14243–14248. [CrossRef] [PubMed]
15. Zhou, J.; Wan, C.; Cheng, J.; Huang, H.; Lovell, J.F.; Jin, H. Delivery strategies for melittin-based cancer therapy. *ACS Appl. Mater. Interfaces* **2021**, *13*, 17158–17173. [CrossRef]
16. Lee, J.A.; Son, M.J.; Choi, J.; Jun, J.H.; Kim, J.-I.; Lee, M.S. Bee venom acupuncture for rheumatoid arthritis: A systematic review of randomised clinical trials. *BMJ Open* **2014**, *4*, e006140. [CrossRef]
17. Jeong, Y.-J.; Shin, J.-M.; Bae, Y.-S.; Cho, H.-J.; Park, K.-K.; Choe, J.-Y.; Han, S.M.; Moon, S.K.; Kim, W.J.; Choi, Y.H.; et al. Melittin has a chondroprotective effect by inhibiting MMP-1 and MMP-8 expressions via blocking NF-κB and AP-1 signaling pathway in chondrocytes. *Int. Immunopharmacol.* **2015**, *25*, 400–405. [CrossRef]
18. Son, D.J.; Lee, J.W.; Lee, Y.H.; Song, H.S.; Lee, C.K.; Hong, J.T. Therapeutic application of anti-arthritis, pain-releasing, and anti-cancer effects of bee venom and its constituent compounds. *Pharmacol. Ther.* **2007**, *115*, 246–270. [CrossRef] [PubMed]
19. Yoon, H.; Kim, M.J.; Yoon, I.; Li, D.X.; Bae, H.; Kim, S.K. Nicotinic acetylcholine receptors mediate the suppressive effect of an injection of diluted bee venom into the GV3 acupoint on oxaliplatin-induced neuropathic cold allodynia in rats. *Biol. Pharm. Bull.* **2015**, *38*, 710–714. [CrossRef]
20. Lim, B.-S.; Moon, H.J.; Li, D.X.; Gil, M.; Min, J.K.; Lee, G.; Bae, H.; Kim, S.K.; Min, B.-I. Effect of bee venom acupuncture on oxaliplatin-induced cold allodynia in rats. *Evid.-Based Complement. Altern. Med.* **2013**, *2013*, 369324. [CrossRef]
21. Varanda, E.A.; Monti, R.; Tavares, D.C. Inhibitory effect of propolis and bee venom on the mutagenicity of some direct-and indirect-acting mutagens. *Teratog. Carcinog. Mutagen.* **1999**, *19*, 403–413. [CrossRef]
22. Hu, H.; Chen, D.; Li, Y.; Zhang, X. Effect of polypeptides in bee venom on growth inhibition and apoptosis induction of the human hepatoma cell line SMMC-7721 in-vitro and Balb/c nude mice in-vivo. *J. Pharm. Pharmacol.* **2006**, *58*, 83–89. [CrossRef] [PubMed]
23. Huh, J.-E.; Baek, Y.-H.; Lee, M.-H.; Choi, D.-Y.; Park, D.-S.; Lee, J.-D. Bee venom inhibits tumor angiogenesis and metastasis by inhibiting tyrosine phosphorylation of VEGFR-2 in LLC-tumor-bearing mice. *Cancer Lett.* **2010**, *292*, 98–110. [CrossRef] [PubMed]
24. Gajski, G.; Garaj-Vrhovac, V. Radioprotective effects of honeybee venom (*Apis mellifera*) against 915-mhz microwave radiation–induced DNA damage in wistar rat lymphocytes: In vitro study. *Int. J. Toxicol.* **2009**, *28*, 88–98. [CrossRef] [PubMed]
25. Zhang, L.; Benz, R.; Hancock, R.E. Influence of proline residues on the antibacterial and synergistic activities of α-helical peptides. *Biochemistry* **1999**, *38*, 8102–8111. [CrossRef]
26. Lam, Y.; Wassall, S.; Morton, C.; Smith, R.; Separovic, F. Solid-state NMR structure determination of melittin in a lipid environment. *Biophys. J.* **2001**, *81*, 2752–2761. [CrossRef]
27. Lam, Y.-H.; Morton, C.; Separovic, F. Solid-state NMR conformational studies of a melittin-inhibitor complex. *Eur. Biophys. J.* **2002**, *31*, 383–388.
28. Ladokhin, A.S.; Selsted, M.E.; White, S.H. Sizing membrane pores in lipid vesicles by leakage of co-encapsulated markers: Pore formation by melittin. *Biophys. J.* **1997**, *72*, 1762–1766. [CrossRef] [PubMed]
29. Saravanan, R.; Bhunia, A.; Bhattacharjya, S. Micelle-bound structures and dynamics of the hinge deleted analog of melittin and its diastereomer: Implications in cell selective lysis by d-amino acid containing antimicrobial peptides. *Biochim. Biophys. Acta (BBA)-Biomembr.* **2010**, *1798*, 128–139. [CrossRef]
30. Asthana, N.; Yadav, S.P.; Ghosh, J.K. Dissection of antibacterial and toxic activity of melittin: A leucine zipper motif plays a crucial role in determining its hemolytic activity but not antibacterial activity. *J. Biol. Chem.* **2004**, *279*, 55042–55050. [CrossRef]
31. Markowska, A.; Markowski, A.R.; Jarocka-Karpowicz, I. The importance of 6-aminohexanoic acid as a hydrophobic, flexible structural element. *Int. J. Mol. Sci.* **2021**, *22*, 12122. [CrossRef] [PubMed]
32. Sun, Z.; Chen, Y.-H.; Wang, P.; Zhang, J.; Gurewich, V.; Zhang, P.; Liu, J.-N. The blockage of the high-affinity lysine binding sites of plasminogen by EACA significantly inhibits prourokinase-induced plasminogen activation. *Biochim. Biophys. Acta (BBA)-Protein Struct. Mol. Enzymol.* **2002**, *1596*, 182–192. [CrossRef]
33. Story, S.C.; Aldrich, J.V. Preparation of protected peptide amides using the Fmoc chemical protocol: Comparison of resins for solid phase synthesis 1. *Int. J. Pept. Protein Res.* **1992**, *39*, 87–92. [CrossRef]
34. Yang, S.-T.; Shin, S.-Y.; Shin, S.-H. The central PXXP motif is crucial for PMAP-23 translocation across the lipid bilayer. *Int. J. Mol. Sci.* **2021**, *22*, 9752. [CrossRef] [PubMed]
35. Lee, H.; Shin, S.-H.; Yang, S. Rationally designed PMAP-23 derivatives with enhanced bactericidal and anticancer activity based on the molecular mechanism of peptide–membrane interactions. *Amino Acids* **2023**, *55*, 1013–1022. [CrossRef] [PubMed]
36. Humphries, R.M.; Ambler, J.; Mitchell, S.L.; Castanheira, M.; Dingle, T.; Hindler, J.A.; Koeth, L.; Sei, K. CLSI methods development and standardization working group best practices for evaluation of antimicrobial susceptibility tests. *J. Clin. Microbiol.* **2018**, *56*, 10–128. [CrossRef] [PubMed]
37. Jahan, I.; Kumar, S.D.; Shin, S.Y.; Lee, C.W.; Shin, S.-H.; Yang, S. Multifunctional properties of BMAP-18 and its aliphatic analog against drug-resistant bacteria. *Pharmaceuticals* **2023**, *16*, 1356. [CrossRef]

38. Lee, H.; Lim, S.I.; Shin, S.-H.; Lim, Y.; Koh, J.W.; Yang, S. Conjugation of cell-penetrating peptides to antimicrobial peptides enhances antibacterial activity. *ACS Omega* **2019**, *4*, 15694–15701. [CrossRef] [PubMed]
39. Yang, S.; Lee, C.W.; Kim, H.J.; Jung, H.-H.; Kim, J.I.; Shin, S.Y.; Shin, S.-H. Structural analysis and mode of action of BMAP-27, a cathelicidin-derived antimicrobial peptide. *Peptides* **2019**, *118*, 170106. [CrossRef]
40. Lee, H.; Yang, S.; Shin, S.-H. Effect of central PxxP motif in amphipathic alpha-helical peptides on antimicrobial activity and mode of action. *J. Anal. Sci. Technol.* **2023**, *14*, 33. [CrossRef]
41. Kim, E.Y.; Kumar, S.D.; Bang, J.K.; Shin, S.Y. Mechanisms of antimicrobial and antiendotoxin activities of a triazine-based amphipathic polymer. *Biotechnol. Bioeng.* **2020**, *117*, 3508–3521. [CrossRef] [PubMed]
42. Lehrer, R.; Barton, A.; Daher, K.A.; Harwig, S.; Ganz, T.; Selsted, M.E. Interaction of human defensins with *Escherichia coli*. Mechanism of bactericidal activity. *J. Clin. Investig.* **1989**, *84*, 553–561. [PubMed]
43. Basak, A.; Abouelhassan, Y.; Zuo, R.; Yousaf, H.; Ding, Y.; Huigens, R.W. Antimicrobial peptide-inspired NH125 analogues: Bacterial and fungal biofilm-eradicating agents and rapid killers of MRSA persisters. *Org. Biomol. Chem.* **2017**, *15*, 5503–5512. [CrossRef] [PubMed]
44. Harrison, J.J.; Stremick, C.A.; Turner, R.J.; Allan, N.D.; Olson, M.E.; Ceri, H. Microtiter susceptibility testing of microbes growing on peg lids: A miniaturized biofilm model for high-throughput screening. *Nat. Protoc.* **2010**, *5*, 1236–1254. [CrossRef]
45. Pandey, B.K.; Ahmad, A.; Asthana, N.; Azmi, S.; Srivastava, R.M.; Srivastava, S.; Verma, R.; Vishwakarma, A.L.; Ghosh, J.K. Cell-selective lysis by novel analogues of melittin against human red blood cells and *Escherichia coli*. *Biochemistry* **2010**, *49*, 7920–7929. [CrossRef]
46. Oren, Z.; Shai, Y. Mode of action of linear amphipathic α-helical antimicrobial peptides. *Pept. Sci.* **1998**, *47*, 451–463. [CrossRef]
47. Overhage, J.; Campisano, A.; Bains, M.; Torfs, E.C.; Rehm, B.H.; Hancock, R.E. Human host defense peptide LL-37 prevents bacterial biofilm formation. *Infect. Immun.* **2008**, *76*, 4176–4182. [CrossRef]
48. Gilbert, P.; Allison, D.; McBain, A. Biofilms in vitro andin vivo: Do singular mechanisms imply cross-resistance? *J. Appl. Microbiol.* **2002**, *92*, 98S–110S. [CrossRef]

biomolecules

MDPI

Article

Synthesis of the Antimicrobial Peptide Murepavadin Using Novel Coupling Agents

Júlia García-Gros [1], Yolanda Cajal [2,3], Ana Maria Marqués [4] and Francesc Rabanal [1,*]

1 Section of Organic Chemistry, Department of Inorganic and Organic Chemistry, Faculty of Chemistry, Universitat de Barcelona, 08028 Barcelona, Spain; juliagarciagros@ub.edu
2 Department of Pharmacy, Pharmaceutical Technology and Physical Chemistry, Faculty of Pharmacy and Food Sciences, Universitat de Barcelona, 08028 Barcelona, Spain; ycajal@ub.edu
3 Institute of Nanoscience and Nanotechnology (IN2UB), Universitat de Barcelona, 08028 Barcelona, Spain
4 Laboratory of Microbiology, Faculty of Pharmacy and Food Sciences, Universitat de Barcelona, 08007 Barcelona, Spain; ammarques@ub.edu
* Correspondence: frabanal@ub.edu

Abstract: The problem of antimicrobial resistance is becoming a daunting challenge for human society and healthcare systems around the world. Hence, there is a constant need to develop new antibiotics to fight resistant bacteria, among other important social and economic measures. In this regard, murepavadin is a cyclic antibacterial peptide in development. The synthesis of murepavadin was undertaken in order to optimize the preparative protocol and scale-up, in particular, the use of new activation reagents. In our hands, classical approaches using carbodiimide/hydroxybenzotriazole rendered low yields. The use of novel carbodiimide and reagents based on OxymaPure® and Oxy-B is discussed together with the proper use of chromatographic conditions for the adequate characterization of peptide crudes. Higher yields and purities were obtained. Finally, the antimicrobial activity of different synthetic batches was tested in three *Pseudomonas aeruginosa* strains, including highly resistant ones. All murepavadin batches yielded the same highly active MIC values and proved that the chiral integrity of the molecule was preserved throughout the whole synthetic procedure.

Keywords: peptide synthesis; antimicrobial cyclic peptide; murepavadin; acylation agents; solid phase; antibiotic; antibacterial activity

check for updates

Citation: García-Gros, J.; Cajal, Y.; Marqués, A.M.; Rabanal, F. Synthesis of the Antimicrobial Peptide Murepavadin Using Novel Coupling Agents. *Biomolecules* **2024**, *14*, 526. https://doi.org/10.3390/biom14050526

Academic Editors: Hyung-Sik Won and Ji-Hun Kim

Received: 5 April 2024
Revised: 18 April 2024
Accepted: 23 April 2024
Published: 27 April 2024

1. Introduction

Peptides are a class of chemical compounds that offer immense potential as therapeutic tools. These biomolecules are highly selective and effective, as they can bind to specific cell surface receptors and trigger intracellular effects while being relatively safe and well tolerated. Consequently, there is a rising interest in therapeutic peptides, and nowadays, more than eighty peptide drugs have already been approved worldwide [1–3]. Since the introduction of solid-phase peptide synthesis (SPPS) by Bruce Merrifield in 1963 [4], this field has experienced a boost in research and development [5]. However, scale-up and production are still complex issues during pharmaceutical development. In fact, small chemical optimization may imply great improvements in yields and purities due to the repetitive nature of the peptide assembly process [3].

In recent decades, a vast arsenal of coupling reagents has been developed for peptide bond formation [6–8], including aminium salts of benzotriazoles, such as 2-(1*H*-benzotriazole-1-yl)-1,1,3,3-tetramethyluronium hexafluorophosphate (HBTU) [9]; phosphonium salts, such as (Benzotriazol-1-yloxy)tris(dimethylamino)phosphonium hexafluorophosphate (BOP) or (Benzotriazol-1-yloxy)tripyrrolidinophosphonium hexafluorophosphate (PyBOP) [10], and carbodiimides, among others. Carbodiimides, in fact, are still the compounds of choice because of their lower cost and good performance in non-hindered peptide bond formation in comparison with more complex reagents.

For solution-phase peptide synthesis, *N*-ethyl-*N′*-(3-(dimethylamino)propyl)carbodiimide (EDC) is commonly used because its urea is highly soluble in aqueous solutions. On the other hand, *N,N′*-diisopropylcarbodiimide (DIC) is preferred in SPPS because the generated urea byproduct is soluble in organic solvents, while the urea of dicylohexylcarbodiimide (DCC) is prone to precipitation. It is well known, though, that carbodiimides can induce a certain degree of epimerization on the alpha-C of the activated acid group [6]. For this reason, additives, such as 1-hydroxybenzotriazole (HOBt) or 1-hydroxy-7-azabenzotriazole (HOAt) [11], are commonly used. These reagents reduce the high reactivity of O-acylisourea by forming intermediate active esters and inhibit side-reactions, such as racemization, through oxazolones or the formation of *N*-acylureas [12].

Unfortunately, additives, such as HOBt, can induce a certain premature cleavage of the peptide chains, especially when using acid-labile trityl-based resins, because of their acidic nature [13]. Moreover, HOBt and HOAt are classified in the Class I category according to the U.S. Department of Transportation (DOT) and United Nations (UN) guidelines due to their explosive character, and hence, their use is restricted [14]. In this sense, ethylcyano(hydroxyimino)acetate (OxymaPure, first described in 1973 by Itoh [15]) was introduced and was shown to perform better than HOBt in terms of yield and epimerization, and more importantly, it also showed better thermal stability [16]. Later, other oxyma-based compounds were developed, including the COMU reagent ((1-cyano-2-ethoxy-2-oxoethylideneaminooxy)-dimethyl-morpholino-carbeniumhexafluorophosphate [17]) or (Z)-ethyl 2-cyano-3-hydroxyacrylate potassium salt (K-Oxyma) [18], among others (Figure 1). The latter is the potassium salt of OxymaPure, a more appropriate choice when dealing with highly acid-labile resins due to the lack of the acid *N*-hydroxy proton (Figure 1) [18].

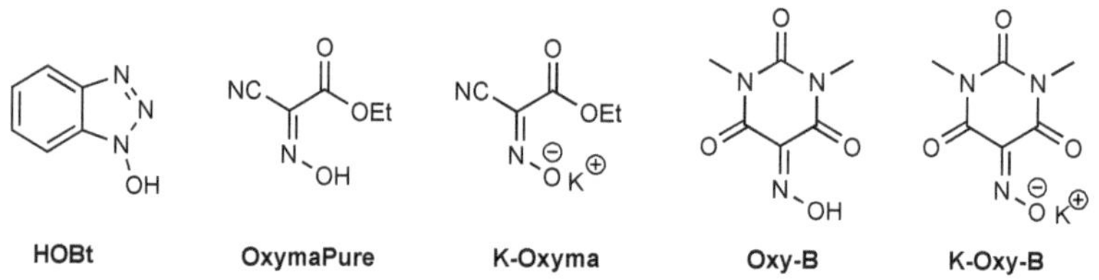

Figure 1. Structures of HOBt and oxyma-based reagents.

However, the combination of DIC with OxymaPure in dimethylformamide (DMF) at 20 °C was demonstrated to lead to the formation of oxadiazole and the harmful volatile HCN [19]. In order to avoid this drawback, the reaction of OxymaPure with carbodiimides was studied. It was found that different sterically hindered *N,N′*-ditertbutylcarbodiimide (DTBC) containing tertiary carbon groups did not produce either oxadiazole or HCN but showed poor reactivity. Also, the primary substituted carbodiimide EDC did not evolve into the formation of these undesirable products but showed nonproductive consumption. In this sense, a hybrid carbodiimide-based reagent, *N,N′*-tertbutylethylcarbodiimide (TBEC), which ensures an HCN-free reaction, was finally found to be the best reagent [20–22].

The problem of antimicrobial resistance is becoming a daunting challenge for human society and healthcare systems around the world. Hence, there is a constant need to develop new antibiotics to fight resistant bacteria, among other important social and economic measures. Our group has been involved in the preparation of cyclic peptide antibiotics to improve their therapeutic window and study their mechanisms of action [5,23–29]. The purpose of this study is to evaluate and test novel coupling reagents to optimize the synthesis of murepavadin, a novel antimicrobial peptide in clinical development, which is highly active against *Pseudomonas aeruginosa*, an infectious bacterial agent considered a serious threat to human health [30].

Murepavadin (Figure 2), previously known as POL7080, is an antimicrobial peptidomimetic first-in-class of the Outer Membrane Protein Targeting Antibiotics (OMPTA), developed initially by Polyphor Ltd. (and now in the portfolio of Basilea Pharmaceutica) [31]. It is a fully synthetic non-branched cyclic peptide composed of 14 amino acids with a sequence related to that of the membranolytic host-defense peptide protegrin-I (PG-I), which contains a β-hairpin conformation stabilized by a DPro-Pro turn dipeptide [32,33]. This cyclic peptide binds to the lipopolysaccharide transport protein D (LptD), an outer membrane (OM) protein involved in the lipopolysaccharide (LPS) biogenesis in Gram-negative bacteria. It inhibits the LPS transport function of LptD, altering the OM and finally causing cell death [34,35]. Murepavadin exhibits a specific and potent bactericidal activity in vitro and in vivo against *Pseudomonas aeruginosa* [36–38]. Unfortunately, the phase III trials of intravenous murepavadin in hospitalized patients with pneumonia showed an unexpectedly high incidence of acute kidney injury. Currently, a clinical phase I trial evaluating an inhaled form of the antibiotic is being evaluated for the treatment of respiratory diseases, particularly cystic fibrosis and non-cystic fibrosis bronchiectasis [39,40].

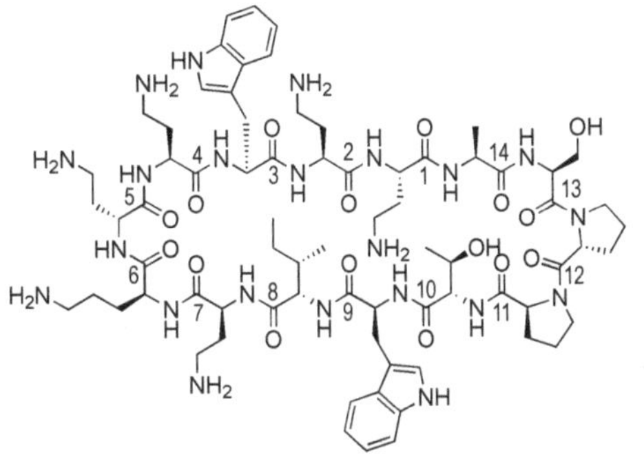

Figure 2. Structure of murepavadin. The sequence consists of 14 amino acids: *cyclo*[Ser-DPro-Pro-Thr-Trp-Ile-Dab-Orn-DDab-Dab-Trp-Dab-Dab-Ala].

2. Materials and Methods

2.1. Chemicals

2-Chlorotrityl chloride resin (2-CTC), trityl chloride resin (Cl-Trt), N-fluorenylmethoxy carbonyl (Fmoc)-protected amino acids, trifluoroacetic acid (TFA), and N-hydroxybenzotria zole (HOBt) were purchased from Fluorochem (Hadfield, UK) and Iris Biotech GmbH (Marktredwitz, Germany). *N,N′*-diisopropylcarbodiimide was from Thermo Fisher Scientific (Waltham, MA, USA). TBEC and Oxyma-B were given by Luxembourg Bio Technologies. Acetonitrile (ACN) HPLC gradient grade was purchased from Labkem (Barcelona, Spain). All chemicals were of the highest available purity. The solvents used were HPLC grade, except for the water, which was doubly distilled and deionized (Milli-Q system, Millipore Corp., Burlington, MA, USA).

2.2. Synthesis of K-Oxy-B

Oxy-B (1 g, 5.4 mmol) was dissolved in 40 mL of H_2O. Then, 5.4 mL of KOH 1 M was slowly added until pH 7 was reached. The mixture was lyophilized, and 1.177 g of a purple/brownish solid (yield of 97%) was obtained. MS analysis: m/z = $[M]^-$ = 184. HPLC analysis: purity of >99%, with relative absorption max. at 235 nm, using a Kinetex® (Phenomenex, Torrance, CA, USA) reversed-phase column (4.6 × 250 mm) of a 5 μm particle diameter and a pore size of 100 Å, with 5–95% gradient of 0.036% TFA/ACN and 0.045% TFA/H_2O over 30 min, flow = 1 mL·min^{-1} (t_R = 8.401 min).

2.3. Peptide Synthesis

Manual solid-phase peptide synthesis was performed following a Fmoc/^{t}Bu protection strategy in polypropylene syringes fitted with a polyethylene disc, which was attached to a vacuum system for the rapid removal of solvents and any excess of reagents. 2-CTC or Cl-Trt resins (1.67 mmol·g^{-1}, 250 mg) were washed with dichloromethane (DCM), DMF, and DCM (2 × 4 mL each). After resin conditioning, 2 eq of Fmoc-Dab(Boc)-OH was added along with 4 eq of DIPEA and the minimum quantity of DCM. The first coupling was left to react for 3 h at room temperature. After that, the resin was washed with DMF and DCM, capped with MeOH (0.8 mL·g^{-1}resin) for 20 min, and washed again with DCM. The loading of the first amino acid residue was assessed by Fmoc quantification. The peptide sequence was assembled by the addition of the Fmoc-protected amino acid (3 eq), coupling reagent (3 eq), additive (3 eq), and the minimum quantity of DMF for 1 h. All couplings yielded ≥99%, as assessed by the Kaiser test. The Fmoc removal was achieved by successive treatments with 20% piperidine/DMF (1 × 1 min, 2 × 10 min). Cleavage of the peptide from the resin was carried out by two successive treatments with hexafluoroisopropanol (HFIP)/DCM (1:4, *v*/*v*, 3 mL·g^{-1} resin) for 1 h. The crude protected peptide was obtained after solvent evaporation under reduced pressure. For cyclization, the resulting solid was dissolved in DMF (2.5 mg·mL^{-1}), and 3 eq HATU, 3 eq HOBt, and 6 eq DIPEA were added. The reaction mixture was stirred, monitored by a ninhydrin test, and after 18 h, the DMF was removed under high vacuum. To remove any excess of coupling agents, the crude product was dissolved in DCM and extracted with ACN/H_2O (1:9, *v*/*v*). The protected peptide was isolated after solvent evaporation. The crude was treated with trifluoroacetic acid (TFA)/triisopropylsilane (TIPS)/H_2O (95:3:2, *v*/*v*/*v*) during 90 min with stirring. Then, the reaction mixture was precipitated in ice-cold diethyl ether (70 mL), centrifuged, and washed two more times with anhydrous Et_2O. The lyophilized peptide was dissolved in ACN/H_2O (1:1, *v*/*v*, 100 mg·mL^{-1}), purified by semipreparative HPLC, and characterized by analytical HPLC and ESI mass spectrometry.

2.4. Minimum Inhibitory Concentration Determination

Minimum inhibitory concentrations (MICs) of the different murepavadin batches were determined by following the Clinical and Laboratory Standards Institute (CLSI) guidelines. Bacteria used in this study were standard isolates from the American Type Culture Collection (ATCC) and German Collection of Microorganisms (DSM) (*P. aeruginosa* ATCC 27853, *P. aeruginosa* DSM 24600, and DSM 25716). Sterile microtiter plates (96 wells of 100 μL) were filled with 50 μL of cation-adjusted Mueller–Hinton broth (MHB) culture medium. Serial 2-fold dilutions of the peptides were arranged in rows ranging from 8 to 0.016 μg·mL^{-1}. The last two columns were used as positive and negative controls, respectively. The bacterial suspensions prepared with an optical density at 600 nm (OD_{600}) of 0.2 were diluted 100-fold, and 50 μL of the resulting suspension was added to each well (excluding the negative control). This resulted in a final concentration of approximately 5 × 10^5 CFU·mL^{-1}. The plates were incubated at 37 °C for 18–20 h, and the MICs were determined. The MIC was defined as the lowest concentration of the antimicrobial agent at which the visible growth of bacteria was prevented. Each determination was carried out in triplicate. To be considered acceptable, the three MIC results have to differ in only one well, and the result is always given as the higher of the three.

3. Results and Discussion

3.1. Murepavadin Synthesis

The synthesis of murepavadin is not described in detail in the literature. The preparation of closely related peptides (i.e., POL7001, L27-11, and L26-19) followed a general Fmoc/^{t}Bu scheme of protection, and cyclization was performed between residues Pro^{11} (C-terminal end) and Thr^{10} (N-terminal, Figure 29) [38,41]. A different approach has been described using a native chemical ligation (NCL)/desulfurization methodology. In this approach, the cyclization site was the Dab-Ala amide bond, as an Ala amino acid is needed for this strategy. Cyclization took place in 30 min and reached a yield of 70% [42].

In our case, we decided to cyclize through the potentially less hindered peptide bond to reduce the risk of epimerization and facilitate amide formation. We avoided β-branched amino acids (Ile, Thr(^{t}Bu)) and, in general, other ^{t}Bu- or Boc- side chain protected amino acids. The chosen bond for cyclization was the amide between Dab and Ala, obtaining yields between 89 and 96%, as described below. Hence, the first amino acid to be attached to the resin was the corresponding Fmoc-Dab(Boc)-OH (Dab[1], as shown in Figure 2).

Overall, the synthesis of murepavadin was undertaken by SPPS following a Fmoc/^{t}Bu scheme of protection on the trityl-type of resins using several acylating agents, as indicated in Table 1 [38]. After the assembly of the linear protected peptide sequence on resin, a mild acidolysis using HFIP/DCM (1:4) was performed in order to obtain the partially protected peptide. The cyclization of the lineal crude was achieved with 3 eq *O*-(7-azabenzotriazol-1-yl)-1,1,3,3-tetramethyl-uronium hexafluorophosphate (HATU), 3 eq HOBt, and 6 eq *N*,*N*-diisopropylethylamine (DIPEA). After cyclization, the crude protected peptide was treated with an acidolysis reagent composed of TFA/TIPS/H_2O (95:3:2, *v*/*v*/*v*) to obtain the totally deprotected cyclic peptide (Scheme 1). The purity of the fully deprotected peptide was assessed by HPLC by the integration of peaks at 220 nm.

Table 1. Yields and purities for each of the syntheses performed (also see Table S1).

Synthesis	Resin	Loading	Coupling Agents	Resin Detachment Yield	Cyclization Yield	Acidolysis Yield	Overall Crude Yield	Crude Purity [a]
A	2-CTC	0.86 mmol/g	3 eq DIC 3 eq HOBt	46%	96%	90%	40%	58%
B	2-CTC	0.86 mmol/g	3 eq DIC 3 eq K-Oxyma	91%	93%	83%	70%	64%
C	Cl-Trt	0.45 mmol/g	3 eq DIC 3 eq HOBt	41%	89%	83%	30%	67%
D	2-CTC	0.63 mmol/g	3 eq TBEC 3 eq K-Oxyma	90%	95%	88%	75%	60%
E	2-CTC	0.69 mmol/g	3 eq TBEC 3 eq Oxy-B	89%	96%	89%	76%	67%
F	2-CTC	0.70 mmol/g	3 eq TBEC 3 eq K-Oxy-B	93%	94%	91%	80%	59%

[a] The HPLC purities were obtained by integrating the peak areas at 220 nm.

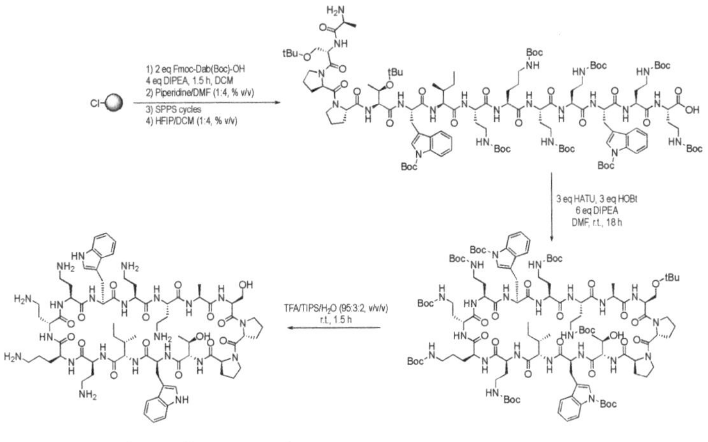

Scheme 1. Synthesis of murepavadin.

Two different trityl-based solid supports (2-CTC and Cl-Trt) were evaluated (Figure 3). In the conditions used, we found that the synthesis performed using 2-CTC resin (Table 1, synthesis A) yielded higher loading in comparison to Cl-Trt (Table 1, synthesis C). Dealing with highly functionalized resins can sometimes be disadvantageous, especially when treating with difficult peptide sequences, as they can lead to uncomplete acylation and make re-coupling of the amino acids necessary [43,44]. However, in the present case, the assembly was quite straightforward, and only a few re-couplings were needed in some of the syntheses performed. According to the results, 2-CTC seems to be a better option than Cl-Trt in terms of loading and overall yield (Tables 1 and 2). Therefore, 2-CTC was the resin of choice in this study.

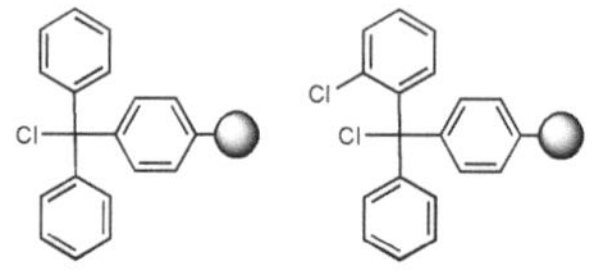

Figure 3. Trityl-based polystyrene solid supports: trityl chloride resin (**left**), 2-chlorotrityl chloride resin (**right**).

Table 2. Purification and global yields for each of the syntheses performed.

Synthesis	Resin	Coupling Agents	Purification Yield	Global Yield
A	2-CTC	3 eq DIC 3 eq HOBt	29%	12%
B	2-CTC	3 eq DIC 3 eq K-Oxyma	40%	28%
C	Cl-Trt	3 eq DIC 3 eq HOBt	45%	14%
D	2-CTC	3 eq TBEC 3 eq K-Oxyma	36%	27%
E	2-CTC	3 eq TBEC 3 eq Oxy-B	39%	30%
F	2-CTC	3 eq TBEC 3 eq K-Oxy-B	34%	27%

When HOBt was used as the additive in carbodiimide (DIC) acylations, a low resin detachment yield was observed in both cases (entries A and C, Table 1). This result could be expected according to the literature since the use of HOBt has been described to cause premature peptide cleavage during assembly on 2-CTC resin due to its acidic character [13]. Similarly, OxymaPure (Luxembourg Bio Technologies, Ness Ziona, Israel) has also been reported to cause the same problem of peptide losses. For this reason, we decided to perform the synthesis using K-Oxyma (a conjugated base of OxymaPure) instead of HOBt or OxymaPure [18]. The resin detachment yield increased from 46 to 91% on the 2-CTC resin (entry B).

We then decided to test the novel protocol involving TBEC. Originally, the TBEC protocol was developed to avoid the formation of oxadiazole and HCN due to the reaction of DIC and OxymaPure [21,22]. In order to avoid losses during the assembly, we used TBEC in combination with K-Oxyma and the newly described additives Oxy-B and its conjugate base K-Oxy-B [18,21,45,46]. According to the literature, the use of K-Oxyma prevents premature peptide detachment from 2-chlorotrityl resin. Our results show that both Oxy-B and K-Oxy-B additives performed satisfactorily from this point of view. All syntheses rendered comparable detachment yields, ranging from 89 to 93% (entries D to F), and much better than the HOBt-based assemblies and similar to DIC/K-Oxyma. This fact could be attributed to the lower acidic character of Oxy-B (pK_a 8.20) in comparison with the higher acidity of HOBt and OxymaPure (the pKa for both is 4.60) [20]. Finally, it can be seen that both Oxy-B and K-Oxy-B performed similarly well. Therefore, there is no apparent need to prepare the corresponding conjugate base of Oxy-B.

In all syntheses, after the acidolysis of the peptidyl resins, the linear protected peptide was cyclized. Macrolactamization was performed in solution using HATU, HOBt, and DIPEA (3:3:6 mole ratio) according to the literature [38]. The cyclization yields ranged from 89 to 96%. It is worth mentioning that this reaction was monitored by ninhydrin since both the linear and cyclic protected peptides did not elute by HPLC using ACN/H_2O mixtures.

Total deprotection was achieved by treatment with TFA/TIPS/H_2O (95:3:2, *v*/*v*/*v*%) to obtain the cyclic deprotected peptide. After precipitation in anhydrous diethyl ether and isolation of the crude peptides, the yields ranged from 83 to 91%.

The assessment of the purity of the different batches was not a straightforward task. As mentioned before, murepavadin contains a DPro-Pro moiety within the sequence. It is well known that proline residues may lead to conformational equilibria due to the possibility of significant populations of both the *cis* and *trans* conformers [47,48]. When assessing purity, we sometimes found out that two peaks with the same m/z ratio were obtained by HPLC-MS (Figure 4d,g). However, if the samples (previously lyophilized) were pre-heated to 50 °C for 30 min or the chromatography was performed using an oven at 50 °C, the coalescence of peaks took place into a single major peak (Figure 4e,f,h). In all cases, the purity was determined by the integration of peaks at 220 nm corresponding to a m/z ratio of a 777.9 mass unit, which corresponds to the $[M+2H^+]^{+2}$ ion, as determined by ESI-MS.

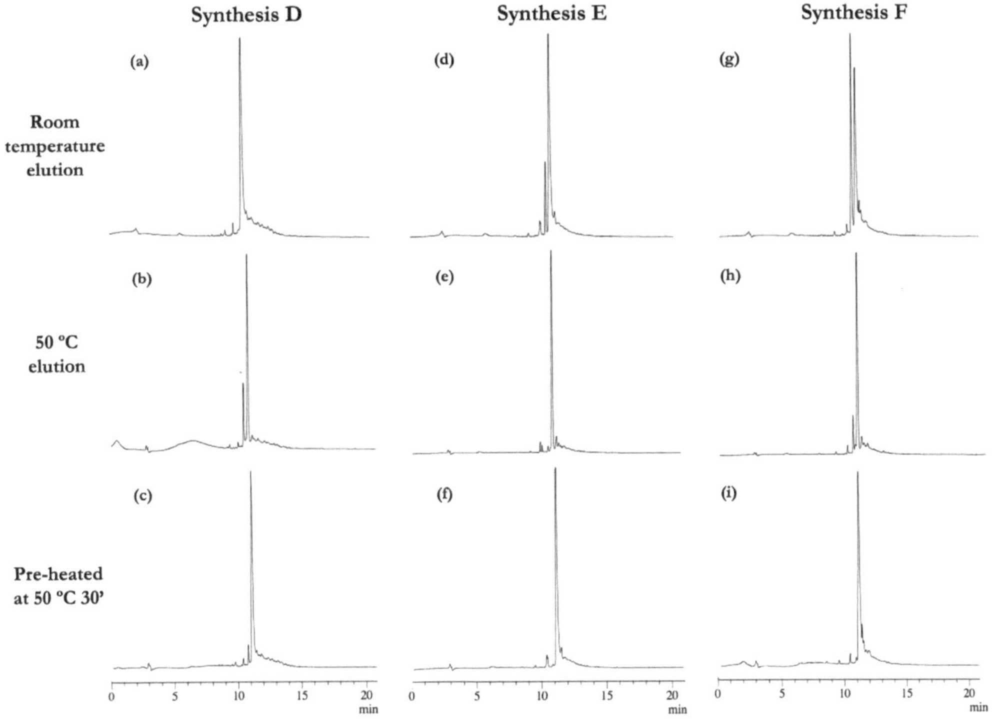

Figure 4. Chromatograms of murepavadin crudes obtained after treating the protected peptide crude with TFA/TIPS/H_2O (95:3:2, *v*/*v*/*v*) using different chromatographic conditions: (**a**) Synthesis D, HPLC 25 °C, (**b**) Synthesis D, HPLC column *T* set to 50 °C, (**c**) Synthesis D, sample pre-heating 50 °C, (**d**) Synthesis E, HPLC 25 °C, (**e**) Synthesis E, HPLC column *T* set to 50 °C, (**f**) Synthesis E, sample pre-heating 50 °C, (**g**) Synthesis F, HPLC 25 °C, (**h**) Synthesis F, HPLC column *T* set to 50 °C, (**i**) Synthesis F, sample pre-heating 50 °C.

The final overall crude yields ranged from 70 to 80% in all cases except those involving the use of HOBt (30–40%). Crude purities went from 58 to 67%. Hence, the use of K-Oxyma, Oxy-B, and K-Oxy-B yielded similar good results. The highest purity (67%) was obtained for the combination of TBEC/Oxy-B in the 2-CTC resin, as shown in Table 1 and Figure 4.

After purification by semipreparative HPLC, all the murepavadin batches were obtained with a purity higher than 99%. As seen in Table 2, global yields of synthesis A and

C were clearly affected by premature loss during the peptide assembly due to the acidic nature of HOBt. In comparison, the syntheses performed using K-Oxyma, Oxy-B, and K-Oxy-B rendered much higher yields (Table 2 and Syntheses B, D, E, and F). As expected, the higher yields and purities obtained for the crudes were reflected in the global yield after purification. Oxy-B is as effective as its conjugate base; hence, there is no need to prepare the potassium salt of Oxy-B (K-Oxy-B) in clear contrast to the pair OxymaPure/K-Oxyma described in the literature. In our hands, the best yield for the total synthesis of murepavadin in the 2-CTC resin was obtained for the acylating agents TBEC/Oxy-B.

3.2. Antimicrobial Activity Determination of the Different Murepavadin Batches

As mentioned before, murepavadin exhibits potent activity against *P. aeruginosa* by targeting the periplasmatic β-jellyroll domain of the LptD protein of this bacteria. It is well known that drug–protein interactions are stereospecific, and studies have shown that murepavadin exerts its antipseudomonal activity by means of a mechanism of action involving a chiral receptor [49,50]. In this sense, we wanted to confirm the chiral integrity of the murepavadin purified batches by assessing their in vitro antibacterial activity. Antimicrobial activity was determined in terms of minimal inhibitory concentrations (MICs) by the broth dilution method and following the CLSI guidelines.

All murepavadin batches were tested against three different *P. aeruginosa* strains. Two of them (DSM 24600 [51] and DSM 25716 [52]) were resistant to ß-lactam antibiotics. *P. aeruginosa* DSM 24600 produces extended-spectrum ß-lactamase (ESBL) and is carbapenem-resistant (Genotype blaVIM-1). *P. aeruginosa* DSM 25716 is resistant to carbapenems (i.e., imipenem) as it expresses a VIM ß-lactamase but it does not produce extended-spectrum ß-lactamases (ESBL).

As seen in Table 3, this cyclic peptide exerts a potent antipseudomonal activity, with *P. aeruginosa* DSM 24600 being the most susceptible strain. The MIC values are in the range of those found in the literature (0.008–0.25 μg·mL^{-1}) [36,38]. No differences were observed between the different batches, which indicates that the chiral integrity of the molecule was preserved in the different syntheses of murepavadin.

Table 3. MIC values (μg·mL^{-1}) for the different batches of murepavadin.

	A	B	C	D	E	F
P. aeruginosa ATCC 27853	0.0625	0.0625	0.0625	0.0625	0.0625	0.0625
P. aeruginosa DSM 24600	0.03125	0.03125	0.03125	0.03125	0.03125	0.03125
P. aeruginosa DSM 25716	0.25	0.25	0.25	0.25	0.25	0.25

4. Conclusions

The preparation of murepavadin, a complex macrocyclic peptide antibiotic, was successfully achieved. Its assembly was accomplished using different resins and coupling reagents. Regarding the resin, 2-CTC was preferred over Cl-Trt, as the loading obtained with this solid support was higher, and the peptide assembly was quite straightforward. When using HOBt in combination with the standard carbodiimide DIC for peptide assembly, low detachment yields were obtained (41–46%), indicating premature cleavage of the peptide chains, probably due to the acidic nature of this additive. The cleavage yield was improved (91%) when the conjugate base of OxymaPure, K-Oxyma, was used with DIC. Also, different oxyma-based additives were used in combination with a relatively new carbodiimide, TBEC, and proved to be as effective as the system DIC/K-Oxyma in terms of cleavage yield (89–93%). The use of K-Oxyma/DIC, Oxy-B/TBEC, and K-Oxy-B/TBEC yielded similar good yields and purities. Oxy-B is as effective as its conjugate base; hence, there is no need to prepare the potassium salt of Oxy-B (K-Oxy-B) in clear contrast to the pair OxymaPure/K-Oxyma. Altogether, the best yield for the total synthesis of murepavadin was obtained using the 2-CTC resin and the acylating agents TBEC/Oxy-B. Chromatographic elution by HPLC at a high temperature (50 °C or pre-heating samples at 50 °C) was necessary for the correct assessment of murepavadin crude purity.

Finally, the antimicrobial activity of the different synthetic batches was tested in three *P. aeruginosa* strains, including highly resistant varieties that consisted of two carbapenem-resistant strains and an ESBL producer. All murepavadin batches yielded the same MIC values, which demonstrates that the chiral integrity of the molecule was preserved throughout the whole synthetic procedure.

Supplementary Materials: The following supporting information can be downloaded at: https://www.mdpi.com/article/10.3390/biom14050526/s1, Table S1: Quantities obtained in each step of the synthesis of murepavadin for the different batches; Figure S1: HPLC and MS analysis of K-Oxy-B; Figures S2–S7: HPLC and MS analysis of murepavadin batches A to F.

Author Contributions: Conceptualization, F.R. and Y.C.; investigation, J.G.-G. and A.M.M.; writing—original draft preparation, J.G.-G. and F.R.; writing—review and editing, F.R., J.G.-G., A.M.M., and Y.C.; funding acquisition, F.R. All authors have read and agreed to the published version of the manuscript.

Funding: This research was funded by the AEI of the Ministry of Science, Innovation and Universities [European project Muryxin, JPI-AMR-2022-066 DRUID call, PCI2023-143362, and PID2021-124342OB-I00]. J.G-G discloses support for the execution of her doctoral thesis from the Agència de Gestió d'Ajuts Universitaris i de Recerca (FISDU 00155, Generalitat de Catalunya) and Grup de Recerca de la Generalitat de Catalunya (2021 SGR 00288).

Institutional Review Board Statement: Not applicable.

Informed Consent Statement: Not applicable.

Data Availability Statement: Dara are contained within the article and Supplementary Materials.

Acknowledgments: We want to thank Josep Martí (Section of Organic Chemistry, UB) for his invaluable support and advice with the ESI-MS analyses. We also acknowledge the generous gift of TBEC and Oxy-B from Luxembourg Biotechnologies.

Conflicts of Interest: The authors declare no conflicts of interest.

References

1. Lau, J.L.; Dunn, M.K. Therapeutic Peptides: Historical Perspectives, Current Development Trends, and Future Directions. *Bioorg. Med. Chem.* **2018**, *26*, 2700–2707. [CrossRef] [PubMed]
2. Al Musaimi, O.; Al Shaer, D.; Albericio, F.; de la Torre, B.G. 2020 FDA TIDES (Peptides and Oligonucleotides) Harvest. *Pharmaceuticals* **2021**, *14*, 145. [CrossRef] [PubMed]
3. Wang, L.; Wang, N.; Zhang, W.; Cheng, X.; Yan, Z.; Shao, G.; Wang, X.; Wang, R.; Fu, C. Therapeutic Peptides: Current Applications and Future Directions. *Signal. Transduct. Target. Ther.* **2022**, *7*, 48. [CrossRef] [PubMed]
4. Merrifield, R.B. Solid Phase Peptide Synthesis. I. The Synthesis of a Tetrapeptide. *J. Am. Chem. Soc.* **1963**, *85*, 2149–2154. [CrossRef]
5. Segovia, R.; Díaz-Lobo, M.; Cajal, Y.; Vilaseca, M.; Rabanal, F. Linker-Free Synthesis of Antimicrobial Peptides Using a Novel Cleavage Reagent: Characterisation of the Molecular and Ionic Composition by NanoESI-HR MS. *Pharmaceutics* **2023**, *15*, 1310. [CrossRef]
6. El-Faham, A.; Albericio, F. Peptide Coupling Reagents, More than a Letter Soup. *Chem. Rev.* **2011**, *111*, 6557–6602. [CrossRef] [PubMed]
7. Al-Warhi, T.I.; Al-Hazimi, H.M.A.; El-Faham, A. Recent Development in Peptide Coupling Reagents. *J. Saudi Chem. Soc.* **2012**, *16*, 97–116. [CrossRef]
8. Albericio, F.; El-Faham, A. Choosing the Right Coupling Reagent for Peptides: A Twenty-Five-Year Journey. *Org. Process Res. Dev.* **2018**, *22*, 760–772. [CrossRef]
9. Carpino, L.A.; Imazumi, H.; El-Faham, A.; Ferrer, F.J.; Zhang, C.; Lee, Y.; Foxman, B.M.; Henklein, P.; Hanay, C.; Wenschuh, H.; et al. The Uronium/Guanidinium Peptide Coupling Reagents: Finally the True Uronium Salts. *Angew. Chem. Int. Ed.* **2002**, *41*, 441–445. [CrossRef]
10. Coste, J.; Lenguyen, D.; Castro, B. PyBOP®: A New Peptide Coupling Reagent Devoid of Toxic by-Product. *Tetrahedron. Lett.* **1990**, *31*, 205–208. [CrossRef]
11. Carpino, L.A.; El-Faham, A.; Minorb, C.A.; Albericio, F. Advantageous Applications of Azabenzotriazole (Triazolopyridine)-Based Coupling Reagents to Solid-Phase Peptide Synthesis. *J. Chem. Soc. Chem. Commun.* **1994**, 201–203. [CrossRef]

12. Carpino, L.A. 1-Hydroxy-7-Azabenzotriazole. An Efficient Peptide Coupling Additive. *J. Chem. Soc. Chem. Commun.* **1970**, *103*, 858. [CrossRef]
13. Spengler, J.; Fernandez-Llamazares, A.I.; Albericio, F. Use of an Internal Reference for the Quantitative HPLC-UV Analysis of Solid-Phase Reactions: A Case Study of 2-Chlorotrityl Chloride Resin. *ACS Comb. Sci.* **2013**, *15*, 229–234. [CrossRef]
14. Wehrstedt, K.D.; Wandrey, P.A.; Heitkamp, D. Explosive Properties of 1-Hydroxybenzotriazoles. *J. Hazard. Mater.* **2005**, *126*, 1–7. [CrossRef] [PubMed]
15. Itoh, M. Racemization Suppression by the Use of Ethyl 2-Hydroximino-2-Cyanoacetate and Its Amide. *Bull. Chem. Soc. Jpn.* **1973**, *46*, 2219–2221. [CrossRef]
16. Subirós-Funosas, R.; Prohens, R.; Barbas, R.; El-Faham, A.; Albericio, F. Oxyma: An Efficient Additive for Peptide Synthesis to Replace the Benzotriazole-Based HOBt and HOAt with a Lower Risk of Explosion. *Chem.—A Eur. J.* **2009**, *15*, 9394–9403. [CrossRef]
17. El-Faham, A.; Albericio, F. COMU: A Third Generation of Uronium-Type Coupling Reagents. *J. Pept. Sci.* **2010**, *16*, 6–9. [CrossRef] [PubMed]
18. Cherkupally, P.; Acosta, G.A.; Nieto-Rodriguez, L.; Spengler, J.; Rodriguez, H.; Khattab, S.N.; El-Faham, A.; Shamis, M.; Luxembourg, Y.; Prohens, R.; et al. K-Oxyma: A Strong Acylation-Promoting, 2-Ctc Resin-Friendly Coupling Additive. *Eur. J. Org. Chem.* **2013**, *28*, 6372–6378. [CrossRef]
19. McFarland, A.D.; Buser, J.Y.; Embry, M.C.; Held, C.B.; Kolis, S.P. Generation of Hydrogen Cyanide from the Reaction of Oxyma (Ethyl Cyano(Hydroxyimino)Acetate) and DIC (Diisopropylcarbodiimide). *Org. Process. Res. Dev.* **2019**, *23*, 2099–2105. [CrossRef]
20. Manne, S.R.; Sharma, A.; Sazonovas, A.; El-Faham, A.; de la Torre, B.G.; Albericio, F. Understanding OxymaPure as a Peptide Coupling Additive: A Guide to New Oxyma Derivatives. *ACS Omega* **2022**, *7*, 6007–6023. [CrossRef]
21. Manne, S.R.; Akintayo, D.C.; Luna, O.; El-Faham, A.; De La Torre, B.G.; Albericio, F. Tert-Butylethylcarbodiimide as an Efficient Substitute for Diisopropylcarbodiimide in Solid-Phase Peptide Synthesis: Understanding the Side Reaction of Carbodiimides with OxymaPure. *Org. Process. Res. Dev.* **2022**, *26*, 2894–2899. [CrossRef]
22. Manne, S.R.; Luna, O.; Acosta, G.A.; Royo, M.; El-Faham, A.; Orosz, G.; De La Torre, B.G.; Albericio, F. Amide Formation: Choosing the Safer Carbodiimide in Combination with OxymaPure to Avoid HCN Release. *Org. Lett.* **2021**, *23*, 6900–6904. [CrossRef] [PubMed]
23. Rabanal, F.; Grau-Campistany, A.; Vila-Farrés, X.; Gonzalez-Linares, J.; Borràs, M.; Vila, J.; Manresa, A.; Cajal, Y. A Bioinspired Peptide Scaffold with High Antibiotic Activity and Low in Vivo Toxicity. *Sci. Rep.* **2015**, *5*, 10558. [CrossRef] [PubMed]
24. Grau-Campistany, A.; Manresa, Á.; Pujol, M.; Rabanal, F.; Cajal, Y. Tryptophan-Containing Lipopeptide Antibiotics Derived from Polymyxin B with Activity against Gram Positive and Gram Negative Bacteria. *Biochim. Biophys. Acta Biomembr.* **2016**, *1858*, 333–343. [CrossRef] [PubMed]
25. Segovia, R.; Solé, J.; Marqués, A.M.; Cajal, Y.; Rabanal, F. Unveiling the Membrane and Cell Wall Action of Antimicrobial Cyclic Lipopeptides: Modulation of the Spectrum of Activity. *Pharmaceutics* **2021**, *13*, 2180. [CrossRef] [PubMed]
26. Rabanal, F.; Cajal, Y. Recent Advances and Perspectives in the Design and Development of Polymyxins. *Nat. Prod. Rep.* **2017**, *34*, 886–908. [CrossRef] [PubMed]
27. Rudilla, H.; Pérez-Guillén, I.; Rabanal, F.; Sierra, J.M.; Vinuesa, T.; Viñas, M. Novel Synthetic Polymyxins Kill Gram-Positive Bacteria. *J. Antimicrob. Chemother.* **2018**, *73*, 3385–3390. [CrossRef] [PubMed]
28. Clausell, A.; Rabanal, F.; Garcia-Subirats, M.; Alsina, M.A.; Cajal, Y. Synthesis and Membrane Action of Polymyxin B Analogues. *Luminescence* **2005**, *20*, 117–123. [CrossRef] [PubMed]
29. Clausell, A.; Rabanal, F.; Garcia-Subirats, M.; Alsina, M.A.; Cajal, Y. Membrane Association and Contact Formation by a Synthetic Analogue of Polymyxin B and Its Fluorescent Derivatives. *J. Phys. Chem. B* **2006**, *110*, 4465–4471. [CrossRef]
30. *Priorization of Pathogens to Guide Discovery, Research and Development of New Antibiotics for Drug-Resistant Bacterial Infections, Including Tuberculosis*; World Health Organization: Geneva, Switzerland, 2017.
31. Martin-Loeches, I.; Dale, G.E.; Torres, A. Murepavadin: A New Antibiotic Class in the Pipeline. *Expert Rev. Anti Infect. Ther.* **2018**, *16*, 259–268. [CrossRef]
32. Shankaramma, S.C.; Athanassiou, Z.; Zerbe, O.; Moehle, K.; Mouton, C.; Bernardini, F.; Vrijbloed, J.W.; Obrecht, D.; Robinson, J.A. Macrocyclic Hairpin Mimetics of the Cationic Antimicrobial Peptide Protegrin I: A New Family of Broad-Spectrum Antibiotics. *ChemBioChem* **2002**, *3*, 1126–1133. [CrossRef]
33. Robinson, J.A.; Shankaramma, S.C.; Jetter, P.; Kienzl, U.; Schwendener, R.A.; Vrijbloed, J.W.; Obrecht, D. Properties and Structure-Activity Studies of Cyclic β-Hairpin Peptidomimetics Based on the Cationic Antimicrobial Peptide Protegrin I. *Bioorg. Med. Chem.* **2005**, *13*, 2055–2064. [CrossRef] [PubMed]
34. Schmidt, J.; Patora-Komisarska, K.; Moehle, K.; Obrecht, D.; Robinson, J.A. Structural Studies of β-Hairpin Peptidomimetic Antibiotics That Target LptD in *Pseudomonas* sp. *Bioorg. Med. Chem.* **2013**, *21*, 5806–5810. [CrossRef] [PubMed]
35. Andolina, G.; Bencze, L.C.; Zerbe, K.; Müller, M.; Steinmann, J.; Kocherla, H.; Mondal, M.; Sobek, J.; Moehle, K.; Malojčić, G.; et al. A Peptidomimetic Antibiotic Interacts with the Periplasmic Domain of LptD from *Pseudomonas aeruginosa*. *ACS Chem. Biol.* **2018**, *13*, 666–675. [CrossRef]
36. Sader, H.S.; Dale, G.E.; Rhomberg, P.R.; Flamm, R.K. Antimicrobial Activity of Murepavadin Tested against Clinical Isolates of *Pseudomonas aeruginosa* from the United States, Europe, and China. *Antimicrob. Agents Chemother.* **2018**, *62*, e00311–e00318. [CrossRef]

37. Werneburg, M.; Zerbe, K.; Juhas, M.; Bigler, L.; Stalder, U.; Kaech, A.; Ziegler, U.; Obrecht, D.; Eberl, L.; Robinson, J.A. Inhibition of Lipopolysaccharide Transport to the Outer Membrane in *Pseudomonas aeruginosa* by Peptidomimetic Antibiotics. *ChemBioChem* **2012**, *13*, 1767–1775. [CrossRef]
38. Srinivas, N.; Jetter, P.; Ueberbacher, B.J.; Werneburg, M.; Zerbe, K.; Steinmann, J.; Van Der Meijden, B.; Bernardini, F.; Lederer, A.; Dias, R.L.A.; et al. Peptidomimetic Antibiotics Target Outer-Membrane Biogenesis in *Pseudomonas aeruginosa*. *Science* **2010**, *327*, 1010–1013. [CrossRef]
39. Díez-Aguilar, M.; Hernández-García, M.; Morosini, M.I.; Fluit, A.; Tunney, M.M.; Huertas, N.; Del Campo, R.; Obrecht, D.; Bernardini, F.; Ekkelenkamp, M.; et al. Murepavadin Antimicrobial Activity against and Resistance Development in Cystic Fibrosis *Pseudomonas aeruginosa* Isolates. *J. Antimicrob. Chemother.* **2021**, *76*, 984–992. [CrossRef]
40. Spexis Reports Solid Safety and Pharmacokinetics Results from First-in-Human Study with Inhaled Murepavadin, a Novel Macrocycle Compound. Available online: https://www.globenewswire.com/news-release/2023/01/09/2584785/0/en/Spexis-reports-solid-safety-and-pharmacokinetics-results-from-first-in-human-study-with-inhaled-murepavadin-a-novel-macrocycle-compound.html (accessed on 16 April 2024).
41. Obrecht, D.; Luther, A.; Bernardini, F.; Zbinden, P. Beta–Hairpin Peptidomimetics. U.S. Patent 20180044380A1, 2018.
42. Chaudhuri, D.; Ganesan, R.; Vogelaar, A.; Dughbaj, M.A.; Beringer, P.M.; Camarero, J.A. Chemical Synthesis of a Potent Antimicrobial Peptide Murepavadin Using a Tandem Native Chemical Ligation/Desulfurization Reaction. *J. Org. Chem.* **2021**, *86*, 15242–15246. [CrossRef] [PubMed]
43. Mueller, L.K.; Baumruck, A.C.; Zhdanova, H.; Tietze, A.A. Challenges and Perspectives in Chemical Synthesis of Highly Hydrophobic Peptides. *Front. Bioeng. Biotechnol.* **2020**, *8*, 162. [CrossRef]
44. Isidro-Llobet, A.; Kenworthy, M.N.; Mukherjee, S.; Kopach, M.E.; Wegner, K.; Gallou, F.; Smith, A.G.; Roschangar, F. Sustainability Challenges in Peptide Synthesis and Purification: From R&D to Production. *J. Org. Chem.* **2019**, *84*, 4615–4628. [CrossRef] [PubMed]
45. Jad, Y.E.; Khattab, S.N.; De La Torre, B.G.; Govender, T.; Kruger, H.G.; El-Faham, A.; Albericio, F. Oxyma-B, an Excellent Racemization Suppressor for Peptide Synthesis. *Org. Biomol. Chem.* **2014**, *12*, 8379–8385. [CrossRef] [PubMed]
46. Jad, Y.E.; Khattab, S.N.; de la Torre, B.G.; Govender, T.; Kruger, H.G.; El-Faham, A.; Albericio, F. EDC·HCl and Potassium Salts of Oxyma and Oxyma-B as Superior Coupling Cocktails for Peptide Synthesis. *Eur. J. Org. Chem.* **2015**, *2015*, 3116–3120. [CrossRef]
47. O'Neal, K.D.; Chari, M.V.; Mcdonald, C.H.; Cook, R.G.; Li-Yuan, Y.-L.; Morrisett, J.D.; Shearer, W.T. Multiple Cis-Trans Conformers of the Prolactin Receptor Proline-Rich Motif (PRM) Peptide Detected by Reverse-Phase HPLC, CD and NMR Spectroscopy. *Biochem. J.* **1996**, *315*, 833–844. [CrossRef]
48. Sui, Q.; Rabenstein, D.L. Cis/Trans Isomerization of Proline Peptide Bonds in the Backbone of Cyclic Disulfide-Bridged Peptides. *Pept. Sci.* **2018**, *110*, e24088. [CrossRef]
49. Upert, G.; Luther, A.; Obrecht, D.; Ermert, P. Emerging Peptide Antibiotics with Therapeutic Potential. *Med. Drug Discov.* **2021**, *9*, 100078. [CrossRef]
50. Zerbe, K.; Moehle, K.; Robinson, J.A. Protein Epitope Mimetics: From New Antibiotics to Supramolecular Synthetic Vaccines. *Acc. Chem. Res.* **2017**, *50*, 1323–1331. [CrossRef]
51. BacDive The Bacterial Diversity Metadatabase. *Pseudomonas aeruginosa* DSM 24600. Available online: https://bacdive.dsmz.de/strain/12803 (accessed on 22 February 2024).
52. BacDive The Bacterial Diversity Metadatabase. *Pseudomonas aeruginosa* DSM 25716. Available online: https://bacdive.dsmz.de/strain/12805 (accessed on 22 February 2024).

biomolecules

MDPI

Article

Analysis of Self-Assembled Low- and High-Molecular-Weight Poly-L-Lysine–Ce6 Conjugate-Based Nanoparticles

Minho Seo [1,†], Kyeong-Ju Lee [1,†], Bison Seo [2], Jun-Hyuck Lee [1], Jae-Hyeon Lee [1], Dong-Wook Shin [2] and Jooho Park [1,2,*]

[1] BK21 Program, Department of Applied Life Science, Konkuk University, Chungju 27478, Republic of Korea
[2] College of Biomedical and Health Science (RIBHS), Konkuk University, Chungju 27478, Republic of Korea
* Correspondence: pkjhdn@kku.ac.kr
† These authors contributed equally to this work.

Abstract: In cancer therapy, photodynamic therapy (PDT) has attracted significant attention due to its high potential for tumor-selective treatment. However, PDT agents often exhibit poor physicochemical properties, including solubility, necessitating the development of nanoformulations. In this study, we developed two cationic peptide-based self-assembled nanomaterials by using a PDT agent, chlorin e6 (Ce6). To manufacture biocompatible nanoparticles based on peptides, we used the cationic poly-L-lysine peptide, which is rich in primary amines. We prepared low- and high-molecular-weight poly-L-lysine, and then evaluated the formation and performance of nanoparticles after chemical conjugation with Ce6. The results showed that both molecules formed self-assembled nanoparticles by themselves in saline. Interestingly, the high-molecular-weight poly-L-lysine and Ce6 conjugates (HPLCe6) exhibited better self-assembly and PDT performance than low-molecular-weight poly-L-lysine and Ce6 conjugates (LPLCe6). Moreover, the HPLCe6 conjugates showed superior cellular uptake and exhibited stronger cytotoxicity in cell toxicity experiments. Therefore, it is functionally beneficial to use high-molecular-weight poly-L-lysine in the manufacturing of poly-L-lysine-based self-assembling biocompatible PDT nanoconjugates.

Keywords: photodynamic therapy; anticancer therapy; bioconjugate; peptide derivatives; nanoparticle

Citation: Seo, M.; Lee, K.-J.; Seo, B.; Lee, J.-H.; Lee, J.-H.; Shin, D.-W.; Park, J. Analysis of Self-Assembled Low- and High-Molecular-Weight Poly-L-Lysine–Ce6 Conjugate-Based Nanoparticles. *Biomolecules* **2024**, *14*, 431. https://doi.org/10.3390/biom14040431

Academic Editor: Mathias O. Senge

Received: 22 February 2024
Revised: 26 March 2024
Accepted: 27 March 2024
Published: 2 April 2024

1. Introduction

Research on tumor-selective anticancer therapies, including photodynamic therapy (PDT), has been ongoing for decades [1,2]. Cancer is a fatal and intractable disease that is difficult to treat, and conventional chemotherapy with cytotoxic anticancer drugs has very little selectivity towards tumors, resulting in severe side effects [3]. Although various targeted anticancer therapies have been developed, only a few are effectively and widely used [4–7]. Among them, PDT is a method of inducing cell death used primarily for treating various cancers, utilizing photosensitizers, light of a specific wavelength, and oxygen [8,9]. Various types of PDT have been developed and are being used to fight the growing problem of antimicrobial resistance or treat different cancers such as pancreatic tumors, skin cancer and head and neck cancer [10–13]. In PDT, the excited photosensitizer directly reacts with cellular substrates to produce free radicals and reactive oxygen species (ROS). These reactive species or radicals interact with cellular components, causing damage to lipids, proteins, and nucleic acids, leading to cell death through necrosis or apoptosis [14,15]. ROS or singlet oxygen causes significant damage to cellular components, especially the lipids in cell membranes and mitochondrial membranes, leading to cell death. Using this principle, various PDTs such as vascular targeting PDT, cellular PDT, or upconversion-based PDT have been developed [16,17].

The combination of nanotechnology and PDT has made notable achievements in cancer therapy [18]. Traditionally, PDT agents have shown very poor physicochemical properties and present the problem of reaching only a small part of the tumor area that requires treatment [17]. However, with the recent integration of PDT agents and nanoparticle technologies, several new methods have been developed that significantly enhance the utility of PDT [19,20]. These PDT-based nanoparticles have demonstrated excellent functionality, improved tumor selectivity, and enhanced physicochemical properties, showing great potential as superior therapeutic agents [21,22]. One of the most commonly used PDT agents in nanoparticles is chlorin e6 (Ce6), which has been studied in combination with various nanomaterials [23].

One method of manufacturing PDT nanoparticles involves using peptides to form self-assembling nanoparticles [9,24]. Self-assembly is of particular interest in nanoparticle manufacturing, and it is not difficult to create self-assembling nanoparticles by using both PDT agents and peptides [25–27]. Through this method, many PDT agents have been developed and widely researched in preclinical studies. While countless combinations of peptides are possible, using poly-L-lysine allows for the utilization of its unique cationic nature and the manufacture of nanoparticles that internalize hydrophobic PDT agents [28,29]. Several types of poly-L-lysine-based nanoparticles have been manufactured by using this method, but effective and widely used poly-L-lysine-based PDT nanoparticles have yet to be developed.

In this study, we manufactured and evaluated two types of nanoparticles capable of self-assembly by using two different poly-L-lysine and Ce6 molecules (Figure 1). In particular, we proved through computer simulation how nanoparticles based on poly-L-lysine self-assemble amphiphilically in solvents. Initially, we synthesized and prepared low-molecular-weight poly-L-lysine molecules, while for high-molecular-weight poly-L-lysine (average molecular weight of 50 kDa), we used materials commonly available as reagents. The self-assembly of these two designed materials in aqueous solutions was evaluated through nanoparticle size and charge measurements. We also evaluated their effect on cell apoptosis and their absorption capabilities to compare which size of poly-L-lysine nanoparticles would be ideal for PDT therapy. This research will serve as a foundational study that can help in the clinical development of many PDT-based nanoparticles currently being developed.

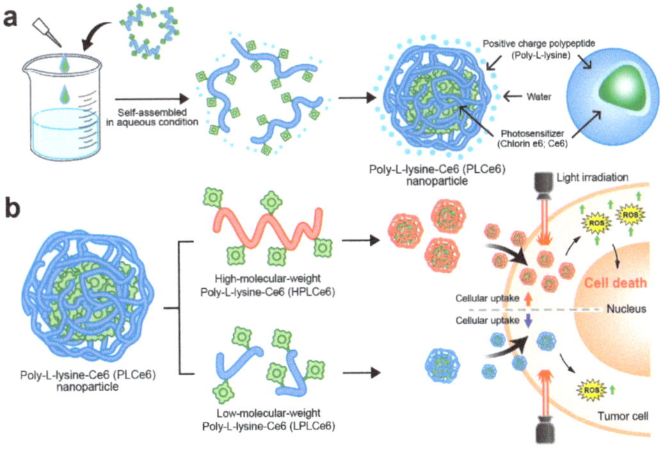

Figure 1. Schematic representation of PLCe6 PDT nanoparticles for cancer treatment through increased cellular uptake. (**a**) PLCe6 can form nanoparticles through self-assembly, based on its amphiphilic drug-based structure; (**b**) upon exposure to visible light, HPLCe6 can induce cytotoxicity due to high cellular uptake, whereas LPLCe6 struggles to induce cytotoxicity due to low cellular uptake.

2. Materials and Methods

2.1. Materials

Antibiotic/antimycotic solution (100×), acetonitrile (ACN), anhydrous dimethyl sulfoxide (DMSO), Dulbecco's modified Eagle's medium (DMEM), 1-ethyl-3-(3-dimethyl aminopropyl)carbodiimide (EDC), ethanol, L-lysine monohydrochloride (Lys), poly-L-lysine hydrobromide (HPL; average molecular weight of 50 kDa), *N*-hydroxysuccinimide (NHS), 2-(*N*-morpholino)ethanesulfonic acid monohydrate (MES monohydrate), phosphate-buffered saline (PBS), trifluoroacetic acid (TFA), and 2-(4-amidinophenyl)-6-indolecarbamidine dihydrochloride (DAPI) were purchased from Sigma-Aldrich (St. Louis, MO, USA). Fetal bovine serum (FBS) was obtained from Gibco (Waltham, MA, USA) and chlorin e6 (Ce6) was obtained from Leap Chem (Hong Kong). An EZ-cytox kit was obtained from DoGenBio (Seoul, Republic of Korea).

2.2. Preparation and Characterization of PL Nanoparticles

Initially, low-molecular-weight poly-L-lysine (LPL) was synthesized by utilizing the amino acid L-lysine with peptide coupling reagents. Specifically, L-lysine (Lys; 50 mg, 273.75 µmol), N-hydroxysuccinimide (NHS; 236.3 mg, 2.05 mmol), and 1-ethyl-3-(3-dimethyl aminopropyl)carbodiimide (EDC; 787.2 mg, 4.11 mmol) were sequentially dissolved in 2-morpholinoethanesulfonic acid (MES) buffer (5 mL, pH 5) and reacted for 24 h. Subsequently, the reaction was quenched by adding 1 N NaOH (1 mL) to adjust the pH to 10, followed by the addition of deionized water (DW) (4 mL) and lyophilization for 2 days. The freeze-dried mixture was then centrifuged at 3000 rpm for 5 min in ethanol to remove the unreacted EDC and NHS molecules, a process repeated four times. The residual organic solvent was removed by using a rotary evaporator, and the final product, LPL, was lyophilized for an additional 2 days. The molecular weight of the synthesized LPL (average molecular weight = 768.1 Da) was confirmed by using matrix-assisted laser desorption/ionization time-of-flight mass spectrometry (MALDI-TOF MS, AXIMA Performance, Kyoto, Japan) by ANYGEN (Gwangju, Republic of Korea).

Next, to fabricate nanoparticles that self-assemble in aqueous solutions, various ratios of Ce6 and LPL (LPL–Ce6 synthesis ratio 1:1, 1:2.5, or 1:5) and HPL (HPL–Ce6 synthesis ratio 1:10, 1:25, or 1:50) were conjugated by using the EDC/NHS reaction. For the synthesis of LPLCe6, LPL (15 mg, 19.53 µmol), Ce6 (11.65 mg, 19.52 µmol), NHS (6.74 mg, 58.56 µmol), and EDC (18.72 mg, 97.65 µmol) were dissolved in DW/DMSO (1:9 *v*/*v*, 6 mL). The solution was stirred at 25 °C for 24 h, purified by centrifugation in cold acetone at 4 °C at 3000 rpm, a step repeated three times, and then lyophilized to obtain LPLCe6 powder.

In the preparation of HPLCe6, HPL (15 mg, 0.3 µmol), Ce6 (1.79 mg, 3.00 µmol), NHS (1.04 mg, 9.04 µmol), and EDC (2.88 mg, 15.02 µmol) were dissolved in DW/DMSO (1:9 *v*/*v*, 6 mL) and stirred at 25 °C for 24 h. The mixture was then purified by centrifugation in cold acetone at 4 °C at 3000 rpm, a step repeated three times, and lyophilized to obtain HPLCe6 powder.

The conjugation of poly-L-lysine and Ce6 was verified by using UV–vis spectroscopy. Ce6, LPLCe6, and HPLCe6 were dissolved in anhydrous DMSO (1 mL), and their absorbance was measured with a SPECTROstar Nano spectrophotometer (BMG Labtech, Ortenberg, Germany). The purified LPLCe6 and HPLCe6 molecules were analyzed by using reverse-phase high-performance liquid chromatography (RP-HPLC) (1200 series, Agilent Technologies, Santa Clara, CA, USA). The RP-HPLC analysis utilized an Eclipse Plus C18 reverse-phase column (4.6 mm × 150 mm, 3.5 µm) with a gradient elution method. The mobile phase consisted of water with 0.1% trifluoroacetic acid (TFA) (90–10%) and acetonitrile with 0.1% TFA (10–90%), at a flow rate of 1 mL/min, with impurities detected by using a UV–vis detector at a wavelength of 405 nm.

2.3. Computer Simulation

Before the simulations, structures of LPLCe6 and HPLCe6 were generated by using the Pep-FOLD 4 website, producing a total of 20 structures each [30]. The structure with the optimal energy value was selected for further analysis. The structure in PDB format was then transferred to the Discovery Studio program, where the Ce6 structure was conjugated to the side chain of lysine. Subsequently, the structure of Lys–Ce6 was modeled with the PDB reader and manipulator in CHARMM-GUI. The combined structure was modeled by using the module for applying covalent bonds. The simulations were conducted by using the GROMACS 2021_2 program [31]. LPLCe6 and HPLCe6 were parameterized with the CHARMM-36m force field, and parameters were generated by using the CHARMM-GUI web server. Solvation was performed by using the Tip3 water model. Neutralization was achieved by adding chloride ions (Cl^-) and sodium ions (Na^+). A time step of 100 ns was employed, with a cutoff of 1.4 nm for short-range van der Waals and electrostatic interactions. Long-range electrostatics were computed by using the particle mesh Ewald method, employing a Fourier spacing of 0.24 nm and fourth-order interpolation. Bonds were constrained by using the LINCS algorithm. Rigid water temperature coupling utilized the v-rescale thermostat, while pressure coupling was managed by the Berendsen barostat during equilibration and the Parrinello—Rahman barostat during sampling. Simulations were conducted at 300 K and 1 bar. After the completion of the 100 ns MD simulation, the GROMACS energy analysis tool was employed to compare the values of Lennard-Jones and Coulomb interactions. These interactions were evaluated not only between solute and solvent but also between the solute molecules themselves. Furthermore, the resulting nanoparticles were imported into the Discovery Studio program in PDB format to analyze molecular interactions with the Analyze Trajectory tool. To evaluate the degree of aggregation for LPLCe6 and HPLCe6, the Protein Aggregation Analyzer in Discovery Studio was utilized, focusing on individual molecules.

2.4. Nanoparticle Analysis

The hydrodynamic size, distribution, and zeta potential of each PLCe6 nanoparticle ratio were measured after dissolving the substances in saline and saline containing 5% FBS at a concentration of 0.5 mg/mL, by using dynamic light scattering (DLS; Zetasizer Nano, Malvern Instruments, Worcestershire, UK). To indirectly verify the formation of particles under conditions mimicking the in vivo environment, we examined the fluorescence changes of LPLCe6 (1 mg/mL) and HPLCe6 (1 mg/mL) in the presence of various concentrations of NaCl (0–0.9%) by using a SpectraMax M2 microplate reader (Molecular Devices, San Jose, USA, λEx = 660 nm, λEm = 710 nm) ($n = 5$).

2.5. Cellular Uptake Study

To assess the endocytosis capability of LPLCe6 and HPLCe6 nanoparticles, murine colorectal carcinoma cells (CT26.WT) were seeded in a 35 mm confocal dish at a density of 5×10^4 cells/well and cultured for 24 h in high glucose Dulbecco's Modified Eagle's Medium (DMEM) supplemented with 10% fetal bovine serum and 1% antibiotic/antimycotic solution. Subsequently, the cells were treated with LPLCe6 and HPLCe6 at a concentration of 10 µg/mL each and incubated at 37 °C for 3 h. Following incubation, the cells were washed once with phosphate-buffered saline (PBS) and fixed with 4% paraformaldehyde for 10 min. After fixation, cells were stained with 4′,6-diamidino-2-phenylindole (DAPI) in the dark for 10 min to visualize the nuclei. The intracellular localization of the nanoparticles was then imaged with an ECLIPSE Ti2 series microscope (Nikon, Tokyo, Japan).

2.6. In Vitro Cytotoxicity Assay of PLCe6 Nanoparticles

Cytotoxicity was assessed by using the EZ-cytox assay. The CT26.WT cells were seeded in a 96-well cell culture plate using high-glucose Dulbecco's modified Eagle's medium (DMEM) supplemented with 10% fetal bovine serum and 1% antibiotic/antimycotic solution, at a density of 1×10^4 cells per well. The cells were allowed to stabilize for 3 h for attachment before treatment with Ce6, LPLCe6, or HPLCe6. Two independent experiments were conducted, one with laser irradiation and one without. In the experiment with laser irradiation, each well was irradiated with a 635 nm laser at an intensity of 20 mW/cm^2 for 1 min, 2 h after treatment. Following an additional 12 or 24 h incubation period, the cells were washed twice with PBS. Subsequently, the cells were incubated in a DMEM medium containing 10% EZ-cytox solution for 1 h. The absorbance at 450 nm and 600 nm was measured with a SPECTROstar Nano spectrophotometer (BMG Labtech, Ortenberg, Germany) (n = 6).

2.7. Statistical Analysis

Statistical analysis was conducted using GraphPad Prism 9 (GraphPad Software 9.5.0). All experimental data were represented as mean ± standard deviation. A one-way ANOVA test was employed for comparison between two groups, and a p-value of less than 0.05 was considered statistically significant (* $p < 0.05$, ** $p < 0.01$, *** $p < 0.001$).

3. Results

3.1. Preparation of Chlorin e6-Conjugated Poly-L-Lysine (PLCe6) Nanoparticles

We synthesized chlorin e6-conjugated poly-L-lysine (PLCe6) nanoparticles to explore the anticancer efficacy associated with the length of poly-L-lysine (PL). Initially, low-molecular-weight poly-L-lysine (LPL) was prepared through chemical conjugation by using the peptide coupling reagent EDC/NHS (Figure 2a). The molecular weight of the resultant LPL was confirmed via MALDI-TOF mass spectrometry (Figure 2b), which revealed an average molecular weight of 768.1 m/z [5Lys + K + 2Cl + H], indicative of the conjugation of five lysine units. Next, amide bonds were formed between the amine groups of PL and the carboxylic acid groups of Ce6 to achieve the conjugation of different lengths of PL with Ce6. The synthesis was carried out while maintaining the pH of the solution at approximately 6 (Figure 2c).

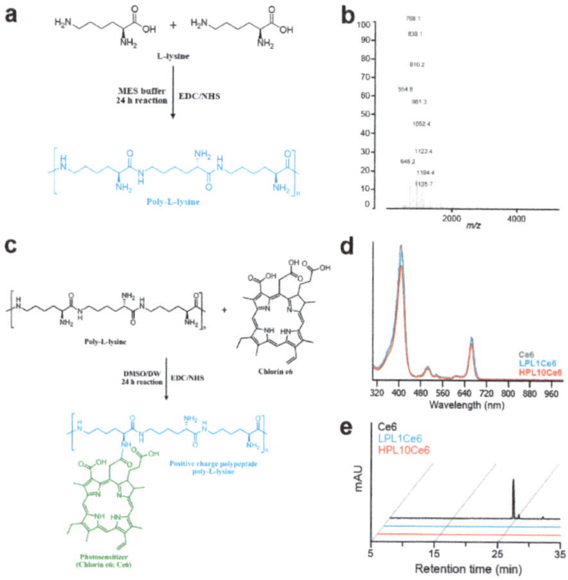

Figure 2. Preparation of LPL and PLCe6. (**a**) Schematic diagram of the structure and chemical synthesis of LPL; (**b**) measurement of the molecular weight of LPL with MALDI-TOF; (**c**) schematic diagram of the structure and chemical synthesis of PLCe6; (**d**) confirmation of the synthesis of LPL1Ce6 and HPL10Ce6 molecules from Ce6 with UV–vis spectroscopy after purification; (**e**) RP-HPLC of Ce6, LPL1Ce6 and HPL10Ce6.

The chemical conjugation of PLCe6 was verified through UV–vis spectroscopy. The synthesized and purified LPL1Ce6 and HPL10Ce6 nanoparticles revealed absorption peaks at 663 or 662 nm (Figure 2d). This shift suggests a change in the molecular structure that affects electron distribution, thus altering the absorption spectrum. Finally, to confirm the complete conjugation of Ce6 to PL without any free Ce6 remaining, reverse-phase high-performance liquid chromatography (RP-HPLC) was employed, showing no detectable free Ce6 (Figure 2e).

3.2. Computer Simulation

In the comparative analysis between LPLCe6 and HPLCe6, it was beneficial to include details on the specific outcomes or insights gained from the in silico experiments. As time progressed, LPLCe6 and HPLCe6 underwent self-assembly in an ion-neutralized solvent model. Nanoparticle formation accelerated around 60 ns, with distinct clustering of nanoparticles observed from approximately 90 ns onwards. At the end of the 100 ns MD simulation, LPLCe6 did not form an assembled structure (Figure 3a). In contrast, HPLCe6 was constructed to form well-defined nanoparticle structures of approximately five molecules (Figure 3b).

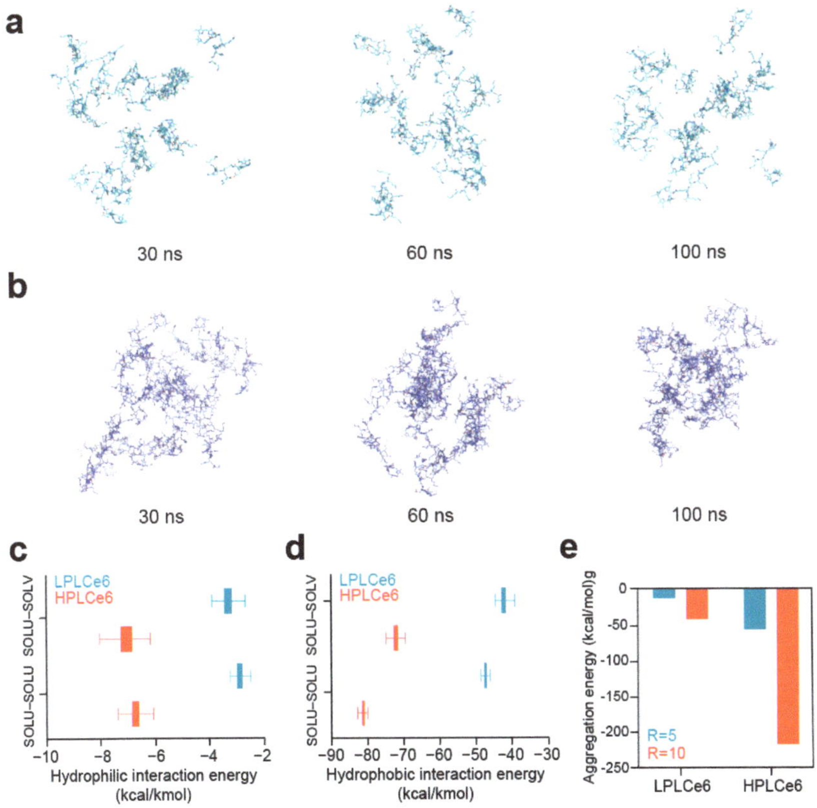

Figure 3. (**a**) LPLCe6 nanoparticle formulation during a 100 ns MD simulation; (**b**) HPLCe6 nanoparticle formulation during a 100 ns MD simulation; (**c**) values for the hydrophilic (Coulomb) interacting energy during the MD simulations of LPLCe6 and HPLCe6; (**d**) hydrophobic (Lennard-Jones) interaction energy during the MD simulations of LPLCe6 and HPLCe6; (**e**) aggregation score for single molecules for HPLCe6 and LPLCe6.

LPLCe6 exhibited relatively low levels of particle cohesion and interaction energy compared to HPLCe6. This is attributed to HPLCe6 comprising 20 Lys amino acids and 4 Ce6 molecules, displaying sufficient amphiphilicity, whereas LPLCe6, composed of 1 Ce6 and 5 lysine molecules, shows relatively low hydrophobicity, making it difficult to exhibit amphiphilicity. Moreover, due to its sufficient molecular size, HPLCe6 can form a 'theoretical' particle as a single molecule. In contrast, LPLCe6, with its smaller molecular size, cannot form a particle shape as a single molecule and requires the aggregation of two or more molecules for interaction (Figure 3c). Even if interactions were formed, it was found that the gap between the hydrophobic and hydrophilic regions was too narrow for smooth particle formation. In summary, the analysis of nanoparticle morphology revealed that in the longer HPLCe6, the hydrophobic Ce6 portion formed a hydrophobic core within the HPLCe6 nanoparticle, while the hydrophilic lysine remained exposed outwardly, interacting with the solvent. Additionally, numerical values for the Lennard-Jones and Coulomb interactions were observed in 100 ns of MD simulation. Lennard-Jones energy is primarily attributed to van der Waals interactions such as London dispersion forces and radius absorption, categorizing them as hydrophobic interactions. Conversely, Coulomb energy mainly encompasses hydrogen bonding, ion interactions, etc., these being classified as hydrophilic interactions. Therefore, the interactions mediated by Ce6 in LPLCe6 and HPLCe6, representing hydrophobic interactions, and those influenced by lysine, indicating hydrophilic interactions, were described with such energy terms.

The interaction energies between solvent and solute were also evaluated in a similar manner to consider the extent of solute–solvent interactions. As a result, the average Lennard-Jones interaction of HPLCe6 was lower than that of HPLCe6 (Figure 3d). The interparticle interaction of LPLCe6, measured at −2.90 Kcal/Kmol, was approximately 2.3 times lower than that of LPLCe6, which stood at −6.75. Additionally, the LPLCe6 interactions with solvent, characterized by LPLCe6 (−3.31), were lower compared to HPLCe6 (−7.07). Furthermore, the average Coulomb interactions of LPLCe6 were also weaker than those of HPLCe6 (Figure 3e). In terms of interparticle interactions, LPLCe6 exhibited values over 1.7 times lower than HPLCe6, with LPLCe6 (−47.45) against LPLCe6 (−81.04). Similarly, solvent–solute interactions showcased values over 1.7 times lower for LPLCe6 (−42.31) compared to HPLCe6 (−72.21). Only HPLCe6 could theoretically form a nanoparticle from a single molecule, accelerating nanoparticle formation. The presence of Lys–Ce6 facilitated aggregation of the poly-L-lysine structure, confirmed through calculations of aggregation scores by using the Analyze Protein Aggregation module. In single molecules, LPLCe6 with only one Ce6 molecule had an average aggregation score of −0.176 for four lysines, whereas HPLCe6 with four Ce6 molecules had a score of −0.619, indicating increased energy due to Ce6's hydrophobicity contrasting with the hydrophilicity of lysine.

3.3. Characterization of PLCe6 Nanoparticles

The optimization of LPLCe6 and HPLCe6 nanoparticles was conducted across various ratios to assess their size, stability, and zeta potential. Due to the amphiphilic nature resulting from the conjugation of the cationic peptide (PL) with the hydrophobic drug (Ce6), PLCe6 nanoparticles demonstrated stability in saline. The diameter of LPLCe6 nanoparticles increased with the amount of Ce6 conjugated to LPL. Specifically, diameters for the ratios (LPL1Ce6, LPL2.5Ce6, and LPL5Ce6) were measured at 474.1 ± 44.1 nm, 789.3 ± 210.7 nm, and 1337 ± 292 nm, respectively, indicating an increase in both diameter and distribution (Figure 4a). Concurrently, the zeta potential showed a gradual decrease to 15.31 ± 0.45, 13.87 ± 1.09, and 11.84 ± 0.62 for each respective ratio, suggesting challenges in nanoparticle formation control due to increased hydrophobic interactions among Ce6 molecules as the Ce6 conjugation ratio rose (Figure 4b). For further experiments, LPL1Ce6 was selected for its relatively higher particle stability and denoted simply as LPLCe6.

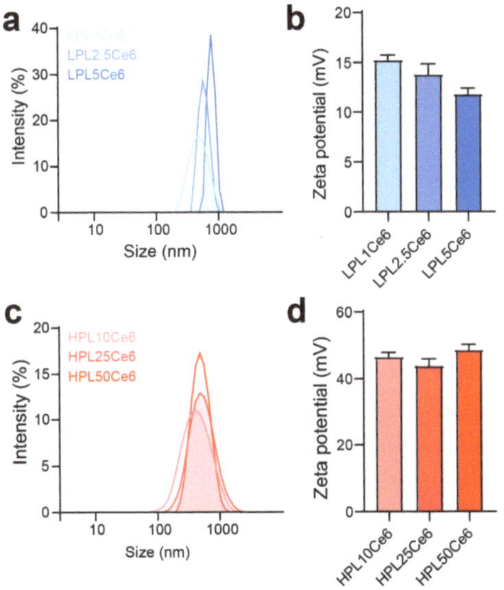

Figure 4. Optimization preparation of PLCe6. (**a**) Size distribution of LPL1Ce6, LPL2.5Ce6, and LPL5Ce6 confirmed through DLS. Results are presented as mean ± SD ($n = 3$). (**b**) Zeta potential of LPL1Ce6, LPL2.5Ce6, and LPL5Ce6. Results are shown as mean ± SD ($n = 3$). (**c**) Size distribution of HPL10Ce6, HPL25Ce6, and PL50Ce6 confirmed through DLS. Results are presented as mean ± SD ($n = 3$). (**d**) Zeta potential of HPL10Ce6, HPL25Ce6, and HPL50Ce6. Results are shown as mean ± SD ($n = 3$).

In contrast, HPLCe6 nanoparticles, across ratios (HPL10Ce6, HPL25Ce6, HPL50Ce6), exhibited diameters of 359.87 ± 37.44 nm, 465.20 ± 32.57 nm, and 481.10 ± 42.07 nm, respectively, showing a gradual increase in diameter with a narrow distribution (Figure 4c). The zeta potentials remained comparatively stable at 46.73 ± 1.24, 44.03 ± 2.15, and 48.75 ± 1.51 for each ratio, indicating that the increase in hydrophobicity ratio did not compromise stability in aqueous solutions, despite the particle size increase (Figure 4d). The smallest nanoparticles, designated as LPL1Ce6 or HPL10Ce6, were LPLCe6 or HPLCe6, respectively. To verify potential particle formation within the body, we additionally measured the sizes of LPLCe6 and HPLCe6 nanoparticles in saline containing 5% FBS. As a result, the average size of LPLCe6 nanoparticles was 1027.1 ± 212.8 nm, while that of HPLCe6 nanoparticles was significantly smaller at 350.8 ± 119.0 nm (Figure S1). These results suggest that HPLCe6 nanoformulates reach an appropriate size in the body, compared with LPLCe6. These results demonstrate that HPLCe6 showed higher particle stability compared to LPLCe6, demonstrating advantageous physicochemical properties for nanoparticle formation.

3.4. Analysis of PLCe6 Nanoparticles

Further investigation into the potential for nanoparticle formation in vivo was conducted by examining the effect of NaCl on fluorescence intensity. For LPLCe6, an increase in NaCl concentration (from 0% to 0.9%) did not significantly alter the fluorescence intensity (Figure 5a). However, HPLCe6 exhibited a notable decrease in fluorescence intensity with increasing NaCl concentrations (Figure 5b). These results indicate that the low fluorescence intensity of nanoparticles in saline is due to a quenching effect resulting from the reduced intermolecular distances among Ce6 molecules. These data suggest that PLCe6 molecules may form nanoparticles by themselves in vivo.

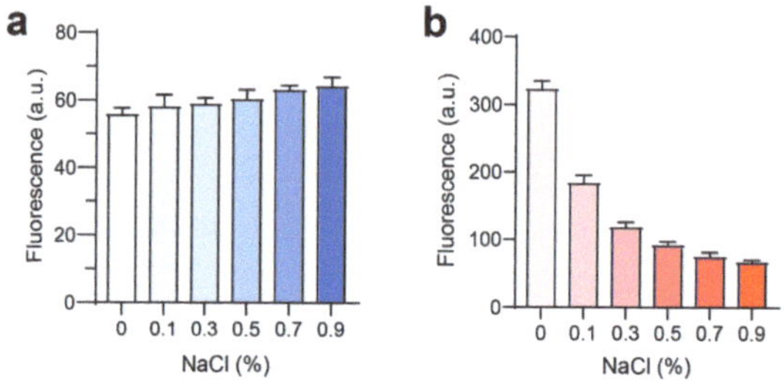

Figure 5. Analysis of PLCe6 nanoparticles under conditions similar to an in vivo environment. (**a**,**b**) Fluorescence intensity of (**a**) LPLCe6 and (**b**) HPLCe6 in an environment similar to in vivo conditions. Results are presented as mean ± SD ($n = 5$).

3.5. Tumor Cell Uptake and Cytotoxicity of PLCe6 Nanoparticles In Vitro

Murine colorectal carcinoma (CT26.WT) cells are widely used cells derived from BALB/c mice and have been receiving attention recently along with cancer immunotherapy; hence, cellular experiments related to cells were conducted using CT26.WT cells. To assess nanoparticle uptake by CT26.WT tumor cells, LPLCe6 and HPLCe6 nanoparticles were administered at a concentration of 10 µg/mL and observed after 3 h. Remarkably, while LPLCe6 nanoparticles exhibited no detectable fluorescence from Ce6 molecules, indicating minimal cell uptake, HPLCe6 nanoparticles demonstrated significant fluorescence intensity within the cytosol (Figure 6a). This observation is attributed to the stronger positive charge of HPLCe6 compared to LPLCe6, indicating that HPLCe6 nanoparticles exhibit superior cellular uptake capabilities relative to LPLCe6. Subsequent analysis focused on the cytotoxic effects of these nanoparticles post laser irradiation. At a concentration of 10 µg/mL, HPLCe6 nanoparticles induced significant cytotoxicity, comparable to that caused by LPLCe6 nanoparticles. LPLCe6 nanoparticles, despite laser irradiation, failed to induce substantial cell apoptosis, likely due to their lower cellular uptake attributed to their weak positive charges. This insufficient uptake, in turn, did not produce significant levels of ROS within the cells, leading to inducing low substantial cell death. Conversely, HPLCe6 nanoparticles, with their strong positive charges, successfully generated intracellular ROS owing to their high uptake by cells, thus inducing cell death (Figures 6b and S2a). No significant cytotoxic effect of them was observed under dark conditions (Figures 6c and S2b). Their phototherapeutic index (PI) was analyzed (Table S1) and the results show that the PI value of HPLCe6 is higher than Ce6. The effectiveness of PDT shown may not be significantly different before and after nanoparticle formation, but, in general, nanoparticle formation will contribute significantly to the improvement of tumor targeting and therapeutic effects [9,22]. These findings underline the enhanced cell uptake and apoptosis-inducing capabilities of HPLCe6 nanoparticles over LPLCe6, highlighting the potential therapeutic advantages of HPLCe6 in targeted cancer treatments.

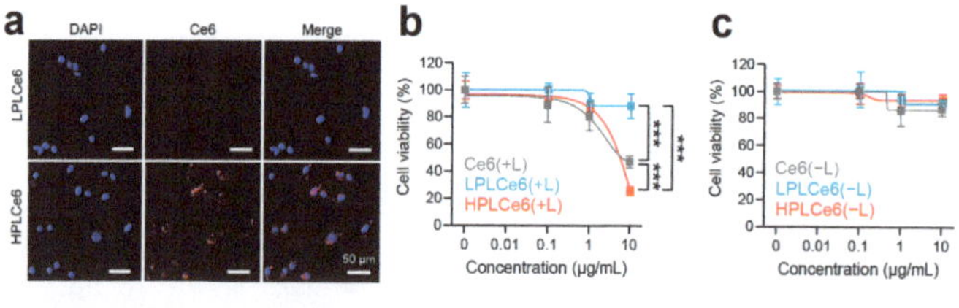

Figure 6. Cellular uptake and cytotoxicity effects of PLCe6 nanoparticles. (**a**) Cellular uptake of PLCe6 nanoparticles in CT26.WT cells treated for 3 h was observed by using fluorescence microscopy (red; Ce6, λEx = 540 nm, λEm = 605 nm, blue; DAPI, λEx = 375 nm, λEm = 460 nm); scale bars = 50 µm for all. (**b**) Cytotoxicity evaluation of Ce6, LPLCe6, and HPLCe6 on CT26.WT cells for 24 h with laser irradiation; (**c**) without laser irradiation ($n = 6$), mean ± SD, *** $p < 0.001$.

4. Discussion

The use of nanomedicine-based photodynamic therapy (PDT) is one of the interesting fields that modern science is paying great attention to, especially with regard to tumor treatment. The clinical use and application of PDT to patients are fraught with various technical challenges, but self-assembling PDT nanoparticles show potential in overcoming these issues [8,32,33]. From this perspective, several peptides and PDT agent-based substances have been synthesized and developed, including poly-L-lysine and PDT conjugates [34,35]. Poly-L-Lysine-based biomolecules with PDT were synthesized a few years ago and evaluated in various forms with therapeutic potentials. The synthesized lysin and PDT conjugates showed different cell absorption and cellular effects depending on the charge, and showed tumor targeting effects in animals [36–38]. Therefore, in this study, the authors have focused on demonstrating how the poly-L-lysine and PDT-based nanoparticles can form and function by using high- and low-molecular-weight poly-L-Lysine and Ce6 conjugates. As a result, this study is the first to show the formation of self-assembling nanoparticles of lysine and Ce6 through computer simulations, among other methods, and observed the conditions of particle formation through various methods. The combination of positively charged lysine and the hydrophobic Ce6 demonstrated successful nanoparticle formation.

In this paper, we prepared and comparatively evaluated particles based on lysine and Ce6 of two different molecular weights. Initially, the authors hypothesized that materials based on low-molecular-weight lysine would be superior due to its compact molecular size. This was because peptides with excessively large molecular weights may limit the functionality as PDT and hinder self-assembled nanoparticle formation in solution. However, the experimental results with LPLCe6 and HPLCe6 nanoparticles showed that the high-molecular-weight Lysine-Ce6 conjugates (HPLCe6 nanoparticles) exhibited better self-assembled nanoparticle formation by themselves. The difference in physicochemical properties was also reflected in cellular absorption and functionality, ultimately indicating that high-molecular-weight conjugates exhibited stronger efficacy as PDT agents. Finally, the phototherapeutic index (PI) using different types of photosensitizers in this study was analyzed and summarized. We presented their therapeutic potential and property for PDT through the analysis of PI for Ce6 and PLCe6 [39]. This research could influence further studies on the formation and evaluation of self-assembled peptide and drug-based nanoparticles for therapy.

5. Conclusions

In this study, two types of poly-L-lysine were prepared and subsequently evaluated concerning their complexation with chlorin e6 (Ce6). The low-molecular-weight poly-L-lysine was synthesized separately, and both peptides were directly chemically bound to Ce6, a PDT agent. As a result, both PDT materials successfully formed self-assembling nanoparticles based on amphiphilicity. Computer simulations were used to predict and evaluate this self-assembly, allowing for an understanding of the self-assembly mechanisms of LPLCe6 and HPLCe6 molecules. While both materials formed particles, the high-molecular-weight lysine-based HPLCe6 nanoparticles showed slightly superior cell permeability and cytotoxicity. This research could significantly influence future studies on the manufacturing of self-assembling PDT nanoparticles.

Supplementary Materials: The following supporting information can be downloaded at https://www.mdpi.com/article/10.3390/biom14040431/s1, Figure S1: the size distribution of HPLCe6 and LPLCe6 nanoparticles, Figure S2: cytotoxicity evaluation of Ce6, LPLCe6, and HPLCe6 on CT26.WT cells for 12 h ($n = 6$), mean ± SD, *** $p < 0.001$, Table S1: photo- and cytotoxicity of Ce6, LPLCe6 and HPLCe6 expressed by IC50 values of the mean ± SD (μg/mL).

Author Contributions: Conceptualization, J.P.; methodology, K.-J.L., B.S. and J.-H.L. (Jun-Hyuck Lee); validation, M.S.; investigation, M.S., K.-J.L., B.S. and J.-H.L. (Jun-Hyuck Lee); resources, J.P.; data curation, M.S. and K.-J.L.; writing—original draft preparation, M.S and J.P.; visualization, M.S. and

J.-H.L. (Jae-Hyeon Lee); supervision, J.P.; project administration, D.-W.S. and J.P.; funding acquisition, J.P. All authors have read and agreed to the published version of the manuscript.

Funding: This study was supported by Konkuk University in 2023.

Data Availability Statement: Data is contained within the article.

Conflicts of Interest: The authors declare no conflicts of interest.

References

1. Dabrowski, J.M.; Arnaut, L.G. Photodynamic therapy (PDT) of cancer: From local to systemic treatment. *Photochem. Photobiol. Sci.* **2015**, *14*, 1765–1780. [CrossRef]
2. Kim, T.E.; Chang, J.E. Recent Studies in Photodynamic Therapy for Cancer Treatment: From Basic Research to Clinical Trials. *Pharmaceutics* **2023**, *15*, 2257. [CrossRef]
3. van der Meel, R.; Sulheim, E.; Shi, Y.; Kiessling, F.; Mulder, W.J.M.; Lammers, T. Smart cancer nanomedicine. *Nat. Nanotechnol.* **2019**, *14*, 1007–1017. [CrossRef]
4. Yang, Y.; Wang, S.; Ma, P.; Jiang, Y.; Cheng, K.; Yu, Y.; Jiang, N.; Miao, H.; Tang, Q.; Liu, F.; et al. Drug conjugate-based anticancer therapy-Current status and perspectives. *Cancer Lett.* **2023**, *552*, 215969. [CrossRef]
5. Fu, Z.W.; Li, S.J.; Han, S.F.; Shi, C.; Zhang, Y. Antibody drug conjugate: The "biological missile" for targeted cancer therapy. *Signal Transduct. Tar.* **2022**, *7*, 93. [CrossRef]
6. Bae, Y.H.; Park, K. Advanced drug delivery 2020 and beyond: Perspectives on the future. *Adv. Drug Deliver. Rev.* **2020**, *158*, 4–16. [CrossRef]
7. Lee, J.H.; Yang, S.B.; Lee, J.H.; Lim, H.; Lee, S.; Kang, T.B.; Lim, J.H.; Kim, Y.J.; Park, J. Doxorubicin covalently conjugated heparin displays anti-cancer activity as a self-assembled nanoparticle with a low-anticoagulant effect. *Carbohydr. Polym.* **2023**, *314*, 120930. [CrossRef]
8. Zhao, N.; Wu, B.Y.; Hu, X.L.; Xing, D. NIR-triggered high-efficient photodynamic and chemo-cascade therapy using caspase-3 responsive functionalized upconversion nanoparticles. *Biomaterials* **2017**, *141*, 40–49. [CrossRef]
9. Um, W.; Park, J.; Ko, H.; Lim, S.; Yoon, H.Y.; Shim, M.K.; Lee, S.; Ko, Y.J.; Kim, M.J.; Park, J.H.; et al. Visible light-induced apoptosis activatable nanoparticles of photosensitizer-DEVD-anticancer drug conjugate for targeted cancer therapy. *Biomaterials* **2019**, *224*, 119494. [CrossRef]
10. Aziz, B.; Aziz, I.; Khurshid, A.; Raoufi, E.; Esfahani, F.N.; Jalilian, Z.; Mozafari, M.R.; Taghavi, E.; Ikram, M. An Overview of Potential Natural Photosensitizers in Cancer Photodynamic Therapy. *Biomedicines* **2023**, *11*, 224. [CrossRef]
11. Zahra, M.; Chota, A.; Abrahamse, H.; George, B.P. Efficacy of Green Synthesized Nanoparticles in Photodynamic Therapy: A Therapeutic Approach. *Int. J. Mol. Sci.* **2023**, *24*, 10931. [CrossRef]
12. Domka, W.; Bartusik-Aebisher, D.; Mytych, W.; Dynarowicz, K.; Aebisher, D. The Use of Photodynamic Therapy for Head, Neck, and Brain Diseases. *Int. J. Mol. Sci.* **2023**, *24*, 11867. [CrossRef]
13. Piksa, M.; Lian, C.; Samuel, I.C.; Pawlik, K.J.; Samuel, I.D.W.; Matczyszyn, K. The role of the light source in antimicrobial photodynamic therapy. *Chem. Soc. Rev.* **2023**, *52*, 1697–1722. [CrossRef]
14. Dolmans, D.E.; Fukumura, D.; Jain, R.K. Photodynamic therapy for cancer. *Nat. Rev. Cancer* **2003**, *3*, 380–387. [CrossRef]
15. Cho, I.K.; Shim, M.K.; Um, W.; Kim, J.H.; Kim, K. Light-Activated Monomethyl Auristatin E Prodrug Nanoparticles for Combinational Photo-Chemotherapy of Pancreatic Cancer. *Molecules* **2022**, *27*, 2529. [CrossRef]
16. Muskovic, M.; Pokrajac, R.; Malatesti, N. Combination of Two Photosensitisers in Anticancer, Antimicrobial and Upconversion Photodynamic Therapy. *Pharmaceuticals* **2023**, *16*, 613. [CrossRef]
17. Park, J.; Lee, Y.K.; Park, I.K.; Hwang, S.R. Current Limitations and Recent Progress in Nanomedicine for Clinically Available Photodynamic Therapy. *Biomedicines* **2021**, *9*, 85. [CrossRef]
18. Abbas, M.; Zou, Q.; Li, S.; Yan, X. Self-Assembled Peptide- and Protein-Based Nanomaterials for Antitumor Photodynamic and Photothermal Therapy. *Adv. Mater.* **2017**, *29*, 1605021. [CrossRef]
19. Jain, M.; Bouilloux, J.; Borrego, I.; Cook, S.; van den Bergh, H.; Lange, N.; Wagnieres, G.; Giraud, M.N. Cathepsin B-Cleavable Polymeric Photosensitizer Prodrug for Selective Photodynamic Therapy: In Vitro Studies. *Pharmaceuticals* **2022**, *15*, 564. [CrossRef]
20. Yang, C.; Fu, Y.; Huang, C.; Hu, D.; Zhou, K.; Hao, Y.; Chu, B.; Yang, Y.; Qian, Z. Chlorin e6 and CRISPR-Cas9 dual-loading system with deep penetration for a synergistic tumoral photodynamic-immunotherapy. *Biomaterials* **2020**, *255*, 120194. [CrossRef]
21. Li, Y.M.; Wu, Q.; Kang, M.M.; Song, N.; Wang, D.; Tang, B.Z. Boosting the photodynamic therapy efficiency by using stimuli-responsive and AIE-featured nanoparticles. *Biomaterials* **2020**, *232*, 119749. [CrossRef] [PubMed]
22. Cho, M.H.; Li, Y.; Lo, P.C.; Lee, H.R.; Choi, Y. Fucoidan-Based Theranostic Nanogel for Enhancing Imaging and Photodynamic Therapy of Cancer. *Nano-Micro Lett.* **2020**, *12*, 47. [CrossRef] [PubMed]
23. Roberts, W.G.; Shiau, F.Y.; Nelson, J.S.; Smith, K.M.; Berns, M.W. In vitro characterization of monoaspartyl chlorin e_6 and diaspartyl chlorin e_6 for photodynamic therapy. *J. Natl. Cancer Inst.* **1988**, *80*, 330–336. [CrossRef] [PubMed]
24. Lu, L.; Zhao, X.; Fu, T.; Li, K.; He, Y.; Luo, Z.; Dai, L.; Zeng, R.; Cai, K. An iRGD-conjugated prodrug micelle with blood-brain-barrier penetrability for anti-glioma therapy. *Biomaterials* **2020**, *230*, 119666. [CrossRef] [PubMed]
25. Bishop, K.J.M. Self-assembly across scales. *Nat. Mater.* **2022**, *21*, 501–502. [CrossRef] [PubMed]

26. Stevens, C.A.; Kaur, K.; Klok, H.A. Self-assembly of protein-polymer conjugates for drug delivery. *Adv. Drug Deliv. Rev.* **2021**, *174*, 447–460. [CrossRef] [PubMed]
27. Shim, M.K.; Park, J.; Yoon, H.Y.; Lee, S.; Um, W.; Kim, J.H.; Kang, S.W.; Seo, J.W.; Hyun, S.W.; Park, J.H.; et al. Carrier-free nanoparticles of cathepsin B-cleavable peptide-conjugated doxorubicin prodrug for cancer targeting therapy. *J. Control Release* **2019**, *294*, 376–389. [CrossRef] [PubMed]
28. Sahu, K.; Sharma, M.; Bansal, H.; Dube, A.; Gupta, P.K. Topical photodynamic treatment with poly-L-lysine-chlorin p6 conjugate improves wound healing by reducing hyperinflammatory response in Pseudomonas aeruginosa-infected wounds of mice. *Lasers Med. Sci.* **2013**, *28*, 465–471. [CrossRef]
29. Patil, N.A.; Kandasubramanian, B. Functionalized polylysine biomaterials for advanced medical applications: A review. *Eur. Polym. J.* **2021**, *146*, 110248. [CrossRef]
30. Maupetit, J.; Derreumaux, P.; Tuffery, P. PEP-FOLD: An online resource for de novo peptide structure prediction. *Nucleic Acids Res.* **2009**, *37*, W498–W503. [CrossRef]
31. Van Der Spoel, D.; Lindahl, E.; Hess, B.; Groenhof, G.; Mark, A.E.; Berendsen, H.J. GROMACS: Fast, flexible, and free. *J. Comput. Chem.* **2005**, *26*, 1701–1718. [CrossRef]
32. Liu, K.; Xing, R.; Zou, Q.; Ma, G.; Mohwald, H.; Yan, X. Simple Peptide-Tuned Self-Assembly of Photosensitizers towards Anticancer Photodynamic Therapy. *Angew. Chem. Int. Ed. Engl.* **2016**, *55*, 3036–3039. [CrossRef]
33. Chung, C.H.; Lu, K.Y.; Lee, W.C.; Hsu, W.J.; Lee, W.F.; Dai, J.Z.; Shueng, P.W.; Lin, C.W.; Mi, F.L. Fucoidan-based, tumor-activated nanoplatform for overcoming hypoxia and enhancing photodynamic therapy and antitumor immunity. *Biomaterials* **2020**, *257*, 120227. [CrossRef]
34. Ma, D.; Lin, Q.M.; Zhang, L.M.; Liang, Y.Y.; Xue, W. A star-shaped porphyrin-arginine functionalized poly(L-lysine) copolymer for photo-enhanced drug and gene co-delivery. *Biomaterials* **2014**, *35*, 4357–4367. [CrossRef]
35. Lee, W.K.; Lee, J.; Lee, J.S. Polyplexes of DNA and Poly(L-lysine) Stabilized by Au Nanoparticles for Targeted Photothermal Therapy. *ACS Appl. Nano Mater.* **2023**, *6*, 8945–8957. [CrossRef]
36. Soukos, N.S.; Hamblin, M.R.; Hasan, T. The effect of charge on cellular uptake and phototoxicity of polylysine chlorin$_{e6}$ conjugates. *Photochem. Photobiol.* **1997**, *65*, 723–729. [CrossRef]
37. Hamblin, M.R.; Miller, J.L.; Rizvi, I.; Ortel, B.; Maytin, E.V.; Hasan, T. Pegylation of a chlorin$_{e6}$ polymer conjugate increases tumor targeting of photosensitizer. *Cancer Res.* **2001**, *61*, 7155–7162.
38. Hamblin, M.R.; Miller, J.L.; Rizvi, I.; Ortel, B. Degree of substitution of chlorin e_6 on charged poly- L-lysine chains affects their cellular uptake, localization and phototoxicity towards macrophages and cancer cells. *J. X-ray Sci. Technol.* **2002**, *10*, 139–152.
39. Mantareva, V.; Iliev, I.; Sulikovska, I.; Durmuş, M.; Genova, T. Collagen Hydrolysate Effects on Photodynamic Efficiency of Gallium (III) Phthalocyanine on Pigmented Melanoma Cells. *Gels* **2023**, *9*, 475. [CrossRef]

biomolecules

MDPI

Communication

Enhancing Stability and Bioavailability of Peptidylglycine Alpha-Amidating Monooxygenase in Circulation for Clinical Use

Yulia Ilina [1,*], Paul Kaufmann [1], Michaela Press [1], Theo Ikenna Uba [2] and Andreas Bergmann [1,2]

1 PAM Theragnostics GmbH, 16761 Hennigsdorf, Germany
2 4TEEN4 Pharmaceuticals GmbH, 16761 Hennigsdorf, Germany
* Correspondence: yulia.ilina@pam-t.com

Abstract: Peptidylglycine alpha-amidating monooxygenase (PAM) is the only enzyme known to catalyze C-terminal amidation, a final post-translational modification step essential for the biological activity of over 70 bioactive peptides, including adrenomedullin (ADM), calcitonin gene-related peptide (CGRP), amylin, neuropeptide Y (NPY), and others. Bioactive (amidated) peptide hormones play crucial roles in various physiological processes and have been extensively explored as therapeutic compounds in clinical and preclinical research. However, their therapeutic viability is limited due to their short half-life and, in most cases, the need for prolonged infusion to maintain effective concentrations. PAM itself has also been considered as a therapeutic compound aiming to increase the level of amidated peptide hormones; however, similarly to peptide hormones, PAM's rapid degradation limits its utility. Here, we present a strategy to enhance PAM stability and bioavailability through PEGylation, significantly extending the enzyme's half-life in circulation assessed in healthy rats. Furthermore, single subcutaneous (s.c.), intramuscular (i.m.), or intraperitoneal (i.p.) administration of PEGylated PAM resulted in a sustained increase in circulating amidating activity, with peak activity observed at 12–24 h post-bolus administration. Notably, amidating activity remained significantly elevated above baseline levels for up to seven days post-administration, with no observable adverse effects. These findings highlight PEGylated PAM's potential as a viable therapeutic compound.

Keywords: peptidylglycine alpha-amidating monooxygenase; C-terminal amidation; peptide hormones; pharmacokinetics; half-life extension

Academic Editors: Hyung-Sik Won and Ji-Hun Kim

Received: 17 December 2024
Revised: 30 January 2025
Accepted: 1 February 2025
Published: 4 February 2025

Citation: Ilina, Y.; Kaufmann, P.; Press, M.; Uba, T.I.; Bergmann, A. Enhancing Stability and Bioavailability of Peptidylglycine Alpha-Amidating Monooxygenase in Circulation for Clinical Use. *Biomolecules* **2025**, *15*, 224. https://doi.org/10.3390/biom15020224

1. Introduction

Peptidylglycine α-amidating monooxygenase (PAM) is a bifunctional enzyme crucial for the C-terminal amidation of peptide hormones—a post-translational modification essential for the biological activity of nearly half of all known peptides. This modification, uniquely catalyzed by PAM, enhances peptide receptor affinity, stabilizes peptides against proteolytic degradation, and is indispensable for their full biological functionality [1,2]. Among the many peptides requiring amidation are adrenomedullin (ADM), calcitonin gene-related peptide (CGRP), amylin, neuropeptide Y (NPY), substance P, pituitary adenylate cyclase-activating polypeptide (PACAP), vasoactive intestinal peptide (VIP), and many others [2–4] (Figure S1).

The amidation process requires the presence of a C-terminal glycine on the peptide substrate. PAM carries out this reaction in two sequential steps mediated by its distinct functional domains. First, the peptidylglycine α-hydroxylating monooxygenase (PHM) domain hydroxylates the C-terminal glycine. Next, the peptidyl-α-hydroxyglycine α-amidating lyase (PAL) domain removes glyoxylate, producing a C-terminal amide [1].

Dysregulation of amidated peptide hormones has been associated with multiple pathologies, including neurodegenerative diseases, cardiovascular conditions, metabolic disorders, and many others [5–10]. The idea of using such peptide hormones as therapeutic compounds is not new, and several attempts have been made in this respect within preclinical and clinical studies. ADM is a multifunctional peptide hormone with potent vasodilatory, anti-inflammatory, and angiogenic properties, playing a critical role in cardiovascular homeostasis and immune regulation. ADM has demonstrated therapeutic potential in inflammatory bowel disease (e.g., refractory ulcerative colitis), cardiovascular diseases (heart failure, myocardial infarction, pulmonary hypertension), vascular cognitive impairment, ischemic stroke, and sepsis [11–15]. VIP displays neuroprotective, anti-inflammatory, and immunomodulatory effects, making it promising for conditions such as Parkinson's, Alzheimer's disease (AD), and autism spectrum disorders, as well as brain injuries [5,6,16]. VIP also showed relevance for treating pulmonary disorders (asthma and COPD) [17] and autoimmune diseases (rheumatoid arthritis, multiple sclerosis) [18]. PA-CAP offers neuroprotection and potentiates as a biomarker for neurological diseases such as Alzheimer's, Parkinson's, and multiple sclerosis [19–22]. PACAP also shows promise in treating retinal degenerations of metabolic origin and rescuing synaptic plasticity in fragile X syndrome [23,24]. In Alzheimer's disease preclinical models, PACAP administration slows down pathology progression, improves cognitive function, and protects against beta-amyloid toxicity [25,26]. Amylin, a pancreatic hormone, has emerged as a potential therapeutic agent for AD and type 2 diabetes (T2D) due to its role in glucose homeostasis and neuroprotection [27]. Studies have shown that amylin and its analogs, such as pramlintide, can reduce AD pathology by decreasing amyloid-β, phospho-tau, and inflammation in animal models [28]. Amylin treatment has also been found to improve cognitive function in AD mouse models [28].

As summarized above, the direct administration of peptide hormones has been explored as a strategy to mitigate disease progression, but its therapeutic applications re-main limited. Subcutaneous administration and inhalation have been explored for peptide hormone delivery, but their success is limited to a few hormones [29,30]. Prolonged intravenous infusion remains the most common method to elevate peptide levels due to their rapid degradation and short half-life [12]. Additionally, gradual adjustment of peptide concentration achieved via infusion is required to prevent adverse effects, such as systemic vasodilation, hypotension, aggregation, etc., which could result from a rapid rise in peptide levels if bolus administration is used [12,31].

Along with dysregulation of peptide hormones, changes in PAM levels have been associated with the emergence or onset of diverse pathologies [32]. Patients suffering from multiple endocrine neoplasia type 1 and pernicious anemia showed a decreased plasma PAM activity in comparison to healthy control subjects [33]. The LoF mutations of PAM have been associated with an increased risk of type 2 diabetes and sarcopenic diabetes, potentially through impacts on insulin granule packaging and secretion from β-cells [34–36]. Notably, reduced PAM activity, when measured in the cerebrospinal fluid of Alzheimer's patients, was significantly lowered compared to that in healthy individuals [37]. Beyond its primary role, Bäck et al. have shown PAM's necessity in the formation of atrial secretory granules [38]. Together, these findings underscore PAM's pivotal role in regulating various physiological and pathophysiological processes, either by modulating peptide hormone levels or serving as a therapeutic compound itself.

Building on this premise, we explored the strategy of enhancing circulating PAM levels to indirectly increase the concentration of amidated peptide hormones by supporting endogenous hormone maturation. Previous work by Kaufmann et al. in 2021 demonstrated that the intravenous bolus administration of unmodified PAM temporarily elevated amidating activity and the circulating levels of amidated adrenomedullin in rats, but its therapeutic potential was constrained by a plasma half-life of only 47 min [39]. To address these limitations, we PEGylated PAM, significantly improving its stability and extending its circulatory half-life to approximately 218 min in rats. PEGylated PAM also showed elevated amidating activity across subcutaneous, intramuscular, and intraperitoneal routes, with peak activity increasing 900–1800% within 12–24 h of a single bolus (225 μg/kg animal weight) in circulation and sustained elevation lasting up to seven days. Safety assessments indicated that PEGylated PAM was well tolerated, with no adverse effects on behavior, weight, or physiological patterns observed. Furthermore, its pharmacokinetic profile, with a lower Cmax and higher AUC than unmodified PAM, may reduce the risk of adverse effects associated with rapid hormone spikes. Finally, this approach provides a stable, clinically viable method to enhance endogenous hormone maturation, offering potential therapeutic benefits for conditions associated with dysregulated peptide hormone levels and/or impaired PAM function.

2. Materials and Methods

2.1. PAM Constructs and PEGylation

For all animals, experiment recombinant human PAM enzyme expressed in HEK293 cells, covering the full-length sequence from Met1 to Ser866 and purchased from SinoBiological (catalog number: 13624-H08H; NP_620176), was used. The resulting constructs are both soluble variants homologous to isoform 3 but exclude the protease-sensitive linker region encompassing amino acids 388 to 494. PAM enzyme was pegylated according to the following PEGylation protocol. Briefly, 10 mg lyophilized PAM was dissolved in 5 mL phosphate-buffered saline (PBS, pH 10). A 20 mM solution of PEG-5000 (MeO-PEG-NHS, Iris Biotech, Marktredwitz, Germany) was prepared by dissolving in 20% DMSO and added to the PAM solution at a 90–120-fold molar excess, equating to a 2.2-fold excess relative to lysine residues within PAM. The mixture was incubated for 180 min at 4 °C with agitation at 100 rpm and quenched subsequently with 500 μL of 1 M unbuffered Tris solution. Separation of PEGylated PAM (PEG-PAM) from free PEG was achieved through size-exclusion chromatography (Superdex 200 16/600-pg, Cytiva Europe GmbH, Freiburg, Germany) with PBS as eluent. Fractions indicative of molecular weights between 160 and 90 kDa were pooled, measured for the amidating activity using the methods described elsewhere [39], sterile-filtered through a 0.2 μm filter, aliquoted, and stored at −80 °C for in vivo application.

2.2. PAM In Vivo Pharmacokinetics

A single intravenous (i.v.) dose of PEG-PAM or unmodified PAM, adjusted to a dose of 72 μg/kg of body weight (approximately 28.8 μg per rat and 2 Units per rat) at 10 mL/kg, was administered for pharmacokinetic assessment. Six male Wistar rats (2.5–3 months old, ≥350 g) were divided into two groups with three animals per group (group A and group B). For group A, blood samples (300 μL whole blood) were collected into Li-heparinized tubes from lateral tail vein under 5 vol.% isofluran at predetermined intervals: pre-administration and at 20, 60, 120, 240, and 300 min post-injection. For group B, blood samples were collected in the same manner as for group A at predetermined intervals: pre-administration and at 40, 80, 180, 240, and 300 min post-injection. Animals were awake between the different blood sampling time points. The samples were processed within 5 min after the blood withdrawal and stored as Li-heparin plasma at −80 °C until further analysis. This animal study was conducted by preclinics Gesellschaft für Präklinische Forschung GmbH (Potsdam, Germany) and the study protocol was approved by the State Office for Occupational Safety, Consumer Protection, and Health of the State of Brandenburg (protocol number 2347-48-2017, sub-experiment 14/21, date of approval 20 March 2018). The animals used in this study were obtained from Charles River Laboratories, Sulzfeld, Germany.

A single subcutaneous (s.c.), intramuscular (i.m.), or intraperitoneal (i.p.) dose of PEG-PAM adjusted to 225 μg/kg body weight (approximately 90 μg per rat and 6 Units per rat) was administered to Sprague Dawley rats with six animals per group. For s.c. and i.p. administrations, the volume applied was 10 mL/kg, while for i.m. administration the volume was fixed at 200 μL per animal. Blood samples (300 μL whole blood) were collected in Li-heparinized tubes under isoflurane anesthesia. Sampling was performed retrobulbarly from the V. saphena and from the V. jugularis at predetermined intervals: pre-administration and at 15 min, 30 min, 60 min, 2 h, 4 h, 8 h, 12 h, 24 h, 3 days, and 7 days post-administration. The sampling was alternated between left and right sides. Samples were processed within 20 min of collection and stored as Li-heparin plasma at −80 °C until further analysis. Rats were anesthetized prior to substance administration and remained anesthetized throughout the experiments. This animal study was conducted in accordance with the German Animal Welfare Act and European Council Directive 86/609/EEC by Bioassay Labor für biologische Analytik GmbH (Heidelberg, Germany) and the study protocol was approved by the Regional Council of Karlsruhe (protocol number 35-9185.81/G192/17, date of approval 26 October 2017). The animals used in this study were obtained from Charles River Wiga GmbH, Sulzfeld, Germany.

The amidating activity was measured as previously described by Kaufmann et al. (2021) [39]. Specific PAM activity was calculated by dividing the measured PAM activity by the PAM quantity, determined using the bicinchoninic acid (BCA) protein assay according to the manufacturer's protocol. Non-compartmental analysis was performed using Phoenix WinNonlin version 8.4 (Certara USA, Inc., Princeton, NJ), calculating the Tmax, Cmax, and AUC. Half-life (t1/2) was determined independently in both groups and the average t1/2 was reported. The activity at each time point was derived by subtracting the mean baseline (t = 0) from the mean measurement at each timepoint. The schematic representation of the study design for both in vivo experiments is shown in Figure 1.

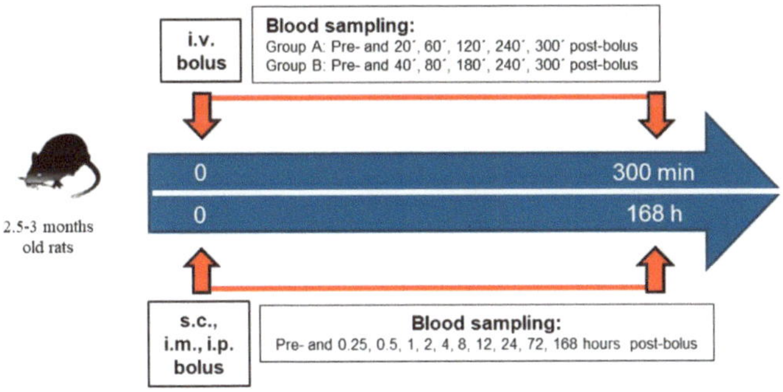

Figure 1. Schematic representation of the experimental setup for assessing the pharmacokinetics and the enrichment of amidating activity of PAM enzyme in circulation after intravenous (i.v.), subcutaneous (s.c.), intramuscular (i.m.), and intraperitoneal (i.p.) administration. The details of this study are described in the Section 2.

3. Results

To enhance PAM stability, we performed PEGylation. Figure S2A shows that the activity of PEGylated PAM was minimally reduced compared to that of non-modified PAM, with a reduction in activity of 4.5% (coefficient of variation (CV)). The PEGylation resulted in a molecular weight shift from approximately 90 kDa to approximately 130 kDa

(Figure S2B), indicating successful PEGylation, as well as covalent attachment of PEG to PAM.

The basic pharmacokinetic parameters are summarized in Tables 1 and S1. The half-life time for PEG-PAM and unmodified PAM was calculated by measuring the half-life in circulation after i.v. bolus administration. To limit blood withdrawal frequency, animals were subdivided into two groups (group A and B) with time-shifted blood withdrawal frequencies as described in Section 2. The baseline amidating activity averaged across all groups was $12.7 \times 10^3 \pm 2.5 \times 10^3$ Units (mean ± standard deviation (SD)). The PEGylation extended the in vivo half-life of PEG-PAM to 223.8 min for group A and to 212.7 min for group B leading to an average 218.2 min, while the mean half-life of unmodified PAM was only 42.3 min (Figure 2A; Tables 1 and S1), consistent with previous reports [39], where the half-life of unmodified PAM in circulation was 47 min. In the case of unmodified PAM, the amidating activity dropped within the baseline range after 100 min after reaching the peak activity (Figures 2A and S3). In contrast, PEG-PAM maintained elevated activity for ca. 6 h post-administration, retaining over 65% of the peak activity in groups A and B (Figures 2A and S3). Additionally, the PEGylation of PAM resulted in a higher AUC (80.9×10^3 h*Units for PEG-PAM compared to 38.3×10^3 h*Units for unmodified PAM (Table 1)) and lower Cmax (18.3×10^3 Units for PEG-PAM vs. 27.9×10^3 Units for unmodified PAM).

Table 1. Pharmacokinetic parameters of PEG-PAM and unmodified PAM following intravenous (i.v.), intramuscular (i.m.), intraperitoneal (i.p.), or subcutaneous (s.c.) bolus administration in rats. Key metrics include t1/2 (half-life), Cmax (maximum concentration in plasma), area under the curve (AUC), baseline (BL) and peak activity, as well as the amidating activity 7 days post-bolus PAM injection; * describes the mean value between groups A and B.

Route	Parameter: Variable	Parameter: Units	PEG-PAM	Unmodified PAM
i.v.	Animals	n/group	6	6
	T1/2 *	min	218.2	42.3
	Cmax *	Units	18.3×10^3	27.9×10^3
	AUC *	h*Units	80.9×10^3	38.3×10^3
	BL activity	Units (mean + SD)	$12.7 \times 10^3 \pm 2.8 \times 10^3$	$12.7 \times 10^3 \pm 2.3 \times 10^3$
i.m.	Animals	n/group	6	
	Cmax	Units	93.9×10^3	
	Tmax	h	24	
	AUC	h*Units	6.5×10^6	
	BL activity	Units	$7.2 \times 10^3 \pm 1.8 \times 10^3$	
	7d post-bolus activity	(mean ± SD)	13,615 ± 1370	
i.p.	Animals	n/group	6	
	Cmax	Units	104.6×10^3	
	Tmax	h	12	
	AUC	h*Units	7.0×10^6	
	BL activity	Units	$5.7 \times 10^3 \pm 0.8 \times 10^3$	
	7d post-bolus activity	(mean ± SD)	$16.2 \times 10^3 \pm 2.0 \times 10^3$	
s.c.	Animals	n/group	6	
	Cmax	Units	50.2×10^3	
	Tmax	h	24	
	AUC	h*Units	4.2×10^6	
	BL activity	Units	$5.4 \times 10^3 \pm 1.2 \times 10^3$	
	7d post-bolus activity	(mean ± SD)	$16.3 \times 10^3 \pm 2.1 \times 10^3$	

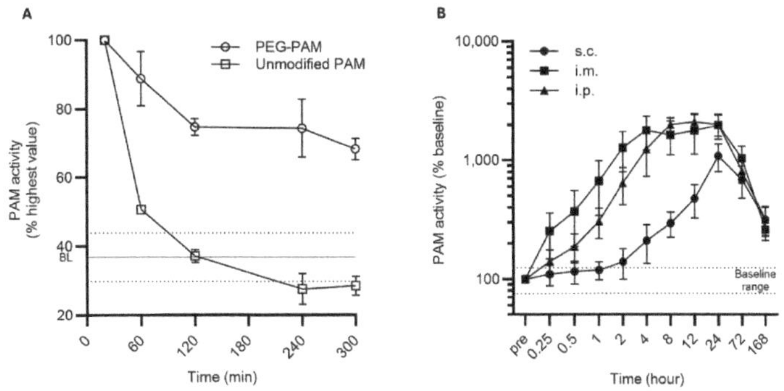

Figure 2. (**A**) Time-resolved decay of relative amidating activity between PEG-PAM and unmodified PAM following intravenous (i.v.) bolus administration (group A). The amidating activity at the 20 min post-bolus time point was set as 100%, with all other values expressed relative to this peak activity. The CV was calculated for the relative baseline values and the CV value was then used to define the upper and lower bounds of the baseline range (dashed lines). BL (solid line)—mean relative baseline value; (**B**) circulating relative amidating activity of PEG-PAM following subcutaneous (s.c.), intramuscular (i.m.), and intraperitoneal (i.p.) administration. The pre-bolus activity values were set to 100%. The CV value was then used to establish the upper and lower bounds of the baseline range (dashed line).

Figure 2B illustrates that PEG-PAM administered via s.c., i.p., and i.m. routes led to prolonged and elevated amidating activity in circulation, surpassing levels observed with i.v. bolus administration. The baseline amidating activity averaged across all groups was $6.1 \times 10^3 \pm 1.5 \times 10^3$ Units (mean ± standard deviation (SD)). The individual baseline levels of amidating activity and further pharmacokinetic parameters per application route are reported in Table 1. Following s.c. administration, PAM activity reached a maximum of 50.2×10^3 Units at 24 h post-bolus, representing a 835% increase from the baseline ($5.4 \times 10^3 \pm 1.2 \times 10^3$ Units); this activity remained elevated at 204% above the baseline at 168 h post-administration. For i.m. administration, PAM activity peaked at 93.9×10^3 Units (an approximate 1200% increase) after 24 h, with sustained activity at 90% above the baseline 168 h post-PEG-PAM administration. The i.p. route produced the highest peak activity of 104.6×10^3 Units (ca. 1730% increase) at 12 h, with levels still 180% above the baseline at 168 h post-PEG-PAM administration. In terms of the AUC, i.p. administration yielded the highest exposure (7.0×10^6 h*Units), followed by i.m. (6.5×10^6 h*Units), with s.c. showing the lowest total exposure (4.2×10^6 h*Units).

No adverse effects were observed in all PAM-treated animals. All animals maintained good clinical condition, displaying normal social interactions with peers, appropriate grooming behavior, regular drinking and eating habits, as well as normal weight development. Sleep patterns also remained unaffected.

4. Discussion

This study presents a comprehensive approach to enhancing circulating amidating activity and substantially increasing the bioavailability of PAM. PEGylation significantly improved the stability and circulatory half-life of PAM, as evidenced by prolonged amidating activity across all tested administration routes (i.v., s.c., i.p., and i.m.).

The pharmacokinetic analysis revealed that PEG-PAM had a markedly extended half-life of approximately 218 min following intravenous administration, compared to 42 min for unmodified PAM. However, this estimate may be conservative, as amidating activity was still elevated above the baseline during the observation period of 6 h post-bolus, suggesting that the actual half-life may be longer. The lower Cmax and higher AUC observed with

PEG-PAM indicate a slower systemic release, potentially mitigating the risks associated with abrupt hormone spikes, such as systemic vasodilation from sudden increases in amidated peptide hormones like adrenomedullin. The comparison of pharmacokinetic parameters (Cmax, Tmax, and AUC) across non-intravenous routes demonstrated that all the tested routes of administration effectively increased endogenous amidating activity and systemic exposure. Subcutaneous administration, in particular, offers a promising route for therapeutic applications due to its practicality for self-administration.

An important question to address is whether PEGylated PAM retains its enzymatic activity in vivo, given that ex vivo measurements of amidating activity using the PAM-AMA assay are conducted under optimal conditions, including an optimal pH range and optimal cofactor concentrations (5 µM copper and 2 mM ascorbate). These conditions differ from the physiological environment in circulation. The optimal pH for PAM activity aligns with the acidic environment of secretory granules (pH 5.0–5.5), which is different from the more basic pH of blood (~7.4). Nonetheless, in the amidating assay previously reported by Kaufmann et al., 2021 [39], conducted at pH 7.5 to approximate physiological conditions, we observed the conversion of glycine-extended adrenomedullin (ADM-Gly; a PAM substrate) into bioactive adrenomedullin (bio-ADM; product of amidation by PAM). This indicates that PAM retains significant enzymatic activity even under non-optimal pH conditions. Furthermore, the retention of the enzymatic activity following exogeneous PAM administration can be inferred from changes in the levels of amidated peptides, such as, e.g., adrenomedullin. As previously demonstrated for unmodified PAM [39], increases in circulating PAM activity correlate well with changes in relative bio-ADM concentrations, even in the absence of exogenous ascorbate. Similarly, after PEG-PAM administration, we observed a consistent trend: elevated PAM activity in circulation was associated with a corresponding increase in bio-ADM levels (Figure S4). However, due to considerable variability among individual rats and resulting large standard deviations, statistical significance was not reached at most time points. Despite this limitation, the observed trend strongly suggests that PEGylated PAM retains enzymatic activity in vivo in circulation after delivery, pointing to the value of further investigation with larger group sizes.

The literature indicates that amidation primarily occurs intracellularly within secretory granules, with mature peptides being released into circulation. However, this reaction does not achieve 100% efficiency. For example, studies have shown that adrenomedullin exists predominantly in its inactive glycine-extended form in circulation, ranging between the 5.6:1 and 2:1 ratios of glycine-extended to bioactive forms in healthy individuals [40,41]. This implies that inactive substrates for PAM are already present in circulation, allowing PEG-PAM to function effectively without the risk of overdosing or excessive hormone activation, enhancing its safety profile. Concerns that PAM activity might be limited to intracellular environments were previously addressed by Kaufmann et al. in 2021 [39], who demonstrated that amidation can also occur in circulation. This finding supports the feasibility of enhancing systemic PAM activity to modulate peptide hormone levels therapeutically.

We observed the differences in baseline amidating activity between experiments involving different administration routes. Animals receiving PEG-PAM intravenously exhibited significantly higher baseline activity compared to those receiving subcutaneous, intramuscular, or intraperitoneal injections. This discrepancy may stem from variations in blood sampling methods; for intravenous administration, blood was collected from the lateral tail vein, whereas for other routes retrobulbar sampling and sampling from V. saphena and V. jugularis were used. Such variations, coupled with the unknown primary source of circulating PAM, could explain the observed differences. Additionally, the use of different rat strains across experiments may have contributed to baseline variability.

Importantly, no adverse effects were detected throughout this study. Animals exhibited normal physiological behaviors, including social interactions, grooming, weight maintenance, and sleep patterns. This favorable safety profile, combined with extended systemic exposure and sustained activity, highlights PEG-PAM's potential as a therapeutic agent for conditions requiring long-term modulation of amidated peptide levels. Nonetheless, comprehensive toxicity and safety assessments remain necessary for further development.

One concern in this study is the use of a His-tagged recombinant protein, which could increase immunogenicity, particularly in the context of long-term PAM applications. Nonetheless, this study establishes a proof of principle, demonstrating for the first time the therapeutic potential of PAM to enhance circulating amidating activity and increase levels of amidated peptide hormones with clinical relevance. For future clinical use, particularly in chronic conditions, the development of an untagged construct will be critical to minimize such immunogenicity concerns, as well as to avoid potential interference of the His-tag with amidating activity, as the His-tag has the capacity to bind copper, an essential cofactor for PAM's enzymatic function. Another significant concern is the broad substrate specificity of PAM, which can activate a wide range of peptide hormones with diverse effects. While an elevation in certain peptide hormones has been shown to have beneficial effects, an increase in others can lead to deleterious outcomes. An increase in bio-ADM supports vascular health by promoting endothelial repair and maintaining vascular homeostasis [42], while elevated GLP-1 enhances insulin secretion, improves glucose regulation, and aids in weight management [43]. Similarly, higher PACAP levels provide neuroprotection by reducing neuronal cell death and offering therapeutic potential in neurological disorders [44]. Likewise, increased amylin contributes to blood glucose control by inhibiting glucagon [45]; cholecystokinin enhances digestion, supporting long-term metabolic balance [46]; and vasopressin helps regulate blood pressure and renal function [47]. Conversely, elevated substance P and CGRP are associated with migraines and pain sensitization [48], while high NPY levels may contribute to obesity and metabolic syndrome [49]. Excessive vasopressin can lead to water retention disorders [50], and chronically elevated gastrin has been linked to hyperplasia and an increased cancer risk [51]. Therefore, before progressing to human applications, the utilization of the drug candidate in regulatory tox and safety studies is mandatory to establish a detailed safety profile. Furthermore, it will be critical to stratify eligible patients by assessing levels of active and inactive peptide hormones (where possible), as well as PAM levels in various pathological conditions, to create a risk–benefit assessment for the target pathology of the treatment. Currently, to our knowledge, adrenomedullin is the only peptide hormone for which both active (bio-ADM) and inactive precursor (ADM-Gly) forms can be directly measured using immunoassays, which are validated and applicable for large-scale human sample processing [40,52]. Developing similar immunoassays for other peptide hormones with various therapeutical properties, e.g., VIP and NPY, would greatly enhance patient classification and help mitigate potential risks associated with PAM therapy.

In summary, PEG-PAM administered via non-intravenous routes achieves prolonged systemic effects without adverse outcomes. These findings lay the groundwork for further studies to explore its long-term pharmacodynamic profile, therapeutic efficacy, and potential applications across diverse disease models.

5. Conclusions

Taken together, our data provide a robust strategy to significantly enhance the stability and bioavailability of PAM, a critical enzyme for the C-terminal amidation of peptide hormones—a reaction essential for their full biological activity. By extending the circulatory half-life of PAM through PEGylation, we demonstrate a novel approach to achieving prolonged systemic amidating activity via subcutaneous, intramuscular, and intraperitoneal administration routes. Remarkably, a single bolus application sustained amidating activity above baseline levels for over a week, with no observed adverse effects. This method minimizes the risks associated with overdosing amidated peptide hormones by utilizing the naturally inactive glycine-extended peptide precursors already present in circulation as substrates. These findings suggest that PEGylated PAM offers a stable, clinically viable solution to enhance endogenous hormone maturation, providing potential therapeutic benefits for conditions associated with dysregulated peptide hormone levels and impaired PAM function. Further studies are needed to explore the long-term pharmacodynamic profile and therapeutic efficacy of PEG-PAM across diverse disease contexts.

6. Patents

This work has resulted in a patent application under international publication number WO 2021/170816 A1 (international application number PCT/EP2021/054869).

Supplementary Materials: The following supporting information can be downloaded at https://www.mdpi.com/article/10.3390/biom15020224/s1, Figure S1: Maturation pathway of peptide hormones; Figure S2: PEGylation of PAM enzyme; Figure S3: Time-resolved decay of relative amidating activity between PEG-PAM and unmodified PAM following intravenous (i.v.) bolus administration (group B); Figure S4: Circulating relative amidating activity of PEG-PAM following intraperitoneal administration and the relative change in bio-ADM concentration; Table S1: Pharmacokinetic parameters of PEG-PAM and unmodified PAM following intravenous bolus administration in rats in group A and group B; Supplementary File S1: Original images for Figure S2B.

Author Contributions: Conceptualization, Y.I., P.K., M.P. and A.B.; research execution incl. data analysis, Y.I., P.K. and M.P.; non-compartmental data analysis, T.I.U.; writing—original draft preparation, Y.I.; writing—review and editing, Y.I. and P.K.; funding acquisition, P.K. and A.B. All authors have read and agreed to the published version of the manuscript.

Funding: This research received no external funding.

Institutional Review Board Statement: The first study was conducted by preclinics Gesellschaft für Präklinische Forschung GmbH (Potsdam, Germany) and approved by the State Office for Occupational Safety, Consumer Protection, and Health of the State of Brandenburg (protocol number 2347-48-2017, sub-experiment 14/21; date of approval 20 March 2018). The second study was conducted in accordance with the German Animal Welfare Act and European Council Directive 86/609/EEC by Bioassay Labor für biologische Analytik GmbH (Heidelberg, Germany) and was approved by the Regional Council of Karlsruhe (protocol number 35-9185.81/G192/17; date of approval 26 October 2017).

Informed Consent Statement: Not applicable.

Data Availability Statement: The original contributions presented in this study are included in the article/Supplementary Materials. Further inquiries can be directed to the corresponding author.

Acknowledgments: The authors gratefully acknowledge Joachim Struck (4TEEN4 Pharmaceuticals GmbH, Hennigsdorf, Germany) for his valuable assistance in proofreading the manuscript.

Conflicts of Interest: Y.I., P.K., M.P. and A.B. are employed by PAM Theragnostics GmbH. A.B. has shares in and is managing director of PAM Theragnostics GmbH. T.I.B. and A.B. are employed by 4TEEN4 Pharmaceuticals GmbH. A.B. is managing director of 4TEEN4 Pharmaceuticals GmbH. A.B. is the inventor of a pending patent application (PCT/EP2021/054869, WO2021/170816).

Abbreviations

The following abbreviations are used in this manuscript:

PAM	peptidylglycine alpha-amidating monooxygenase
ADM	adrenomedullin
CGRP	calcitonin gene-related peptide
NPY	neuropeptide Y
VIP	vasoactive intestinal peptide
PACAP	pituitary adenylate cyclase-activating polypeptide
T2D	type 2 diabetes
COPD	chronic obstructive pulmonary disease
CV	coefficient of variation
AUC	area under the curve
Cmax	maximum analyte concentration in plasma
Tmax	time to reach maximum analyte concentration
BL	baseline
i.v.	intravenous
i.m.	intramuscular
i.p.	intraperitoneal

References

1. Kumar, D.; Mains, R.E.; Eipper, B.A. 60 YEARS OF POMC: From POMC and α-MSH to PAM, molecular oxygen, copper, and vitamin C. *J. Mol. Endocrinol.* **2016**, *56*, T63–T76. [CrossRef]
2. Vishwanatha, K.S.; Mains, R.E.; Eipper, B.A. Peptidylglycine Amidating Monoxygenase (PAM). In *Handbook of Biologically Active Peptides*; Academic Press: Cambridge, MA, USA, 2013; Volume 3, pp. 1780–1788. [CrossRef]
3. Eipper, B.A.; Mains, R.E. Peptide α-Amidation. *Annu. Rev. Physiol.* **1988**, *50*, 333–344. [CrossRef] [PubMed]
4. Eipper, B.A.; Stoffers, D.A.; Mains, R.E. The biosynthesis of neuropeptides: Peptide alpha-amidation. *Annu. Rev. Neurosci.* **1992**, *15*, 57–85. [CrossRef] [PubMed]
5. Gonzalez-Rey, E.; Chorny, A.; Fernandez-Martin, A.; Varela, N.; Delgado, M. Vasoactive intestinal peptide family as a therapeutic target for Parkinson's disease. *Expert Opin. Ther. Targets* **2005**, *9*, 923–929. [CrossRef]
6. White, C.M.; Ji, S.; Cai, H.; Maudsley, S.; Martin, B. Therapeutic Potential of Vasoactive Intestinal Peptide and its Receptors in Neurological Disorders. *CNS Neurol. Disord. Drug Targets* **2012**, *9*, 661–666. [CrossRef] [PubMed]
7. Adeghate, E.; Ponery, A.S.; Sharma, A.K.; El-Sharkawy, T.; Donáth, T. Diabetes mellitus is associated with a decrease in vasoactive intestinal polypeptide content of gastrointestinal tract of rat. *Arch. Physiol. Biochem.* **2001**, *109*, 246–251. [CrossRef] [PubMed]
8. Duarte-Neves, J.; de Almeida, L.P.; Cavadas, C. Neuropeptide Y (NPY) as a therapeutic target for neurodegenerative diseases. *Neurobiol. Dis.* **2016**, *95*, 210–224. [CrossRef] [PubMed]
9. Li, C.; Wu, X.; Liu, S.; Zhao, Y.; Zhu, J.; Liu, K. Roles of Neuropeptide Y in Neurodegenerative and Neuroimmune Diseases. *Front. Neurosci.* **2019**, *13*, 869. [CrossRef] [PubMed]
10. Han, P.; Liang, W.; Baxter, L.C.; Yin, J.; Tang, Z.; Beach, T.G.; Caselli, R.J.; Reiman, E.M.; Shi, J. Pituitary adenylate cyclase–activating polypeptide is reduced in Alzheimer disease. *Neurology* **2014**, *82*, 1724–1728. [CrossRef] [PubMed]
11. Ashizuka, S.; Kuroishi, N.; Nakashima, K.; Inatsu, H.; Kita, T.; Kitamura, K. Adrenomedullin: A novel therapy for intractable Crohn's disease with a loss of response to infliximab. *Intern. Med.* **2019**, *58*, 1573–1576. [CrossRef]
12. Kita, T.; Kitamura, K. Translational studies of adrenomedullin and related peptides regarding cardiovascular diseases. *Hypertens. Res.* **2022**, *45*, 389–400. [CrossRef] [PubMed]
13. Wong, H.K.; Cheung, T.T.; Cheung, B.M.Y. Adrenomedullin and cardiovascular diseases. *JRSM Cardiovasc. Dis.* **2012**, *1*, 1–7. [CrossRef] [PubMed]
14. Ihara, M.; Washida, K.; Yoshimoto, T.; Saito, S. Adrenomedullin: A vasoactive agent for sporadic and hereditary vascular cognitive impairment. *Cereb. Circ. Cogn. Behav.* **2021**, *2*, 100007. [CrossRef] [PubMed]
15. Yoshimoto, T.; Saito, S.; Omae, K.; Tanaka, K.; Kita, T.; Kitamura, K.; Fukuma, K.; Washida, K.; Abe, S.; Ishiyama, H.; et al. Efficacy and safety of adrenomedullin for acute ischemic stroke (AMFIS): A phase 2, randomized, double-blinded, placebo-controlled, clinical trial. *eClinicalMedicine* **2024**, *77*, 102901. [CrossRef] [PubMed]
16. Delgado, M.; Varela, N.; Gonzalez-Rey, E. Vasoactive intestinal peptide protects against β-amyloid-induced neurodegeneration by inhibiting microglia activation at multiple levels. *Glia* **2008**, *56*, 1091–1103. [CrossRef] [PubMed]
17. Wu, D.; Lee, D.; Sung, Y.K. Prospect of vasoactive intestinal peptide therapy for COPD/PAH and asthma: A review. *Respir. Res.* **2011**, *12*, 45. [CrossRef] [PubMed]

18. Gomariz, R.; Martinez, C.; Abad, C.; Leceta, J.; Delgado, M. Immunology of VIP: A Review and Therapeutical Perspectives. *Curr. Pharm. Des.* **2001**, *7*, 89–111. [CrossRef] [PubMed]
19. Reglodi, D.; Vaczy, A.; Rubio-Beltrán, A.E.; MaassenVanDenBrink, A. Protective effects of PACAP in ischemia. *J. Headache Pain* **2018**, *19*, 19. [CrossRef]
20. DToth, D.; Reglodi, D.; Schwieters, L.; Tamas, A. Role of endocrine PACAP in age-related diseases. *Front. Endocrinol.* **2023**, *14*, 1118927. [CrossRef]
21. Reglodi, D.; Helyes, Z.; Nemeth, J.; Vass, R.A.; Tamas, A. PACAP as a Potential Biomarker: Alterations of PACAP Levels in Human Physiological and Pathological Conditions. In *Pituitary Adenylate Cyclase Activating Polypeptide—PACAP*; Current Topics in Neurotoxicity; Springer: Berlin/Heidelberg, Germany, 2016; Volume 11, pp. 815–832. [CrossRef]
22. Yang, R.; Jiang, X.; Ji, R.; Meng, L.; Liu, F.; Chen, X.; Xin, Y. Therapeutic potential of PACAP for neurodegenerative diseases. *Cell. Mol. Biol. Lett.* **2015**, *20*, 265–278. [CrossRef] [PubMed]
23. Gábriel, R.; Pöstyéni, E.; Dénes, V. Neuroprotective Potential of Pituitary Adenylate Cyclase Activating Polypeptide in Retinal Degenerations of Metabolic Origin. *Front. Neurosci.* **2019**, *13*, 1031. [CrossRef]
24. Ciranna, L.; Costa, L. Pituitary Adenylate Cyclase-Activating Polypeptide Modulates Hippocampal Synaptic Transmission and Plasticity: New Therapeutic Suggestions for Fragile X Syndrome. *Front. Cell. Neurosci.* **2019**, *13*, 524. [CrossRef] [PubMed]
25. Rat, D.; Schmitt, U.; Tippmann, F.; Dewachter, I.; Theunis, C.; Wieczerzak, E.; Postina, R.; Leuven, F.; Fahrenholz, F.; Kojro, E. Neuropeptide pituitary adenylate cyclase-activating polypeptide (PACAP) slows down Alzheimer's disease-like pathology in amyloid precursor protein-transgenic mice. *FASEB J.* **2011**, *25*, 3208–3218. [CrossRef] [PubMed]
26. Han, P.; Tang, Z.; Yin, J.-X.; Beach, T.; Reiman, E.; Shi, J. PACAP Deficit in Alzheimer's Disease and Protection Against Beta-Amyloid Toxicity (I11-1.010). *Neurology* **2014**, *82* (Suppl. S10). [CrossRef]
27. Lutz, T.A.; Meyer, U. Amylin at the interface between metabolic and neurodegenerative disorders. *Front. Neurosci.* **2015**, *9*, 216. [CrossRef] [PubMed]
28. Zhu, H.; Xue, X.; Wang, E.; Wallack, M.; Na, H.; Hooker, J.M.; Kowall, N.; Tao, Q.; Stein, T.D.; Wolozin, B.; et al. Amylin receptor ligands reduce the pathological cascade of Alzheimer's disease. *Neuropharmacology* **2017**, *119*, 170–181. [CrossRef]
29. Nagata, S.; Yamasaki, M.; Kitamura, K. Anti-Inflammatory Effects of PEGylated Human Adrenomedullin in a Mouse DSS-Induced Colitis Model. *Drug Dev. Res.* **2017**, *78*, 129–134. [CrossRef]
30. von der Hardt, K.; Kandler, M.; Chada, M.; Cubra, A.; Schoof, E.; Amann, K.; Rascher, W.; Dötsch, J. Brief adrenomedullin inhalation leads to sustained reduction of pulmonary artery pressure. *Eur. Respir. J.* **2004**, *24*, 615–623. [CrossRef] [PubMed]
31. Geven, C.; Kox, M.; Pickkers, P. Adrenomedullin and adrenomedullin-targeted therapy as treatment strategies relevant for sepsis. *Front. Immunol.* **2018**, *9*, 292. [CrossRef]
32. Merkler, D.J.; Hawley, A.J.; Eipper, B.A.; Mains, R.E. Peptidylglycine α-amidating monooxygenase as a therapeutic target or biomarker for human diseases. *Br. J. Pharmacol.* **2022**, *179*, 3306–3324. [CrossRef]
33. Kapuscinski, M.; Green, M.; Sinha, S.N.; Shepherd, J.J.; Shulkes, A. Peptide α-amidation activity in human plasma: Relationship to gastrin processing. *Clin. Endocrinol.* **1993**, *39*, 51–58. [CrossRef]
34. Sheng, B.; Wei, H.; Li, Z.; Wei, H.; Zhao, Q. PAM variants were associated with type 2 diabetes mellitus risk in the Chinese population. *Funct. Integr. Genom.* **2022**, *22*, 525–535. [CrossRef] [PubMed]
35. Thomsen, S.K.; Raimondo, A.; Hastoy, B.; Sengupta, S.; Dai, X.-Q.; Bautista, A.; Censin, J.; Payne, A.J.; Umapathysivam, M.M.; Spigelman, A.F.; et al. Type 2 diabetes risk alleles in PAM impact insulin release from human pancreatic β-cells. *Nat. Genet.* **2018**, *50*, 1122–1131. [CrossRef] [PubMed]
36. Giontella, A.; Åkerlund, M.; Bronton, K.; Fava, C.; Lotta, L.A.; Baras, A.; Overton, J.D.; Jones, M.; Bergmann, A.; Kaufmann, P.; et al. Deficiency of Peptidylglycine-alpha-amidating Monooxygenase, a Cause of Sarcopenic Diabetes Mellitus. *J. Clin. Endocrinol. Metab.* **2024**. [CrossRef]
37. Wand, G.S.; May, C.; May, V.; Whitehouse, P.J.; Rapoport, S.I.; Eipper, B.A. Alzheimer's disease: Low levels of peptide alpha-amidation activity in brain and CSF. *Neurology* **1987**, *37*, 1057. [CrossRef]
38. Bäck, N.; Luxmi, R.; Powers, K.G.; Mains, R.E.; Eipper, B.A. Peptidylglycine α-amidating monooxygenase is required for atrial secretory granule formation. *Proc. Natl. Acad. Sci. USA* **2020**, *117*, 17820–17831. [CrossRef] [PubMed]
39. Kaufmann, P.; Bergmann, A.; Melander, O. Novel insights into peptide amidation and amidating activity in the human circulation. *Sci. Rep.* **2021**, *11*, 15791. [CrossRef]
40. Kaufmann, P.; Ilina, Y.; Press, M.; Bergmann, A. Sandwich immunoassay for adrenomedullin precursor and its practical application. *Sci. Rep.* **2024**, *14*, 28091. [CrossRef] [PubMed]
41. Kitamura, K.; Kato, J.; Kawamoto, M.; Tanaka, M.; Chino, N.; Kangawa, K.; Eto, T. The intermediate form of glycine-extended adrenomedullin is the major circulating molecular form in human plasma. *Biochem. Biophys. Res. Commun.* **1998**, *244*, 551–555. [CrossRef] [PubMed]
42. Kato, J.; Tsuruda, T.; Kita, T.; Kitamura, K.; Eto, T. Adrenomedullin: A Protective Factor for Blood Vessels. *Arterioscler. Thromb. Vasc. Biol.* **2005**, *25*, 2480–2487. [CrossRef]

43. Müller, T.; Finan, B.; Bloom, S.; D'Alessio, D.; Drucker, D.; Flatt, P.; Fritsche, A.; Gribble, F.; Grill, H.; Habener, J.; et al. Glucagon-Like Peptide 1 (GLP-1). *Mol. Metab.* **2019**, *30*, 72–130. [CrossRef]
44. Manecka, D.L.; Boukhzar, L.; Falluel-Morel, A.; Lihrmann, I.; Anouar, Y. PACAP signaling in neuroprotection. In *Pituitary Adenylate Cyclase Activating Polypeptide—PACAP*; Springer: Cham, Switzerland, 2016; pp. 549–561. [CrossRef]
45. Scherbaum, W.A. The role of amylin in the physiology of glycemic control. *Exp. Clin. Endocrinol. Diabetes* **1998**, *106*, 97–102. [CrossRef] [PubMed]
46. Desai, A.J.; Dong, M.; Harikumar, K.G.; Miller, L.J. Cholecystokinin-induced satiety, a key gut servomechanism that is affected by the membrane microenvironment of this receptor. *Int. J. Obes. Suppl.* **2016**, *6*, S22–S27. [CrossRef] [PubMed]
47. Den Ouden, D.T.; Meinders, A.E. Vasopressin: Physiology and clinical use in patients with vasodilatory shock: A review. *Neth. J. Med.* **2005**, *63*, 4–13. [PubMed]
48. Jang, M.; Park, J.; Kho, H.; Chung, S.; Chung, J. Plasma and saliva levels of nerve growth factor and neuropeptides in chronic migraine patients. *Oral Dis.* **2011**, *17*, 187–193. [CrossRef] [PubMed]
49. Ailanen, L.; Ruohonen, S.T.; Vähätalo, L.H.; Tuomainen, K.; Eerola, K.; Salomäki-Myftari, H.; Röyttä, M.; Laiho, A.; Ahotupa, M.; Gylling, H.; et al. The metabolic syndrome in mice overexpressing neuropeptide Y in noradrenergic neurons. *J. Endocrinol.* **2017**, *234*, 57–72. [CrossRef] [PubMed]
50. Ranieri, M.; Di Mise, A.; Tamma, G.; Valenti, G. Vasopressin–aquaporin-2 pathway: Recent advances in understanding water balance disorders. *F1000Research* **2019**, *8*, 149. [CrossRef]
51. Fossmark, R.; Qvigstad, G.; Martinsen, T.C.; Hauso, Ø.; Waldum, H.L. Animal Models to Study the Role of Long-Term Hypergastrinemia in Gastric Carcinogenesis. *J. Biomed. Biotechnol.* **2011**, *2011*, 975479. [CrossRef]
52. Weber, J.; Sachse, J.; Bergmann, S.; Sparwaßer, A.; Struck, J.; Bergmann, A. Sandwich Immunoassay for Bioactive Plasma Adrenomedullin. *J. Appl. Lab. Med.* **2017**, *2*, 222–233. [CrossRef] [PubMed]

biomolecules MDPI

Article

Generation of Rapid and High-Quality Serum by Recombinant Prothrombin Activator Ecarin (RAPClot™)

Kong-Nan Zhao [1,*,†], Goce Dimeski [2,3,4], Paul Masci [1,†,‡], Lambro Johnson [1], Jingjing Wang [1], John de Jersey [3], Michael Grant [5] and Martin F. Lavin [1,6,*]

1 Australian Institute of Biotechnology and Nanotechnology, The University of Queensland, Brisbane, QLD 4072, Australia; lambro.johnson@uq.edu.au (L.J.); jingjing.wang2@uq.net.au (J.W.)
2 Chemical Pathology, Princess Alexandra Hospital, Woolloongabba, Brisbane, QLD 4102, Australia; goce.dimeski@health.qld.gov.au
3 School of Chemistry and Molecular Biosciences, The University of Queensland, Brisbane, QLD 4072, Australia; j.dejersey@uq.edu.au
4 School of Medicine, University of Queensland, Brisbane, QLD 4072, Australia
5 Q-Sera Pty Ltd., Level 9, 31 Queen St, Melbourne, VIC 3000, Australia; michael.grant@q-sera.com
6 Centre for Clinical Research, The University of Queensland, Brisbane, QLD 4029, Australia
* Correspondence: k.zhao@uq.edu.au (K.-N.Z.); m.lavin@uq.edu.au (M.F.L.); Tel.: +61-7-3343-1291 (K.-N.Z.); +61-7-3346-6045 (M.F.L.)
† These authors contributed equally to this work.
‡ Deceased.

Abstract: We recently reported the potential application of recombinant prothrombin activator ecarin (RAPClot™) in blood diagnostics. In a new study, we describe RAPClot™ as an additive to develop a novel blood collection prototype tube that produces the highest quality serum for accurate biochemical analyte determination. The drying process of the RAPClot™ tube generated minimal effect on the enzymatic activity of the prothrombin activator. According to the bioassays of thrombin activity and plasma clotting, γ-radiation (>25 kGy) resulted in a 30–40% loss of the enzymatic activity of the RAPClot™ tubes. However, a visual blood clotting assay revealed that the γ-radiation-sterilized RAPClot™ tubes showed a high capacity for clotting high-dose heparinized blood (8 U/mL) within 5 min. This was confirmed using Thrombelastography (TEG), indicating full clotting efficiency under anticoagulant conditions. The storage of the RAPClot™ tubes at room temperature (RT) for greater than 12 months resulted in the retention of efficient and effective clotting activity for heparinized blood in 342 s. Furthermore, the enzymatic activity of the RAPClot™ tubes sterilized with an electron-beam (EB) was significantly greater than that with γ-radiation. The EB-sterilized RAPClot™ tubes stored at RT for 251 days retained over 70% enzyme activity and clotted the heparinized blood in 340 s after 682 days. Preliminary clinical studies revealed in the two trials that 5 common analytes (K, Glu, lactate dehydrogenase (LD), Fe, and Phos) or 33 analytes determined in the second study in the γ-sterilized RAPClot™ tubes were similar to those in commercial tubes. In conclusion, the findings indicate that the novel RAPClot™ blood collection prototype tube has a significant advantage over current serum or lithium heparin plasma tubes for routine use in measuring biochemical analytes, confirming a promising application of RAPClot™ in clinical medicine.

Keywords: prothrombin activator; RAPClot™ prototype tube; γ-radiation; enzymatic activity; blood clotting; serum; biochemical analytes

Citation: Zhao, K.-N.; Dimeski, G.; Masci, P.; Johnson, L.; Wang, J.; de Jersey, J.; Grant, M.; Lavin, M.F. Generation of Rapid and High-Quality Serum by Recombinant Prothrombin Activator Ecarin (RAPClot™). *Biomolecules* **2024**, *14*, 645. https://doi.org/10.3390/biom14060645

Academic Editors: Hyung-Sik Won and Ji-Hun Kim

Received: 8 April 2024
Revised: 20 May 2024
Accepted: 20 May 2024
Published: 30 May 2024

1. Introduction

It is well documented that laboratory blood tests impact at least 70% of the patient care decisions starting from diagnosis, treatment, and management to discharge [1,2]. Over the past two decades, there have been additional changes in the tubes used for blood collection for laboratory tests to improve the accuracy of results. This includes the introduction of thrombin as a clotting agent [3,4], a new cell plasma separator device to decrease cell remnants in the plasma of lithium heparin plasma [4] and new anticoagulant combinations to prevent glucose consumption by cells [5].

Currently, there are a number of tubes that produce either serum or plasma for analyte testing. The most frequently used fluid–serum or plasma tubes are as follows: (a) serum tubes with or without gel separator and either with silica or thrombin as the procoagulant which require time to clot and do not always provide fully clotted samples in patients on anticoagulants and (b) lithium heparin tubes suitable for immediate centrifugation to improve the turn-around-times of results (TAT). Both of these types of tubes have well-documented problems in producing desirable high-quality samples [6–9]. The vast majority of results in chemical pathology and serology testing are obtained from serum. There are only a few analytes that require plasma samples [10,11].

Although rapid analysis is achieved with plasma, the presence of clotting factors and higher concentrations of remnant cellular material post-separation of the cells from plasma can alter the integrity and stability of the sample upon short or prolonged storage, compromising the accuracy of many critical analytes [12]. It has also been reported that the presence of anticoagulants in plasma collection tubes can introduce interfering factors, such as enzyme inhibitors, fibrinogen and cations [13,14], and fibrins, such as with the Beckman troponin assay [15]. The alternative, serum, represents a cleaner, higher-quality sample type when blood is fully clotted before centrifugation. However, the standard commercially available serum tubes, primarily using silica particles for the coagulation of blood, require long clotting times (30 min) for healthy individuals and longer times (over 60 min) for patients on anticoagulants, whose samples may only achieve partial or no clotting at all (Dimeski PhD Thesis) [3,7,12,16,17]. The use of rapid serum tubes (RST) containing bovine thrombin is a well-established technology for serum preparation [3,4]. The drawback of these tubes is their high costs and inability to clot blood from many anticoagulated patients [3,4].

To overcome the above-described issues, we have employed snake venom prothrombin activators (PAs) for the rapid preparation of consistently high-quality serum in both normal individuals and in blood from anticoagulated patients [18,19]. PAs utilize prothrombin in the blood samples to generate rapid and sustained levels of human thrombin, and more thrombin is produced than the amount used in commercially available thrombin tubes [18,19]. We have established this using PAs purified from the venoms of *Oxyuranus scutellatus* (OsPA) and *Pseudonaja textilis* (PtPA) added to blood collection tubes to efficiently coagulate blood from normal and several anticoagulated samples [18,19]. While these venoms contain relatively large amounts of PAs [20,21], it was apparent that their use in commercial tubes was not optimal due to supply considerations associated with procuring venom from snakes. Although venom-sourced proteins can be produced to a high purity, it was desirable to develop a recombinant form of snake venom PA for more consistent quality generation and in sufficient quantity, which could be manufactured in a controlled environment of high purity in any quantity with quality assured. The PA ecarin from the saw-scaled viper (*Echis carinatus*) was selected because unlike OsPA and PtPA, it is synthesized as a single polypeptide chain and is subject to a lesser amount of post-translational modification [22,23]. Ecarin has a very different structure than OsPA and PtPA which consist of active factor Xa- and factor Va-like proteins in a stable complex, homologous with the human prothrombinase complex [23,24]. Ecarin is a metalloproteinase and like all snake venom PAs is minimally or not affected by any regulatory components of the mammalian coagulation–fibrinolysis system including activated protein C and antithrombin III (ATIII) [23,25], making it ideal for rapid clotting of blood including anticoagulated blood, producing high-quality serum for analysis.

Recently, we reported that a codon-optimized form of ecarin was successfully cloned for expression in mammalian cells at high yield [23]. It was demonstrated that the recombinant ecarin enzyme could efficiently clot normal blood and blood spiked with high concentrations of anticoagulants including heparin and had great potential as an additive to blood collection tubes to produce high-quality serum for analyte testing in diagnostic medicine [23]. Here, we describe an experimental approach to develop a novel type of RAPClot™ prototype tube for future application in analyte determination in diagnosis.

2. Materials and Methods

2.1. RAPClot™ Prototype Tubes and Commercial Blood Collection Tubes

Firstly, Greiner-Bio-One (GBO,) white-top no-additive plain blood collection tubes (GBO Vacuette® Catalogue No 4566001, Kremsmünster, Austria) were used to prepare RAPClot™ prototype tubes for laboratory experiments. Twenty microliter of 0.24% surfactant (Dow Corning silicone hydrophilic surfactant (Catalogue No SH3771 H, Midland, MI, USA)) was used to coat the bottom of the tubes and then they were dried. Becton Dickinson (BD) red-top no-additive plain blood collection tubes (BD Vacutainer® Catalogue No 366406, Franklin Lakes, NJ, USA) and Greiner BCA Fast Clot tubes (GBO Vacutainer® Catalogue No 456313, Kremsmünster, Austria) were also used in some experiments where indicated.

RAPClot™ concentrate was added to 20 µL of the patented protective formulation consisting of a colloid, Gelofusine™ (succinylated gelatin 4%-GF, Catalogue No 210317641, Sydney, Australia) with a stabilizing sugar which was added to the surfactant-coated tubes and dried using an air–nitrogen dryer (Brisbane, Australia). Dried prototype tubes treated with γ-radiation at ~25–27.8 kGy were labelled as RAP+Ir, with untreated tubes labelled as RAP-Ir (Supplementary Table S1). In tubes designated "wet", an aliquot of RAPClot™ concentrate was added to the blood collection tube without drying prior to adding the blood sample.

Three types of BD commercially available blood collection tubes that included BD standard serum separator tube (SST, Catalogue No 367974) with silica as clot activator, BD rapid serum tubes containing bovine thrombin (RST Catalogue No 368771), and BD Vacutainer® PST™ tube (PST Catalogue No 367962) (Brisbane, Australia) were used in clinical trials.

2.2. Study Design

To use RAPClot™ as an additive to develop a novel type of blood collection tube for clinical diagnosis, we designed and carried out different types of experiments in the laboratory. (A). Formulation development experiments: Different colloids such as lactulose, dextran, Polyvinylpyrrolidone, voluven, and sorbitol were initially tested for developing an optimal RAPClot™ formulation which is particularly helpful for clotting anticoagulant-blood, especially heparin-blood, to produce high-quality serum (Supplementary Figure S2). Finally, six RAPClot™ formulations were designed for developing RAPClot™ prototype tubes for further experiments (Supplementary Tables S1 and S2). (B). γ-radiation and Electron-beam (E-beam) sterilization experiments: RAPClot™ prototype tubes prepared in different formulations were dried in nitrogen air at room temperature. The RAPClot™ prototype tubes were then divided into two groups, one group of the tubes was sterilized by either γ-radiation (Supplementary Tables S1 and S2) or *E-beam* with a typical dose range of 25–30 kGy, and the other group was used as control without γ-radiation and E-beam sterilization. Both types of the prototype tubes were assayed for the activity of RAPClot™ by S2238 assay and blood clotting assay. (C). Shelf-life experiments of RAPClot™ prototype tubes: Currently, most blood collection tubes on the market have at least a 12-month shelf-life (Ref). Thus, the prototype tubes whether they were dry-only or sterilized by γ-radiation/E-beam were also divided into two groups, which were, respectively, stored under two temperature conditions—room temperature (RT) and higher temperatures (50 °C) that could cause reductions in draw volume up to two years. (D). Small clinical trials: Trial 1 was designed to recruit five volunteers for assessing the capacity of the γ-sterilized RAPClot™ prototype tubes in clotting both fresh and heparinized blood and its effects on the determination of five important analytes. Trial 2 was designed to determine all 33 analytes in sera produced by RAPClot™ tubes from the five volunteers, compared to those produced by three commercial blood collection tubes.

2.3. Clotting of Whole Blood Samples in Blood Collection Tubes

Either fresh whole blood was added directly to tubes or for recalcified citrated whole blood, 50 μL of 1 M $CaCl_2$ was added followed by 3.95 mL of citrated whole blood (total sample volume 4 mL). The tubes were recapped immediately after the timer was started and gently tilted every 15 s for 5–6 times to monitor clotting. Clotting start times were estimated visually and recorded when the clotting was first observed and when a firm clot formed as defined by the clot staying in place upon the inversion of the tube as previously reported [18,19]. For experiments using anticoagulated blood, fresh whole or recalcified citrated whole blood was spiked with commercial sodium heparin solution (DBL™ heparin sodium injection BP, C84593, Pfizer, New York, NY, USA) and dosed as above.

2.4. Plasma Clotting Assay

The recalcified citrated plasma clotting assay was performed using a Hyland-Clotek instrument as described previously [19].

2.5. Thrombelastography (TEG) of Recalcified Citrated Whole Blood

The TEG® Haemostasis Analyser 5000 series (Haemscope Corporation, Niles, IL, USA) was used as per manufacturer recommendations and as described elsewhere [26]. The TEG assay captures four important parameters (R time, K time, α-angle, and MA value). The R-value represents the time until the first evidence of a clotting; the K value is the time from the end of R until the clot reaches 20 mm, representing the speed of clot formation; the α-angle is the tangent of the curve made as the K is reached, and MA is a reflection of clot strength [27]. The details of the TEG assay were the same as described previously [18,19].

2.6. S2238 Chromogenic Bioassay for RAPClot™ Prototype Tube

RAPClot™ was assayed in a single reaction mixture containing prothrombin and the thrombin-specific substrate S2238 (Cat No 00082032439, Werfen, Barcelona, Spain). The coupled reactions, prothrombin to thrombin and S2238 to pNA, monitored at 410 nm, result in the non-linear progress curves of absorbance vs. time. These were analyzed by fitting second-order polynomials to give the RAPClot™ activity in mUs defined as nmol thrombin/min, and the assay was also carried out to monitor the recovery of RAPClot™ in RAPClot™ prototype tubes [28].

2.7. Statistical Analysis

The Excel-2403 (Formula-Statistical program) software was used for all analyses with Student's two-tailed *t*-test and one-way analysis of variance being employed. The patients and sample numbers together with numerical values including the mean ± standard deviation are included. p values < 0.05 or $p < 0.01$ were used to present the significance levels.

2.8. Human Research Ethics

The study was conducted in accordance with the Declaration of Helsinki. Human research ethics approval for this study involving blood collection from volunteers and patients was obtained from Metro South Human Research Ethics Committee and The University of Queensland Human Ethics Committee: HREC Reference number: HREC/08/QPAH/005. Most recent date of approval on 21 March 2017. The supply of human blood for research with ethics approval was obtained from the Australian Red Cross Service (ARCBS), Brisbane, Australia.

3. Results

3.1. Establishment of Stabilizing Formulation to Develop RAPClot™ Prototype Tube

To be commercially viable as a procoagulant in blood collection tubes, RAPClot™ must retain its activity over standard industry manufacturing and storage stability conditions [29,30]. We initially observed that wet RAPClot™, dissolved in Hepes or Gelofusine (GF) patented buffer and added to GBO or BD plain tubes (Figure 1A), coated with either of the two silicone surfactants DC3771 or L7-9245 (Dow Corning, Midland, MI, USA) had similar blood clotting times that varied from 92 to 98 s (Figure 1A). By comparison, control tubes without RAPClot™ took longer than 30 min to clot (Figure 1A). Whole blood clotting was shown to depend on the concentration of RAPClot™ without any influence by the surfactant (Supplementary Figure S1). To establish a stabilizing formulation for developing RAPClot™ prototype tubes coated with or without the surfactant DC3771, the RAPClot™ was dried in the tubes in both the GF and Hepes buffers under standard laboratory conditions (Figure 1B). The clotting activity of the air-dried RAPClot™ in the GF buffer was comparable in time to that observed with the wet RAPClot™ in both the GBO and BD tubes and the surfactant had no effect on the clotting (Figure 1B). However, when the Hepes buffer was used instead of the GF buffer, the clotting activity of the air-dried form was markedly reduced (Figure 1B). These findings suggested that the RAPClot™ tested in the GF buffer whether it was wet or air-dried in different tube types has great potential for development as a rapid serum prototype tube. We also tested bovine serum Albumin (BSA, Sigma-Aldrich, St Louis, MO, USA), Polyvinylpyrrolidone (PVP, Merck, Darmstadt, Germany), Voluven™ (a starch-based plasma volume expander) (Fresenius Kabi Ltd., Sydney, Australia), dextran, and several stabilizing sugars (sorbitol sucrose, trehalose and mannitol) that might play an important role in stabilizing RAPClot™ (Supplementary Figure S2). The results show that the addition of different compounds had some effects on activity with a combination of Gelofusine and 10% stabilizing sugar having the most significant effect on stabilizing activity. We employed the GF stabilizing formulation with RAPClot™ and dried the tubes by nitrogen and vacuum-desiccator air-dry to determine the drying process impact on the enzymic activity of RAPClot™. The use of the S2238 chromogenic bioassay showed that the process of drying had no effect on the RAPClot™ activity compared with the wet RAPClot™ solution (Figure 1C). In the next experiment, RAPClot™ at 0.15 mU/tube was added with the identified stabilizing formulation to the tubes that were dried by vacuum-desiccator air-drying, with results showing no loss of the blood clotting activity consistent with the results from the S2238 assay (Figure 1D). The results again confirmed that our patented GF formulation (Patent No, WO2016061611A1) was suitable for developing RAPClot™ blood collection prototype tubes for the generation of high-quality serum. We defined the quality of the serum based on the visual lack of cellular material and red blood cell hang-up, lack of fibrin strands as well as fibrinogen (Supplementary Figures S3 and S4). This shows the quality of the serum produced in the RAPClot™ tubes compared to four other commercial tubes. In addition, the determination of five key analytes was comparable to those measured in a commercial blood collection tube in a small clinical trial. This also agrees with the data obtained in another clinical trial showing that the serum quality produced by the RAPClot™ prototype tube does not interfere with the determination of 33 different biochemical analytes (Supplementary Table S3).

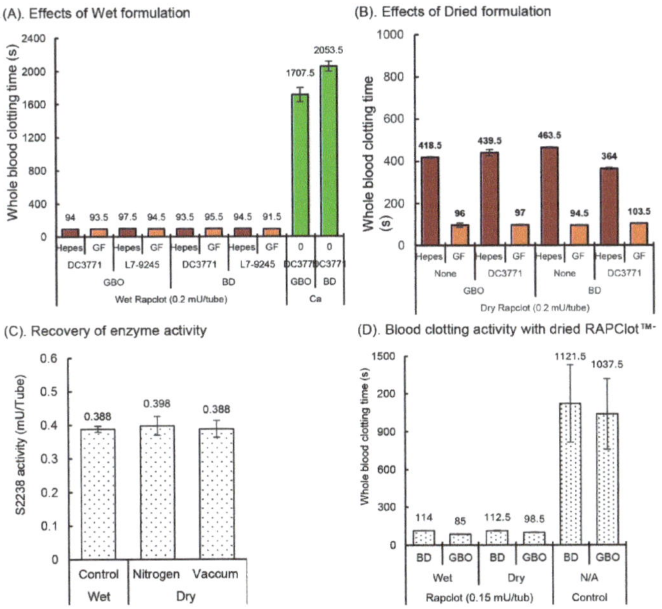

Figure 1. Effects of exogenous conditions on the development of RAPClot™ -prototype blood collection tube. (**A**). The comparison of RAPClot™ –Hepes working solution with RAPClot™ –Gelofusine working solution in the presence of the surfactants DC3771 or L7-9245 when clotting 4 mL recalcified citrated whole blood. (**B**). The activity of air-dried RAPClot™ prepared from Hepes and Gelofusine solutions with or without the surfactant DC3771 in clotting 4 mL recalcified citrated whole blood. (**C**). The S2238 activity of wet RAPClot™ (0.4 mU/tube) in GBO plain blood collection tube at 4 °C for 48 h, compared with those of dried RAPClot™ in GBO plain blood collection tube by nitrogen-drying for 2 h, then stored at RT for 46 h and vacuum-desiccator air-dried for 24 h, then stored at RT for 24 h. At 48 h post preparation, the activity of RAPClot™ in the three groups of the RAPClot™ -containing tubes was analyzed in a single reaction mixture containing prothrombin and the thrombin-specific substrate S2238 ($n = 6$). (**D**). The activity of RAPClot™ (0.15 mU/tube) in stabilizing formulation in both the BD and GBO plain tubes vacuum-desiccator air-dried in clotting 4 mL of recalcified citrated whole blood. The error bars represent the standard deviation (SD).

3.2. *γ-Radiation Sterilization of the RAPClot™ Prototype Tube*

The RAPClot™ prototype tubes (0.33 mU/tube) were prepared in four formulations (Supplementary Table S1) and treated with or without γ-radiation (25.34 kGy) as the sterilizing agent to determine the effect on the enzymatic activity (Figure 2A). We observed that the RAPClot™ in formulation A (S-A, lead formulation) did not lose activity after drying; however, the activity was reduced by 8–15% in the other three formulations (S-B, S-C and S-D) compared with the wet solution acting as the control (Figure 2A). Subsequently, the γ-radiation treatment reduced the RAPClot™ activity by 26% in the tubes dried with formulation A and 32–38% in the other three formulations (Figure 2A), providing further evidence that our preferred formulation (A) was the most suitable for developing RAPClot™ prototype tubes. Next, we prepared RAPClot™ 0.4 mUnit/4 mL blood prototype tubes with formulation A to which we added an increasing concentration of BSA followed by sterilization with γ-radiation (27.8 kGy) and compared these to the RAPClot™ in the Hepes buffer with the addition of lactulose and BSA (Supplementary Table S2 and Supplementary Figure S5B,C; Figure 2B). Using a plasma clotting assay (Supplementary Figure S6), the activity of the RAPClot™ tubes without sterilization decreased from 97% to 76% (21% decrease) with the increasing concentration of BSA while that for the tubes treated with γ-radiation decrease ranged from 69% to 66% (Figure 2B). In comparison with the S2238 enzymatic assay, the untreated RAPClot™ tubes' decrease ranged from 79% to 66% with increasing concentrations of BSA while those treated with γ-radiation had a decrease range of 55% to 50% (Figure 2B). Thus, the decrease with added BSA was of the same order for both clotting and enzyme activity assays in each case, revealing that the two assays are correlated (r = 0.9404**, Figure 2C). A related set of data comparing clotting times to the S2238 activity with increasing BSA protein in the Hepes buffer also showed a similar relationship (Figure 2B). The effect of the heparin anticoagulant on the RAPClot™ tubes using recalcified citrated whole blood on day 15 post-radiation showed clotting was achieved in <2.5 min without heparin and in the presence of 8 U/mL heparin clotting was achieved in <5 min (Figure 2D). All the RAPClot™ tubes generated clearly high-quality serum without latent clotting occurring at 24 h after centrifugation (Figure 2E). These results suggest that the RAPClot™ prototype tubes using formulation A (GF + 10% *wsv* stabilizing sugar) retained the highest blood clotting and S2238 activity after the γ-radiation sterilization at a dose of 27.8 kGy.

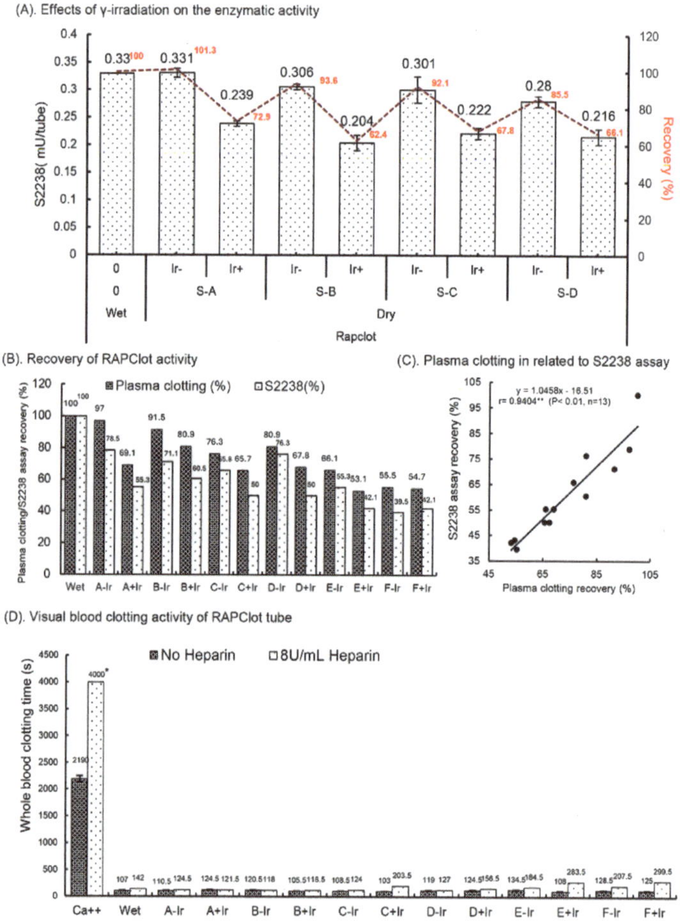

Figure 2. *Cont.*

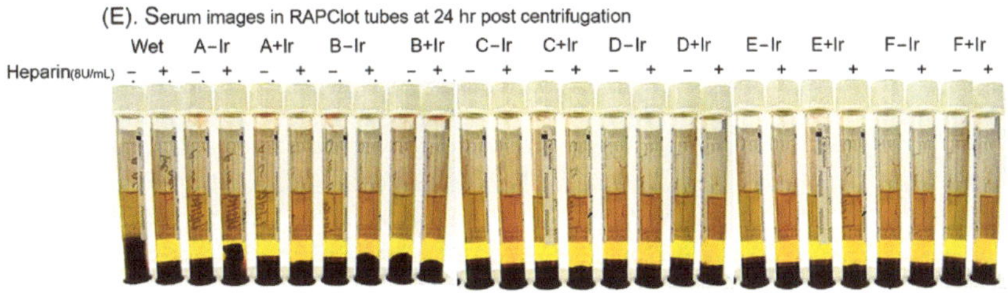

Figure 2. Effects of γ-radiation on the enzymatic activity of the RAPClot™ -containing prototype tubes prepared in different formations in GBO white-top plain tube. (**A**). The recovery (%) of the enzyme activity of the RAPClot™ -prototype tubes (0.33 mU/tube) in four formulations (S-A, S-B, S-C, and S-D) with or without γ-radiation (25.34 kGy) at day 4 post-radiation (n = 3) (see also Supplementary Table S1). (**B**). The activity recovery (%) of the RAPClot™ -prototype tubes (0.26 mU/tube) in six formulations with or without γ-radiation (27.8 kGy) at day 14 post-radiation in clotting recalcified citrated plasma, compared with the S2238 assay (n = 2) (Supplementary Table S2). (**C**). The activity recovery (%) of plasma clotting correlated with the S2238 assay for the RAPClot™ -prototype tubes with γ-radiation (27.8 kGy). r = 0.9404 ($p < 0.01$, n = 13)) representing a highly significant linear relationship between two assays. ** indicates that $p < 0.01$. (**D**). The activity of the RAPClot™ -prototype tubes prepared in six formulations (**A–E**, see Supplementary Table S2) with or without γ-radiation (27.8 kGy) at day 14 post-radiation in clotting recalcified citrated whole blood spiked with or without heparin at 8 U/mL. Note: * indicates no clotting occurred (n = 2). (**E**). Serum images that were generated from normal and heparinized blood (8 U/mL) clotted in the RAPClot™ prototype tubes with or without sterilization by γ-radiation 24 h after centrifugation (n = 2) (Supplementary Table S2). The error bars represent the standard deviation (SD).

3.3. *TEG Assay for the γ-Radiation-Sterilized RAPClot™ Blood Prototype Tubes*

Based on the results obtained from the studies of γ-radiation-sterilized RAPClot™ prototype tubes in six formulations (Figure 2), the patented formation was used with the stabilizing sugar to prepare a new set of RAPClot™ prototype tubes containing two relatively lower doses of RAPClot™ tubes with 0.15 mU/tube (Figure 3) and 0.3 mU/tube (Supplementary Figures S7 and S8). The newly produced RAPClot™ prototype tubes with or without γ-radiation at 25.7 kGy were stored at RT for testing blood clotting stabilities by the TEG assay at three time points over a two-month period (64 days) (Figure 3 and Supplementary Figure S6). The TEG assay generates four whole blood clotting parameters: R time, K time, angle-α, and MA values (Figure 3A–D and Supplementary Figure S8). As expected, the γ-radiation-treated prototype tubes showed slightly longer R times compared with the RAPClot™ wet control and the prototype tubes at 0.15 mU/tube without γ-radiation (Figure 3A). The R times were, however, similar with the heparinized blood at the three time points up to 64 days, indicating that the γ-irradiated tubes could retain the higher enzymatic activity in clotting the non-heparinized blood although they clotted the heparinized blood (4 U/mL), except in one sample where the result was 260 s at day 9 (Figure 3A) which was still within the reported clotting range of 263–496 s [31]. In a similar experiment using tubes as above with a dose of 0.3 mU/tube RAPClot™, the TEG R times improved with (4 U/mL) heparinized blood for up to 64 days (Supplementary Figure S8). The γ-radiation-sterilized RAPClot™ prototype tubes containing 0.15 mU/tube generated K times for clotting the non-heparinized blood at the three time points similar to the RAPClot™ wet control and the non-irradiated prototype tubes (Figure 3B). Both RAPClot™ wet control and non-γ-radiation-sterilized (Dry-IR) prototype tubes had similar K times for clotting the heparinized blood over the 64 day period with the range of 55–160 s (Figure 3B). However, the γ-radiation-sterilized (Dry+IR) RAPClot™ prototype tubes produced a larger variation with the K times for clotting heparinized blood over the time course, with a time of 150 s at day 30 (Figure 3B), but showed an improved performance in the 0.3 mU-containing tubes (Supplementary Figure S5B). Both angle-α and MA values obtained from the TEG assay for the RAPClot™ prototype tubes are shown in Figure 3C,D. The Dry+IR RAPClot™ prototype tubes clotted heparinized blood producing a greater variation in angle-α and MA values, the lowest angle-α of 26.5 (<30) and MA value of 14.8 being on day 9 (Figure 3C,D), which were unacceptable for the propagation phase of coagulation and overall stability of the clot. However, the Dry+IR RAPClot™ prototype tubes containing 0.3 mU RAPClot™/tube clotted the heparinized blood at 4 U/mL with a significant increase in angle-α (46.5) and MA value (40.1) on day 9 (Supplementary Figure S8), suggesting that a relatively higher dose of the RAPClot™ (>0.3 mU/tube) is required for the consistent clotting of heparinized blood to produce a solid blood clot with larger angle-α and higher mA values. Both the wet and Dry-IR RAPClot™ tubes produced satisfactory angle-α and MA values in clotting both non-heparinized and heparinized blood samples (Figure 3C,D and Supplementary Figure S8).

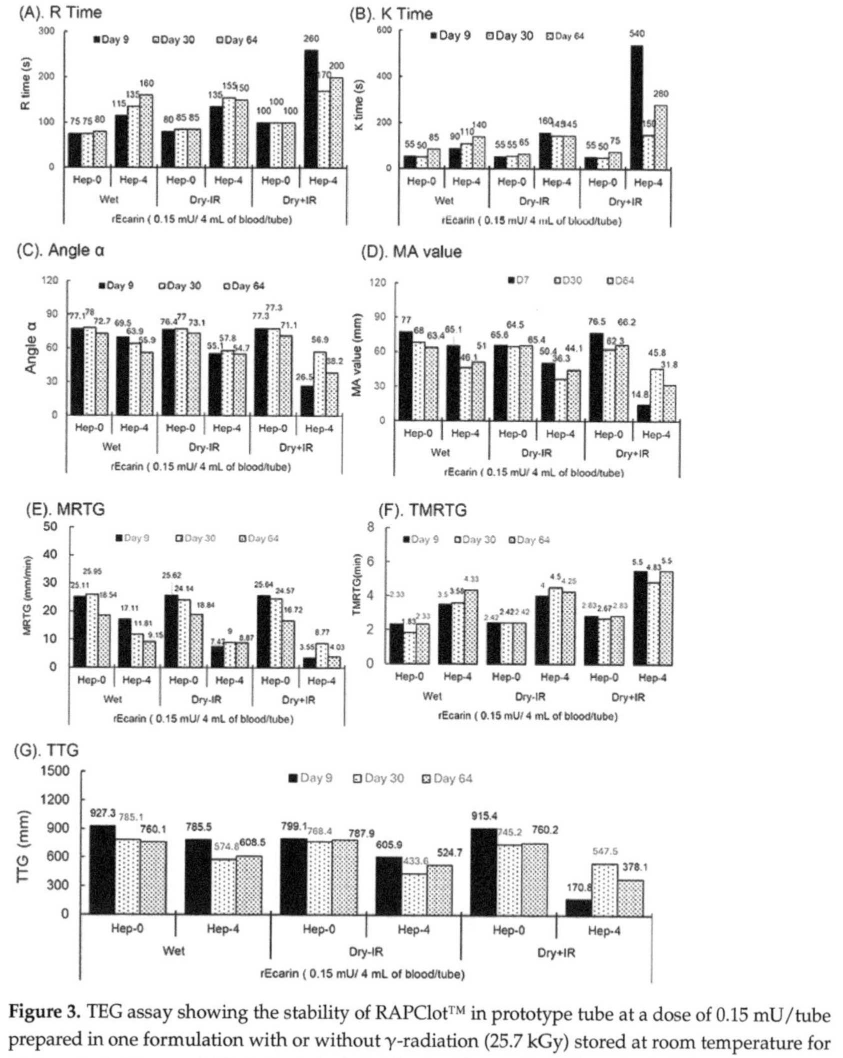

Figure 3. TEG assay showing the stability of RAPClot™ in prototype tube at a dose of 0.15 mU/tube prepared in one formulation with or without γ-radiation (25.7 kGy) stored at room temperature for 64 days in clotting recalcified citrated whole blood with or without heparin (4 U/mL). (**A**). R time, (**B**). K time, (**C**). α angle value, (**D**). MA value, (**E**). MRTG (maximum rate of thrombin generation), (**F**). TMRTG (time to maximum rate of thrombus generation), and (**G**). TTG (total thrombus generation.

The TEG demonstrated the maximum rate of thrombus generation (MRTG) values in mm/min for the individual RAPClot™ prototype tubes over the two-month period (Figure 3E and Supplementary Figure S8). The results showed that the 0.15 mU/tube wet, Dry-IR, and Dry+IR tubes produced similar MRTG values in clotting non-heparin blood, although the MRTG values (16.72–18.84) at day 64 were significantly lower than those (25.11–25.62) at day 9 and (24.14–25.95) day 30 (Figure 3E and Supplementary Figure S8). Correspondingly, all the tubes had very short TMRTG with a range of 2.33–2.83 min except the wet tube at day 30 which had only 1.83 min (Figure 3E,F; Supplementary Figure S8). Furthermore, the results showed that all the wet and Dry-IR, especially RAP+IR, RAPClot™ tubes produced significantly lower MRTG values in clotting heparinized blood and the MRTG values for the Dry+IR tubes were only 3.55–8.77 at day 64 (Figure 3F, Supplementary Figure S8). In addition, all the wet, RAP-IR, and RAP+IR sterilized RAPClot™ tubes had a high total thrombus generation (TTG) of 745.2–927.3 mm in clotting non-heparin blood but had a large variation in TTG (170.8–785.5 in clotting the heparinized blood, with the RAP+IR RAPClot™ tubes having the lowest TTG (Figure 3G and Supplementary Figure S8). All the results revealed that heparin inhibited the MRTG, leading to prolonging the TMRTG and producing low TTG, suggesting that a relatively higher dose of RAPClot™ is required for developing the dry+γ-radiation RAPClot™ prototype tubes able to clot blood containing high concentrations of heparin.

3.4. *Shelf Life (Blood Clotting Stability) of the Sterilized RAPClot™ Prototype Tube*

Next, we investigated the potential shelf life of the sterilized RAPClot™ prototype tube. We prepared RAPClot™ -unirradiated prototype tubes (0.4 mU/tube) stored at room temperature (RT) for periods of up to 486 days to investigate their blood clotting activities (Figure 4A). The RAPClot™ tubes clotted efficiently recalcified citrated whole blood with or without heparin (8 U/mL) over the time course (Figure 4A). This was most apparent for the 0.4 mU/tube RAPClot™ tubes which clotted heparinized blood (8 U/mL) significantly faster than 300 s at day 486 (Figure 4A). Further experimentation showed that the RAPClot™ tubes containing 0.4 mU/tube still efficiently clotted both heparinized and non-heparinized blood after 3 years of storage (Supplementary Figure S9). Two further batches of RAPClot™ prototype tubes (no radiation) were prepared and stored at both RT and 50 °C for 147 days (Figure 4B, left panel) and 286 days (Figure 4B, right panel), respectively. The 50 °C stored RAPClot™ tubes for 147 days (Figure 4B, left panel) and 286 days (Figure 4B, right panel) had very high activity in clotting heparinized blood (8 U/mL), with the clotting times of 194.5 and 133 s, respectively, comparable to the RT-stored tubes (Figure 4B). The results revealed that RAPClot™ appears to be stable at high temperatures and retains its activity in clotting high-dose heparinized blood. Furthermore, it demonstrated that the RAPClot™ prototype tubes containing a lower dose (0.26 mU/tube), which were sterilized with γ-radiation (27.8 kGy) and stored at RT, still exhibited high blood clotting capability up to day 373 (Figure 4C). After 12 months at RT, these tubes clotted heparinized blood (8 U/mL) in 342.5 s, only slightly longer than 320.5 s for non-irradiated tubes and 327 s for γ-radiation-sterilized tubes in clotting non-heparinized blood (Figure 4C). These results demonstrated that γ-radiation is useful for sterilizing RAPClot™ prototype tubes that maintain high blood clotting activity for greater than 12 months of storage.

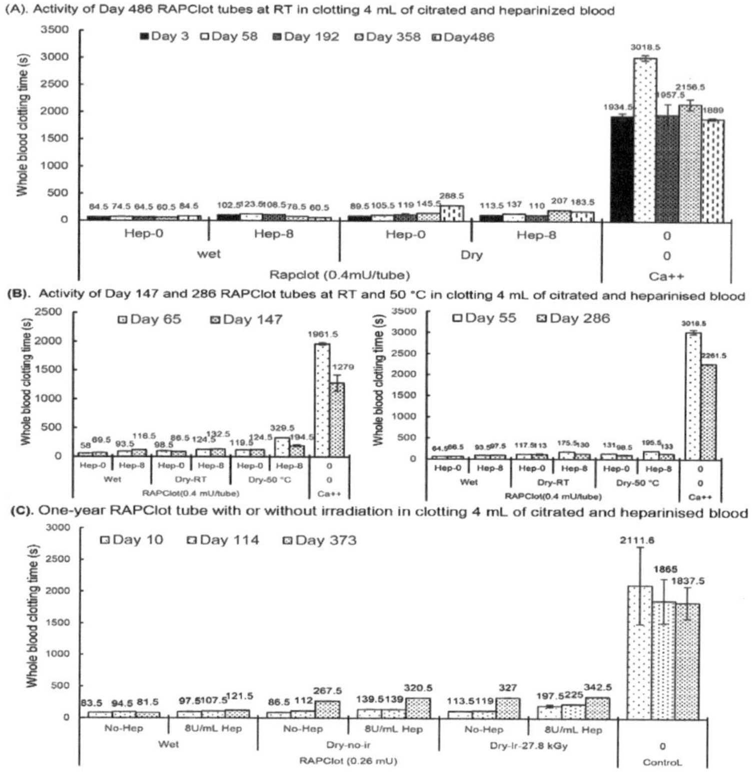

Figure 4. Blood clotting activity of the RAPClot™ prototype tubes with or without γ-radiation that were stored at room temperature (RT) or 50 °C in the long term. (**A**). The activity of the RAPClot™ prototype tubes stored at RT for 486 days in clotting 4 mL recalcified citrated whole blood with or without heparin (8 U/mL). (**B**). The activity of the RAPClot™ prototype tubes (0.4 mU/tube) stored at RT or 50 °C for 147 days (left panel) or 286 days (right panel) in clotting 4 mL recalcified citrated whole blood with or without heparin (8 U/mL). (**C**). The activity of the RAPClot™ prototype tubes (0.26 mU/tube) with or without γ-radiation (27.8 kGy) that were stored at RT for 373 days in clotting 4 mL recalcified citrated whole blood with or without 8 U/mL heparin. The error bars represent the standard deviation (SD).

3.5. Stability of RAPClot™ Prototype Tube Sterilized by Electron-Beam (E-Beam)

The effect of electron-beam (E-beam) radiation at a dose of 25 kGy was investigated on the enzymatic activity of the RAPClot™ prototype tubes, compared with that of γ-radiation (Figure 5). The S2238 assay showed a recovery of >90% enzymatic activity with the E-beam treatment, significantly higher than that of 59.5% with the γ-radiation treatment (Figure 5A). The next experiment was to compare the effects of E-beam with that of γ-radiation on the blood clotting activity of the RAPClot™ prototype tubes (Figure 5B). Exposure to E-beam radiation caused approximately a 10% loss of blood clotting activity, compared with a 40% loss for γ-radiation treatment (Figure 5B), consistent with the S2238 assay results (Figure 5A). The enzyme and blood clotting activities of the RAPClot™ prototype tubes were determined to contain a higher dose (0.9 mU/tube) with E-beam sterilization post storage at both RT and 50 °C conditions for 251 days, compared with those of the wet RAPClot™ prototype tubes stored at 4 °C and the dry-only RAPClot™ prototype tubes at RT and 50 °C (Figure 5C). The S2238 assays showed that the wet RAPClot™ prototype tubes (Wet 4 °C) retained over 86% of the enzymatic activity at 4 °C for 251 days, significantly lower than 93% of the enzymatic activity in the RAPClot™ prototype tubes (Dry-RT) at

RT (Figure 5C). The 50 °C storage for the RAP prototype tubes (Dry-50 °C) caused the loss of approximately 22% of the enzymatic activity at day 251 compared with the RAP-RT tubes, similar to that of the E-beam-sterilized RAPClot™ prototype tubes (Dry-EB RT) (Figure 5C). The E-beam sterilization plus 50 °C storage caused the RAPClot™ prototype tubes (Dry-EB-50 °C) to decrease activity by ~50% over this time period (Figure 5C). The blood clotting activities of the RAPClot™ tubes with different treatments under different storage conditions paralleled those of the S2238 assay (Figure 5C). The E-beam-sterilized RAPClot™ prototype tubes at 50 °C storage (Dry-EB-50 °C) clotted 6 mL of recalcified citrated whole blood only at 109 s and the heparinized blood at 8 U/mL faster than 3 min (174.5 s) (Figure 5C). Furthermore, we prepared four sets of RAPClot™ prototype tubes (A1, A2, B1, and B2) containing high dose (0.9 mU/tube) and one set of low dose RAPClot™ prototype tubes (0.4 mU/tube) as a positive control in protective formulations (Figure 5D). All the RAPClot™ tubes after the E-beam sterilization (25 kGy) were stored at RT for 682 days and then used to clot recalcified citrated whole blood with or without heparin (8 U/mL) (Figure 5D). All the A1, A2, B1, and B2 tubes showed high blood clotting activities, clotting the non-heparinized blood within 2–3 min and the heparinized blood (8 U/mL) in ~4 min (Figure 5D). The positive control RAPClot™ tubes (0.4 mU/tube) clotted the non-heparinized blood at 4 min and the heparinized blood (8 U/mL) slightly over 5 min with high-quality serum produced (339.5) (Figure 5D). The data suggest that the E-beam sterilization retains 30% higher clotting activity in the RAPClot™ prototype tubes compared to the gamma-radiation which showed a clotting activity of ~5 min after storage at RT for nearly two years.

3.6. Initial Clinical Study of RAPClot™ Rapid Serum Prototype Tubes

In a small clinical study, the activity of the γ-sterilized RAPClot™ prototype tubes (0.4 mU/4 mL blood) in clotting both fresh and recalcified citrated whole blood from five volunteers was determined (Figure 6). The average clotting times for fresh whole blood for the SST tubes were 455.0 $\pm$ 42 s, for the RAP-Ir tubes only 142.5 $\pm$ 42 s, for the RAP+Ir tubes 188.5 $\pm$ 31.6 s, and for the RAP+Ir+HEP (8 U heparin/mL) 139 $\pm$ 36.3 s (Figure 6A). The average clotting times of recalcified citrated whole blood for the RAP+Ir tubes was 95.2 $\pm$ 5 s and for the RAP+Ir+HEP was 107.6 $\pm$ 10 s (Figure 6B), providing further support that RAPClot™ with γ-radiation clotted efficiently not only recalcified citrated whole blood, but also heparinized blood at 8 U/mL. Furthermore, TEG demonstrated a similar clotting pattern to that of visual clotting in the RAP+Ir tubes with or without heparin (Figure 6C,D). The TEG images are provided here for two volunteers who are representative of all five individuals (Figure 6C,D). RAP+Ir and RAP+Ir+HEP produced R and K times that were 45 and 50 s for volunteer 1 and 50 and 50 s for volunteer 2 while Ca^+ alone had 870 and 480 s for volunteer 1 blood and 590 and 215 s for volunteer 2 (Figure 6C,D). The study showed that significantly greater angle-α, which measures the speed of clot formation, was obtained in RAP+Ir (79.6 and 77.5) and RAP+Ir+HEP (68.7 and 67.2) compared with Ca^+ alone (25.4 and 47.3) (Figure 6C,D). MA values in RAP+Ir (75.9 and 59.2), which determines clot strength, were substantially higher, compared with those in Ca^+ alone (40.0 and 52.6) and RAP+Ir+HEP (35.7 and 35.5) (Figure 6C,D). Figure 6E shows that the average R time of the five volunteers was 641.5 s in Ca^+, which was significantly decreased to 54.4 s in RAP+Ir and 95 s in RAP+Ir+HEP. Similarly, the K time was 262.4 s in Ca^+, which was significantly decreased to 63 s in RAP+Ir and 113.2 s in RAP+Ir+HEP (Figure 6F). Angle-α was significantly increased in RAP+Ir (75.3) and RAP+Ir+HEP (64.5) compared with Ca^+ (43.6) (Figure 6G). The MA value was increased in RAP+Ir (59.3), compared with those in Ca^+ (47.2) and in RAP+Ir+HEP (38.2) (Figure 6H), suggesting further that RAPClot™ improved substantially the clot strength in normal blood, with a decrease in clot strength in the presence of heparin. Figure 6I shows the V-curves from two participants. V-curves generated by RAP+Ir are similar to those by RAP+Ir+HEP, but significantly different from that by Ca^+ alone (Figure 6I). The average MRTG of the five participants was 22.5 mm/min in RAP+Ir, significantly higher than those both in RAP+Ir+HEP (13.3 mm/min) and Ca^+

alone (5.6 mm/min) (Figure 6J). The MRTG in RAP+Ir+HEP was also significantly higher in Ca^+ (Figure 6J). On average, RAP+Ir had a TMRTG (1.9 min) significantly shorter than RAP+Ir+HEP (3.3 min) and Ca^+ (13.7 min) (Figure 6K). Total thrombus generation (TTG) in RAP+Ir was significantly higher than that in RAP+Ir+HEP, but no significant difference was statistically obtained between RAP+Ir and Ca^+ and between RAP+Ir+HEP and Ca^+ (Figure 6L).

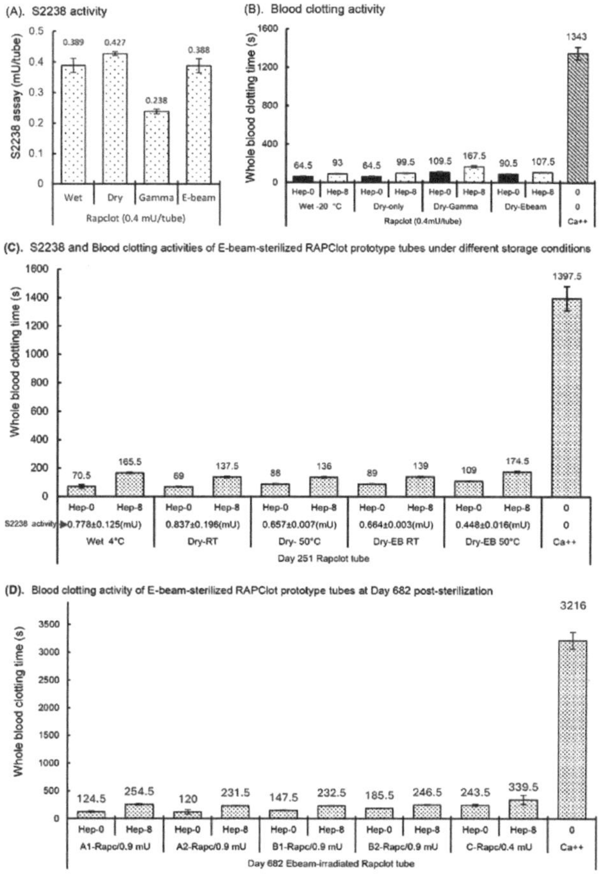

Figure 5. Enzymatic and blood clotting activities of the RAPClot™ prototype tubes with E-beam radiation. (**A**) The S2238 assay showed the recovery of enzyme activity of the RAPClot™ prototype tubes with the E-beam treatment compared with those with γ-radiation at day 7 post-radiation (n = 4). (**B**). The activity of the RAPClot™ prototype tubes with the E-beam treatment in clotting recalcified citrated whole blood (4 mL of blood/tube), compared with those with γ-radiation at day 7 post treatment (n = 2). (**C**). The enzymatic and blood clotting activities of the RAPClot™ prototype tubes (0.9 mU of RAPClot™ was added to one tube at day 0. Its enzymatic and blood clotting activities were measured at day 251 post E-beam sterilization) in clotting recalcified citrated whole blood (6 mL of blood/tube) with or without heparin (8 U/mL) (n = 3). Blue arrow indicates enzymatic activity of the individual RAPClot™ tubes based on S2238 assay at Day 251 post-E-beam sterilization. (**D**). The blood clotting activities of the RAPClot™ prototype tubes at day 682 post E-beam sterilization in clotting recalcified citrated whole blood (4 mL of blood/tube) with or without heparin (8 U/mL) (n = 2). Tube A1, A2, B1, and B2 contained 0.9 mU of the RAPClot™ prototype tube at day 0. As a positive control, the amount of RAPClot™ at 0.4 mU/tube was reduced from 0.9 mU/tube to achieve optimal conditions. The error bars represent the standard deviation (SD).

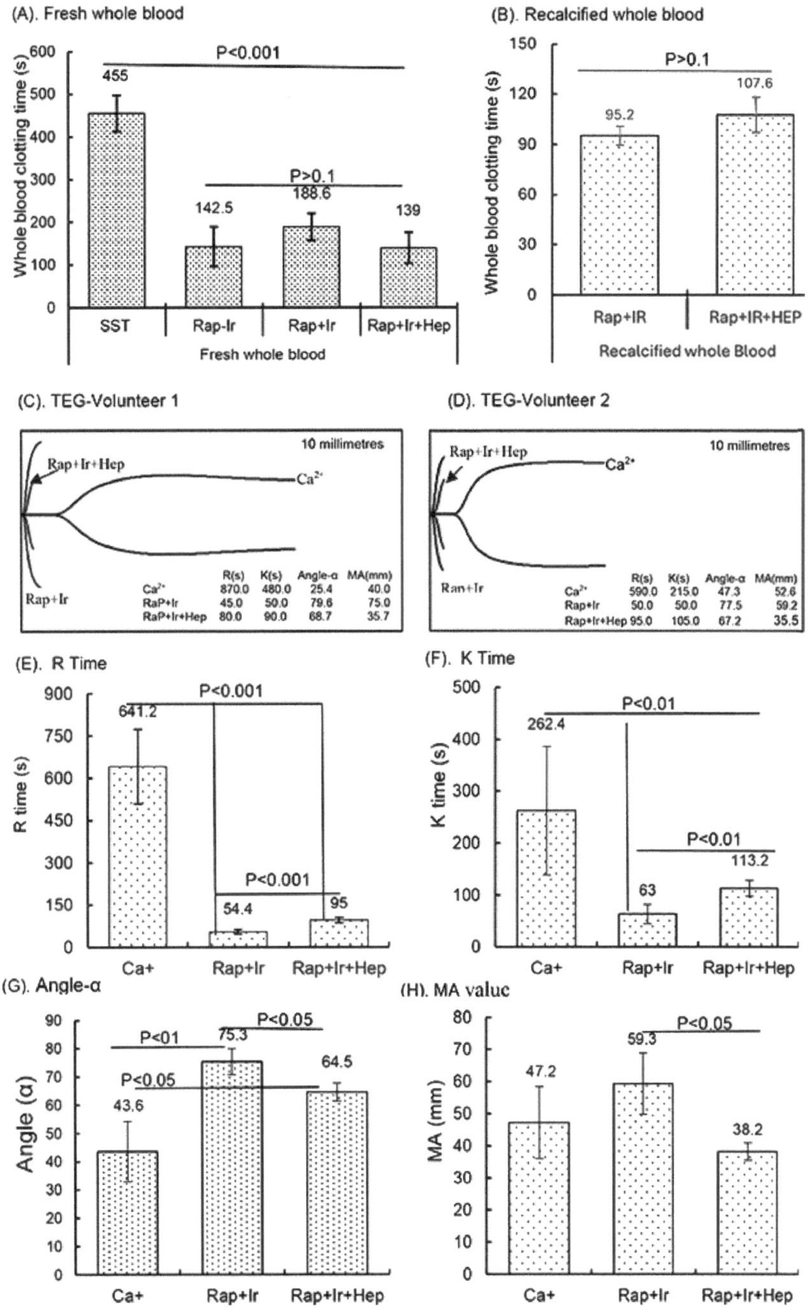

Figure 6. *Cont.*

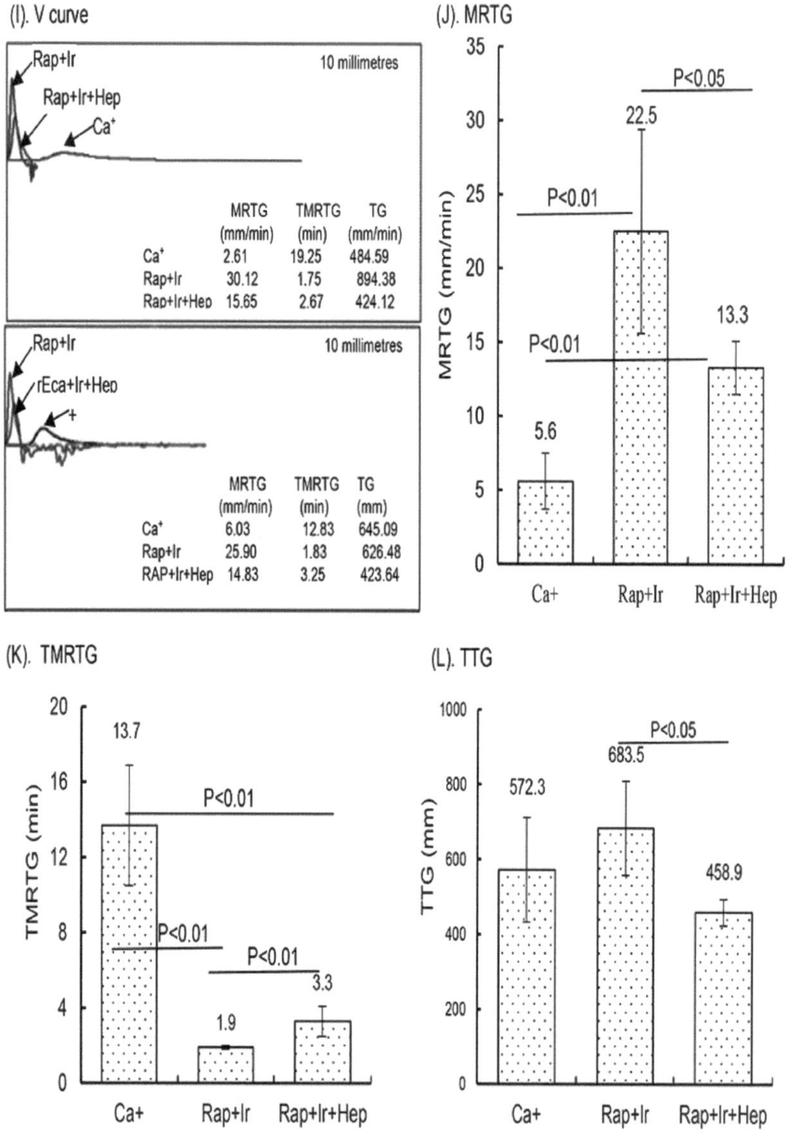

Figure 6. Clinical blood clotting trial with the RAPClot™ tubes using the five participants. The activity of the RAPClot™ tube in clotting fresh whole blood and recalcified citrated whole blood samples from the five volunteers by visual clotting and TEG assays. A total of 0.26 mU of RAPClot™ was used to add into one GBO plain tube for preparing the RAPClot™ prototype tube with or without γ-radiation as described in the Material and Methods Section. (**A**). The visual clotting activity of the BD SST tube (SST), RAPClot™ prototype tube without radiation treatment (Rap-Ir), and RAPClot™ prototype tube treated with r-radiation (Rap+Ir) in clotting fresh whole blood and the RAPClot™ prototype tube treated with γ-radiation (Rap+Ir+Hep) in clotting fresh whole blood containing

heparin at 8 U/mL. (**B**). The activity of RAPClot™ prototype tubes with r-radiation treatment in clotting recalcified citrated whole blood without (Rap+Ir) or with heparin at 8 U/mL (Rap+Ir+Hep). The data are the mean ± standard deviation (X ± SD) from the 5 volunteers. (**C**,**D**). Parallel to the visual clotting assay shown in (**B**), the thromboelastography (TEG) assay shows two representative images of RAPClot™ in clotting recalcified citrated whole blood samples from the three types of tubes (Ca^+, Rap+Ir, and Rap+Ir+Hep) from 2 volunteers out of the 5 volunteers, revealing significantly different thromboelastographic traces of the RAPClot™ prototype tubes from Ca^+-only tubes in clotting recalcified citrated whole blood and different TEG parameters (R times, K time, α angle values, and MA values) showing in inserted squares. (**E–H**). TEG assay shows four parameters (R times, K time, α angle values, and MA values) of the RAPClot™ prototype tubes in clotting recalcified citrated whole blood from five participants. The data are the x ± SD of the four parameters from the five participants in three types of tubes in the duplicate assay (n = 10). $p < 0.05$, $p < 0.01$, and $p < 0.001$ represent that the difference between the two types of tubes was statistically significantly different, respectively. $p > 0.1$ represents that the difference between the two types of tubes was not statistically different. (**I**). Two representative V-curves derived from the TEG assay for two volunteers (see Figure 1C,D) showing significantly different thrombin generation of the RAPClot™ prototype tubes in clotting recalcified citrated whole blood with or without heparin. (**J**). The mean ± SD of the maximum rate of thrombin generation (MRTG) at mm/min of the recalcified citrated whole blood from the 5 participants clotted in three types of tubes in the TEG assay in duplicate (n = 10). (**K**). The mean ± SD of the time to the maximum rate of thrombus generation (TMRTG) (min) (n = 10). (**L**). The mean ± SD of the total thrombus generation (TTG) (n = 10). $p < 0.05$, and $p < 0.01$ represent that the difference between the two types of tubes was significantly different, respectively. The error bars represent the standard deviation (SD).

3.7. Analyte Measurements from Sera Produced in RAPClot™ Rapid Serum Prototype Tubes

We next determined the levels of commonly measured analytes (potassium (K), glucose (Glu), lactate dehydrogenase (LD), iron (Fe), and phosphate (Phos)) known to be affected by clotting and cell lyses during the clotting process, and remnant cells on top of the blood gel "buffy coat" or cells in contact with the serum in gel-free tubes post centrifugation [3]. Blood was collected from the five participants and serum was produced by the three 0.4 mUnit RAPClot™ prototype tubes (RAP-Ir, RAP+Ir, and RAP+Ir+HEP), and compared with that generated by the commercial SST tube (Figure 7). As shown in Figure 7, the values for the five analytes examined were similar in the sera of the five volunteers' fresh blood produced in four blood collection tubes with p values > 0.05. Furthermore, in a separate clinical trial with five volunteers, we compared 33 analyte measurements in the sera generated from the RAP+Ir and RAP+Ir+HEP (8 U/mL) prototype tubes, compared with those from the three commercial blood collection tubes (SST, RST, and PST tubes) (Supplementary Table S3). The results showed that there was very good agreement between the analyte concentrations determined among the variation in all the 33 analytes measured among the five tubes (Supplementary Table S3). These results suggest that the presence of RAPClot™ in the prototype blood collection tubes does not interfere with analyte determination.

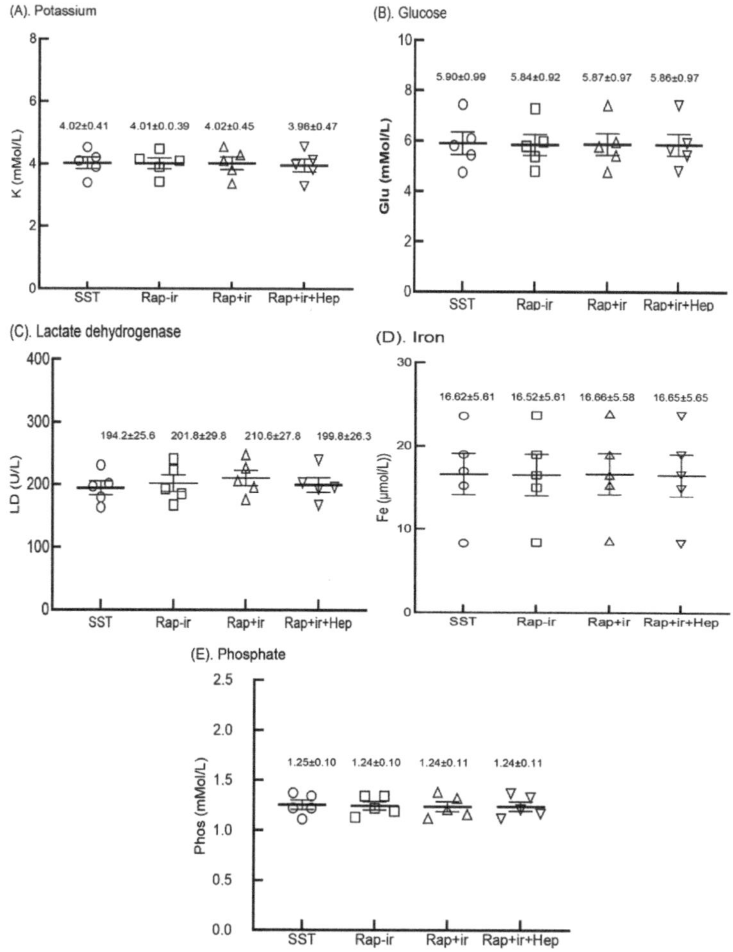

Figure 7. Five analytes in the sera of the five volunteers' fresh blood clotted in the BD SST tube (SST), RAPClot™ prototype tube without γ-radiation (Rap-Ir), and RAPClot™ prototype tube treated with γ-radiation (Rap+Ir) in clotting fresh whole blood and RAPClot™ prototype tube treated with γ-radiation (Rap+Ir+Hep) in clotting heparinized fresh whole blood (8 U/mL) in the clinical trial as shown in Figure 6A. (**A**). Potassium (K) (p = 0.9999, >0.05), (**B**). glucose (Glu) (p = 0.9997, >0.05), (**C**). lactate dehydrogenase (LD) (p = 0.8191, >0.05), (**D**). iron (Fe) (p = 0.9997, >0.05), and (**E**). phosphate (Phos) (p = 0.9966, >0.05). The data inserted in the individual sub-figures are the mean ± standard deviation (SD) of the five volunteers, respectively (n = 5). The data analysis results did not show that the concentrations of the individual analytes among the four tubes were statistically different (p > 0.05). The error bars represent the standard deviation (SD).

4. Discussion

Blood collection tube components starting with the tube wall, and including rubber stoppers, lubricants, anticoagulants, separator gels, clot activators, and surfactants, can all affect the quality of the sample generated and subsequently the accuracy and precision of laboratory tests [32]. Surfactants are usually low-viscosity silicone-based fluids used to coat collection tubes to enhance the spreadability of blood in tubes during blood clotting and act as a release agent to ensure the clean separation of clotted blood from the walls during centrifugation, reducing "clots hang up". In this study, we used several surfactants to coat both GBO and BD plain blood collection tubes which were used for testing the blood clotting activity of RAPClot™ consistent with published studies. In this study, the surfactant used was 20 μL of DC3771 at the concentrations of 0.25–0.5% used for preparing per RAPClot™ prototype tube in which the findings showed that it did not affect either the S2238 assay or blood clotting activities for the assay of 31 analytes.

Hepes buffer has been widely used for protein purification and extraction as a stabilizer of different proteins [33–36]. In the present study, Hepes was used for preparing the RAPClot™ aqueous working solution which retained a high level of blood clotting activity. However, when it was used for drying RAPClot™ under different temperature conditions in two types of commercial plain tubes (GBO and BD), the blood clotting activity was significantly reduced whether the tubes were coated with or without surfactant. In contrast, the use of Gelofusine (GF) for preparing and drying the RAPClot™ working solution in both the GBO and BD tubes retained both high enzymatic and blood clotting activities. Therefore, GF was selected for use in the RAPClot™ prototype tubes. It was subsequently found that the inclusion of 10% stabilizing sugar in the GF buffer optimized the recovery and stability of the RAPClot™ tubes and was selected for further studies to optimize the prototype formulation performance.

A requirement for blood collection tubes is that they can be stored for periods in excess of 12 months in order to eliminate stability issues. Gamma-radiation (γ-radiation) is a method of choice and was first used for sterilizing disposable medical products in the 1960s [37,38]. Since then, over 50% of the disposable medical products manufactured in developed countries have been radiation-sterilized at doses varying from 17 to 50 kGy [38–40]. Here, we used γ-radiation at the doses of 25–27.5 kGy to sterilize the RAPClot™ prototype tubes. Even at the highest dose, we revealed a recovery of approximately 42% of the enzymatic activity and 53% of the plasma clotting activity in the RAPClot™ tube. While it is evident that the metalloproteinase is sensitive to γ-radiation, the use of the GF formulation limits the loss of activity and retains the usefulness of RAPClot™ as an important additive to blood collection tubes to enhance clotting to produce quality serum. The γ-radiation-sterilized RAPClot™ prototype tubes prepared in all six formations on day 14 post-radiation were capable of clotting heparinized blood at a high dose of 8 U/mL within 5 min even at concentrations as low as 0.26 mU/tube. These data demonstrated that γ-radiation is acceptable for sterilizing RAPClot™ prototype tubes. More recently, E-beam radiation has also been employed to sterilize pharmaceutical packaging products [41]. It operates by directing a continuous flow of electrons through the articles being sterilized [42]. We also used E-beam at 25 kGy to sterilize RAPClot™ prototype tubes, finding that the tubes retained up to 80% of the enzyme activity based on the S2238 assay, revealing that this form of sterilization is an effective technology for developing the RAPClot™ prototype tubes.

The standard shelf life for blood collection tubes is 12 months from the time of manufacture [29,30]. Thus, in introducing any new blood collection tube into the market, this is an important consideration for its commercial viability. Our results showed that RAPClot™ is stable in blood collection tubes prepared using a protective formulation and sterilized with both Y-radiation and E-beam exposure. RAPClot™ stored in blood collection tubes at room temperature in either wet or dried form (evacuated) was stable for periods of up to 3 years. The activity was comparable in both citrated and heparinized (8 U/mL) blood and it was capable of withstanding temperatures of 50 °C for periods as long as 286 days. The capacity to produce quality serum in the presence of anticoagulants is a big advantage over the RST tube and Greiner BCA Fast Clot tube [4] to which thrombin is added and have been found not to be suitable for serum preparation for patients on anticoagulants, especially heparin [3]. The activity of the RAPClot™ tube was also maintained when exposed to sterilization conditions at levels used commercially. While the more conventional method of exposure to γ-radiation sterilization reduced activity by 50%, exposure to E-beam radiation only had minimal effects on its activity.

The results presented here demonstrate that RAPClot™ can be used to produce RAPClot™ rapid serum prototype tubes that can meet the requirement of a new standard blood collection tube to clot blood samples including high-dose heparinized blood (8 U/mL) within 5 min post-γ-radiation or E-beam sterilization with a potential for long-term storage stability at RT. Further clinical testing of spray-dried and irradiated RAPClot™ rapid serum tubes is warranted.

While the RAPClot™ tube possessed the major characteristics required for a suitable serum tube, it was also important that the presence of RAPClot™ did not lead to any interference with analytes tested in a clinical setting. Accordingly, we carried out two clinical trials with five volunteers to test whether there was any interference with biochemical analytes in these tubes. In the initial trial, the concentrations of five commonly measured analytes: K, Glu, LD, Fe, and Phos by the three RAPClot™ tubes (RAP-Ir, RAP+Ir, and RAP+Ir+HEP) were equal to those generated by the commercial SST tube. In a separate clinical trial with the five participants, the concentrations of 33 biochemistry markers in sera were generated from the two RAPClot™ tubes, which were not clinically different to those generated from the commercial SST, RST, and PST tubes. In fact, the K and Gluc in the serum from heparinized blood were closer to lithium heparin plasma. These data provide strong evidence that the RAPClot™ prototype tube is suitable for routine laboratory use in both non- and heparin-anticoagulated blood samples.

5. Conclusions

In conclusion, we have developed a novel blood collection tube (RAPClot™ rapid serum prototype tube) that produces quality serum for analyte determination. We established a stabilizing formulation that upon spray-drying as an additive in commercial plain tubes and radiation using standard commercial methods and levels retained RAPClot™ enzyme and blood clotting activities when stored over periods of time required for commercial viability including samples with very high concentrations of heparin. The experimental data have demonstrated that a RAPClot™ containing clotting tube is a commercially competitive product and has the potential to be the standard tube, eliminating the need for the various serum/plasma tubes, e.g., SST, RST, BCA Fast, PST (gel or plasma separator device), Na fluoride, and FC Mix due to its ability to clot all anticoagulated samples within five minutes and consistently produce the highest quality serum and significantly minimize sample quality related result errors with optimal TAT.

Supplementary Materials: The following supporting information can be downloaded at: https://www.mdpi.com/article/10.3390/biom14060645/s1, Figure S1. Effects of surfactants used for coating GBO white top plain blood collection tube on the activity of RAPClot™ in clotting wet recalcified citrated whole blood; Figure S2. Activity of RAPClot™ (0.2 mU/tube) prepared in Hepes buffer containing 10% lactulose (10% lac) plus BSA (0.5% and 4%), dextran (0.5% and 4% Dex), Polyvinylpyrrolidone (4% *PVP*), voluven (4% Voluv) and sorbitol (4% Sorb), respectively, compared with that prepared in Gelofusine containing 10% lactulose (10% lac); Figure S3. Effects of BSA as an additional component used for developing RAPClot™ blood clotting formulation on the activity of the wet RAPClot™ in clotting recalcified citrated whole blood; Figure S4. Activity of RAPClot™ recovered from the RAPClot™ prototype tubes prepared in six formulations with or without γ-radiation (27.8 kGy) according to plasma clotting and S2238 assays; Figure S5. TEG® 5000 Thrombelastograph® Hemostasis System; Figure S6. TEG assay showing the stability of RAPClot™ prototype-tube at dose of 0.30 mU/tube propared in one formuation with or without gamma radiation (25.7 kGy) stored for 64 days at room temperature in clotting the recalcified citrated whole bloods; Figure S7. Activity of three-years RAPClot™ -prototype tubes in clotting 4 mL of recalcified citrated whole blood with or without heparin at 8 U/mL; Table S1: RAPClot™ prototype tubes prepared in different formulations with or without γ-radiation were used for S2238 assay (Figure 2A); Table S2: RAPClot™ prototype tubes prepared in six formulations with or without γ-radiation were used for S2238, plasma and blood clotting assay (Figure 2B–D; Figure S4); Table S3: Thirty-three analytes measured in serum generated from five blood collection tubes: SST, RST, RAPClot™, RAPClot™ +Heparin(8 U/mL) and PST prepared at 0 h after collection in the second trial. The data are the mean ± standard deviation (SD) of participants respectively (n = 5).

Author Contributions: M.F.L., J.d.J., M.G., P.M., G.D. and K.-N.Z. conceived the study; L.J. and J.W. performed the S2238 assay. P.M. and K.-N.Z. performed the blood clotting and TEG assay. K.-N.Z. and M.F.L. wrote the manuscript with assistance from L.J., G.D. and M.G. All authors have read and agreed to the published version of the manuscript.

Funding: We appreciate all financial support of Q-Sera for funding for the project "QSera: a novel serum collection tube" grant number T10473-D01/AG-027735.

Institutional Review Board Statement: HREC reference number: HREC/08/QPAH/005, approval on 21 March 2017, see Section 2.8.

Informed Consent Statement: Not applicable.

Data Availability Statement: We confirm that the data supporting the findings of this study are available within the article and its Supplementary Materials.

Acknowledgments: We wish to thank the Australian Red Cross Blood Service (ARCBS) and Princess Alexandra Hospital, Brisbane, Qld, Australia for the provision of blood for the experiments.

Conflicts of Interest: K.-N.Z., P.M., L.J., J.d.J. and M.F.L. are employed by The University of Queensland, Australia. GD is employed by Princess Alexandra Hospital, Woolloongabba, Brisbane, QLD 4102. They have Inventor Share Option Scheme in Q-Sera. The remaining authors declare that the research was conducted in the absence of any commercial or financial relationships that could be construed as a potential conflict of interest. Q-Sera in affiliation and funding had no role in the design of the study; in the collection, analyses, or interpretation of data; in the writing of the manuscript, or in the decision to publish the results.

References

1. Forsman, R.W. Why is the laboratory an afterthought for managed care organizations? *Clin. Chem.* **1996**, *42*, 813–816. [CrossRef] [PubMed]
2. Hallworth, M.J. The '70% claim': What is the evidence base? *Ann. Clin. Biochem.* **2011**, *48*, 487–488. [CrossRef] [PubMed]
3. Dimeski, G.; Masci, P.P.; Trabi, M.; Lavin, M.F.; de Jersey, J. Evaluation of the Becton-Dickinson rapid serum tube: Does it provide a suitable alternative to lithium heparin plasma tubes? *Clin. Chem. Lab. Med.* **2010**, *48*, 651–657. [CrossRef] [PubMed]
4. Dimeski, G.; Johnston, J.; Masci, P.P.; Zhao, K.N.; Brown, N. Evaluation of the Greiner Bio-One serum separator BCA Fast Clot tube. *Clin. Chem. Lab. Med.* **2017**, *55*, 1135–1141. [CrossRef] [PubMed]
5. Dimeski, G.; Yow, K.S.; Brown, N.N. Evaluation of the accuracy of the Greiner Bio-One FC Mix Glucose tube. *Clin. Chem. Lab. Med.* **2017**, *55*, e96–e98. [CrossRef]
6. Kumura, T.; Hino, M.; Yamane, T.; Tominaga, K.; Tatsumi, N. DX-9065a, a specific factor Xa inhibitor, as a universal anticoagulant for blood collection tubes. *Clin. Chim. Acta* **2000**, *294*, 27–35. [CrossRef] [PubMed]
7. Bowen, R.A.; Remaley, A.T. Interferences from blood collection tube components on clinical chemistry assays. *Biochem. Med.* **2014**, *24*, 31–44. [CrossRef] [PubMed]
8. Bowen, R.A.; Sattayapiwat, A.; Gounden, V.; Remaley, A.T. Blood collection tube-related alterations in analyte concentrations in quality control material and serum specimens. *Clin. Biochem.* **2014**, *47*, 150–157. [CrossRef] [PubMed]
9. Aziz, N.; Butch, A.W.; Ryner, T.C.; Martinez-Maza, O.; Detels, R. The influence of EDTA Vacutainer blood collection tube on the level of blood interleukin-1 receptor antagonist. *J. Immunol. Methods* **2019**, *464*, 114–118. [CrossRef]
10. Vignali, D.A.; Collison, L.W.; Workman, C.J. How regulatory T cells work. *Nat. Rev. Immunol.* **2008**, *8*, 523–532. [CrossRef]
11. Lee, H.J.; Kim, Y.T.; Park, P.J.; Shin, Y.S.; Kang, K.N.; Kim, Y.; Kim, C.W. A novel detection method of non-small cell lung cancer using multiplexed bead-based serum biomarker profiling. *J. Thorac. Cardiovasc. Surg.* **2012**, *143*, 421–427. [CrossRef] [PubMed]
12. Dimeski, G.; Solano, C.; Petroff, M.K.; Hynd, M. Centrifugation protocols: Tests to determine optimal lithium heparin and citrate plasma sample quality. *Ann. Clin. Biochem.* **2011**, *48*, 218–222. [CrossRef]
13. Kumura, T.; Hino, M.; Yamane, T.; Tatsumi, N. Hirudin as an anticoagulant for both haematology and chemistry tests. *J. Autom. Methods Manag. Chem.* **2000**, *22*, 109–112. [CrossRef] [PubMed]
14. Kumura, T.; Hino, M.; Yamane, T.; Tatsumi, N. Argatroban as an anticoagulant for both hematologic and chemical tests. *J. Clin. Lab. Anal.* **2000**, *14*, 136–140. [CrossRef] [PubMed]
15. Pretorius, C.J.; Dimeski, G.; O'Rourke, P.K.; Marquart, L.; Tyack, S.A.; Wilgen, U.; Ungerer, J.P. Outliers as a cause of false cardiac troponin results: Investigating the robustness of 4 contemporary assays. *Clin. Chem.* **2011**, *57*, 710–718. [CrossRef] [PubMed]
16. Aoki, N.; Sakata, Y.; Ichinose, A. Fibrin-associated plasminogen activation in alpha 2-plasmin inhibitor deficiency. *Blood* **1983**, *62*, 1118–1122. [CrossRef] [PubMed]
17. Cuhadar, S.; Atay, A.; Koseoglu, M.; Dirican, A.; Hur, A. Stability studies of common biochemical analytes in serum separator tubes with or without gel barrier subjected to various storage conditions. *Biochem. Med.* **2012**, *22*, 202–214. [CrossRef]
18. Zhao, K.N.; Dimeski, G.; de Jersey, J.; Johnson, L.A.; Grant, M.; Masci, P.P.; Lavin, M.F. Rapid serum tube technology overcomes problems associated with use of anticoagulants. *Biochem. Med.* **2019**, *29*, 030706. [CrossRef] [PubMed]

19. Zhao, K.N.; Dimeski, G.; de Jersey, J.; Johnson, L.A.; Grant, M.; Masci, P.P.; Lavin, M.F. Next-generation rapid serum tube technology using prothrombin activator coagulant: Fast, high-quality serum from normal samples. *Clin. Chem. Lab. Med.* **2019**, *57*, 483–497. [CrossRef]
20. Kini, R.M. The intriguing world of prothrombin activators from snake venom. *Toxicon* **2005**, *45*, 1133–1145. [CrossRef]
21. Speijer, H.; Govers-Riemslag, J.W.; Zwaal, R.F.; Rosing, J. Prothrombin activation by an activator from the venom of Oxyuranus scutellatus (*Taipan snake*). *J. Biol. Chem.* **1986**, *261*, 13258–13267. [CrossRef] [PubMed]
22. Nishida, S.; Fujita, T.; Kohno, N.; Atoda, H.; Morita, T.; Takeya, H.; Kido, I.; Paine, M.J.; Kawabata, S.; Iwanaga, S. cDNA cloning and deduced amino acid sequence of prothrombin activator (ecarin) from Kenyan Echis carinatus venom. *Biochemistry* **1995**, *34*, 1771–1778. [CrossRef] [PubMed]
23. Zhao, K.N.; Masci, P.; Dimeski, G.; Johnson, L.; Grant, M.; de Jersey, J.; Lavin, M.F. Potential Application of Recombinant Snake Prothrombin Activator Ecarin in Blood Diagnostics. *Biomolecules* **2022**, *12*, 1704. [CrossRef] [PubMed]
24. Kini, R.M.; Rao, V.S.; Joseph, J.S. Procoagulant proteins from snake venoms. *Haemostasis* **2001**, *31*, 218–224. [CrossRef] [PubMed]
25. Moore, G.W.; Jones, P.O.; Platton, S.; Hussain, N.; White, D.; Thomas, W.; Rigano, J.; Pouplard, C.; Gray, E.; Devreese, K.M.J. International multicenter, multiplatform study to validate *Taipan snake* venom time as a lupus anticoagulant screening test with ecarin time as the confirmatory test: Communication from the ISTH SSC Subcommittee on Lupus Anticoagulant/Antiphospholipid Antibodies. *J. Thromb. Haemost.* **2021**, *19*, 3177–3192. [CrossRef]
26. Ungerstedt, J.S.; Kallner, A.; Blomback, M. Measurement of blood and plasma coagulation time using free oscillating rheometry. *Scand. J. Clin. Lab. Investig.* **2002**, *62*, 135–140. [CrossRef] [PubMed]
27. Swallow, R.A.; Agarwala, R.A.; Dawkins, K.D.; Curzen, N.P. Thromboelastography: Potential bedside tool to assess the effects of antiplatelet therapy? *Platelets* **2006**, *17*, 385–392. [CrossRef] [PubMed]
28. Johnson, L.A.; de Jersey, J.; Masci, P.P.; Zhao, K.N.; Bennett, N.C.; Dimeski, G.; Grant, M.; Lavin, M.F. Progress Curve Analysis of the one stage chromogenic assay for ecarin. *Anal. Biochem.* **2020**, *608*, 113907. [CrossRef]
29. Gros, N.; Klobucar, T.; Gaber, K. Accuracy of Citrate Anticoagulant Amount, Volume, and Concentration in Evacuated Blood Collection Tubes Evaluated with UV Molecular Absorption Spectrometry on a Purified Water Model. *Molecules* **2023**, *28*, 486. [CrossRef]
30. Weikart, C.M.; Breeland, A.P.; Wills, M.S.; Baltazar-Lopez, M.E. Hybrid Blood Collection Tubes: Combining the Best Attributes of Glass and Plastic for Safety and Shelf life. *SLAS Technol.* **2020**, *25*, 484–493. [CrossRef]
31. Ni, L.; Xue, P.; An, C.; Yu, X.; Qu, J.; Yao, Y.; Li, Y. Establishment of Normal Range for Thromboelastography in Healthy Middle-Aged and Elderly People of Weihai in China. *J. Healthc. Eng.* **2021**, *2021*, 7119779. [CrossRef] [PubMed]
32. Bowen, R.A.; Vu, C.; Remaley, A.T.; Hortin, G.L.; Csako, G. Differential effect of blood collection tubes on total free fatty acids (FFA) and total triiodothyronine (TT3) concentration: A model for studying interference from tube constituents. *Clin. Chim. Acta* **2007**, *378*, 181–193. [CrossRef] [PubMed]
33. Le Guevel, X.; Daum, N.; Schneider, M. Synthesis and characterization of human transferrin-stabilized gold nanoclusters. *Nanotechnology* **2011**, *22*, 275103. [CrossRef] [PubMed]
34. Muinao, T.; Deka Boruah, H.P.; Pal, M. Diagnostic and Prognostic Biomarkers in ovarian cancer and the potential roles of cancer stem cells—An updated review. *Exp. Cell Res.* **2018**, *362*, 1–10. [CrossRef]
35. Brudar, S.; Hribar-Lee, B. Effect of Buffer on Protein Stability in Aqueous Solutions: A Simple Protein Aggregation Model. *J. Phys. Chem. B* **2021**, *125*, 2504–2512. [CrossRef] [PubMed]
36. Tan, M.; Ding, Z.; Chu, Y.; Xie, J. Potential of Good's buffers to inhibit denaturation of myofibrillar protein upon freezing. *Food Res. Int.* **2023**, *165*, 112484. [CrossRef] [PubMed]
37. Darmady, E.M.; Hughes, K.E.; Burt, M.M.; Freeman, B.M.; Powell, D.B. Radiation sterilization. *J. Clin. Pathol.* **1961**, *14*, 55–58. [CrossRef] [PubMed]
38. Cook, A.M.; Berry, R.J. Microbial contamination on disposable hypodermic syringes prior to sterilization by ionizing radiation. *Appl. Microbiol.* **1968**, *16*, 1156–1162. [CrossRef] [PubMed]
39. Emerson, J.F.; Abbaszadeh, Y.; Lo, J.N.; Tsinas, Z.; Pettersson, J.; Ward, P.; Al-Sheikhly, M.I. Sterilizing photocurable materials by irradiation: Preserving UV-curing properties of photopolymers following E-beam, gamma, or X-ray exposure. *J. Mater. Sci. Mater. Med.* **2017**, *28*, 185. [CrossRef]
40. Gomes, A.D.; de Oliveira, A.A.R.; Houmard, M.; Nunes, E.H.M. Gamma sterilization of collagen/hydroxyapatite composites: Validation and radiation effects. *Appl. Radiat. Isot.* **2021**, *174*, 109758. [CrossRef]
41. Silindir, M.; Ozer, Y. The effect of radiation on a variety of pharmaceuticals and materials containing polymers. *PDA J. Pharm. Sci. Technol.* **2012**, *66*, 184–199. [CrossRef] [PubMed]
42. Semmler, E.; Novak, W.; Allinson, W.; Wallis, D.; Wood, N.; Awakowicz, P.; Wunderlich, J. Plasma Decontamination: A Case Study on Kill Efficacy of Geobacillus stearothermophilus Spores on Different Carrier Materials. *PDA J. Pharm. Sci. Technol.* **2016**, *70*, 256–271. [CrossRef] [PubMed]

biomolecules

Article

The Adipokinetic Hormone (AKH) and the Adipokinetic Hormone/Corazonin-Related Peptide (ACP) Signalling Systems of the Yellow Fever Mosquito *Aedes aegypti*: Chemical Models of Binding

Graham E. Jackson [1], Marc-Antoine Sani [2,*], Heather G. Marco [3], Frances Separovic [2,4] and Gerd Gäde [3]

1 Department of Chemistry, University of Cape Town, Private Bag, Rondebosch 7701, South Africa; graham.jackson@uct.ac.za
2 Bio21 Institute, University of Melbourne, Melbourne, VIC 3010, Australia; fs@unimelb.edu.au
3 Department of Biological Sciences, University of Cape Town, Private Bag, Rondebosch 7701, South Africa; heather.marco@uct.ac.za (H.G.M.); gerd.gade@uct.ac.za (G.G.)
4 School of Chemistry, University of Melbourne, Melbourne, VIC 3010, Australia
* Correspondence: msani@unimeb.edu.au

Abstract: Neuropeptides are the main regulators of physiological, developmental, and behavioural processes in insects. Three insect neuropeptide systems, the adipokinetic hormone (AKH), corazonin (Crz), and adipokinetic hormone/corazonin-related peptide (ACP), and their cognate receptors, are related to the vertebrate gonadotropin (GnRH) system and form the GnRH superfamily of peptides. In the current study, the two signalling systems, AKH and ACP, of the yellow fever mosquito, *Aedes aegypti*, were comparatively investigated with respect to ligand binding to their respective receptors. To achieve this, the solution structure of the hormones was determined by nuclear magnetic resonance distance restraint methodology. Atomic-scale models of the two G protein-coupled receptors were constructed with the help of homology modelling. Thereafter, the binding sites of the receptors were identified by blind docking of the ligands to the receptors, and models were derived for each hormone system showing how the ligands are bound to their receptors. Lastly, the two models were validated by comparing the computational results with experimentally derived data available from the literature. This mostly resulted in an acceptable agreement, proving the models to be largely correct and usable. The identification of an antagonist versus a true agonist may, however, require additional testing. The computational data also explains the exclusivity of the two systems that bind only the cognate ligand. This study forms the basis for further drug discovery studies.

Keywords: *Aedes aegypti*; adipokinetic hormone; corazonin hormone; molecular modelling; yellow fever mosquito; peptide signalling

Citation: Jackson, G.E.; Sani, M.-A.; Marco, H.G.; Separovic, F.; Gäde, G. The Adipokinetic Hormone (AKH) and the Adipokinetic Hormone/Corazonin-Related Peptide (ACP) Signalling Systems of the Yellow Fever Mosquito *Aedes aegypti*: Chemical Models of Binding. *Biomolecules* **2024**, *14*, 313. https://doi.org/10.3390/biom14030313

Academic Editors: Hyung-Sik Won and Ji-Hun Kim

Received: 15 January 2024
Revised: 27 February 2024
Accepted: 1 March 2024
Published: 6 March 2024

1. Introduction

Three neuropeptide signalling systems exist in invertebrates, where the mature peptides and their cognate G protein-coupled receptors (GPCRs) are, respectively, structurally similar. Collectively, these signalling systems are related to the vertebrate gonadotropin-releasing hormone (GnRH) system, giving rise to the concept of a large peptide superfamily [1–4]. The aforementioned invertebrate neuropeptide systems are the adipokinetic hormone (AKH)/red pigment-concentrating hormone (RPCH) family, the corazonin (Crz) family, and the structurally intermediate family known as the adipokinetic hormone/corazonin-related peptide (ACP) family (see a recent review by Marco et al. [5]). In the current study, we focus on members of the GnRH superfamily in the medically relevant pest insect, the mosquito *Aedes agypti*, hence, a description of the GnRH superfamily will be restricted here to insects.

AKHs are primarily or exclusively produced in neurosecretory cells of the corpus cardiacum (CC), and a major function is the mobilisation of energy reserves stored in the fat body, thus providing an increase in the concentration of diacylglycerols, trehalose, or proline in the haemolymph for locomotory active phases. Accordingly, the AKH receptor (AKHR) transcripts are predominantly found in fat body tissue, where the AKH activates the enzymes glycogen phosphorylase and triacylglycerol lipase, respectively [6–8]. As with most endocrine regulatory peptides, additional functions, such as inhibition of anabolic processes (protein and lipid syntheses), involvement in oxidative stress reactions, and egg production inter alia are known, making AKH a truly pleiotropic hormone [9,10].

Crz is mainly synthesised in neuroendocrine cells of the pars lateralis of the protocerebrum and released into circulation via the CC [11]. Although originally described as a potent cardio-stimulatory peptide [12], Crz does not generally fulfil this role but is known for other functions, such as involvement in the release of pre-ecdysis and ecdysis-triggering hormones, reduction of silk spinning rates in the silk moth, pigmentation events (darkening) of the epidermis in locusts as they transition to the gregarious phase, and regulation of caste identity in an ant species [13–16].

The functional role of ACP is less clear. Previous studies had not found a clear-cut function for this peptide in *Anopheles gambiae* and *Rhodnius prolixus* [17,18] until work by Zhou et al. [19] claimed that ACP in male crickets (*Gryllus bimaculatus*) regulates the concentration of carbohydrates and lipids in the haemolymph. This, however, could not be verified in independent experiments (H.G. Marco and G. Gäde, unpublished observations). In 2021, Hou et al. [20] reported the involvement of ACP in the regulation of lipid use during long-distance flight in *Locusta migratoria*, specifically in the oxidation and transport of fatty acids in the flight muscles. Most recently, a surprising sex-specific role of ACP in adult *A. aegypti* was put forward by Afifi et al. [21]: in adult female mosquitos, abdominal glycogen content decreased upon ACP injection, whereas no increase in free carbohydrates was found in the haemolymph. In contrast, ACP had the opposite effect in adult mosquito males: no change in the abdominal glycogen content but an elevation of circulating carbohydrates was observed. There is, thus, a need for further investigation into the ACP signalling system to ascertain the extent of functional overlap with the AKH system.

In the current study, we aimed to address this information gap by examining the AKH and ACP signalling systems of *A. aegypti* which is an infamous disease vector for pathogens, such as yellow fever virus (estimated to cause 200,000 cases of disease and 30,000 deaths each year, with 90% occurring in Africa [22]), Dengue fever, chikungunya, and Zika, as the latest addition to the spectrum of arboviruses, all of which summarily are responsible for a great number of painful infections and death of people following virus transmission from a mosquito bite [23]. *A. aegypti* was selected as a test case since there is already a fair amount of data available from partial investigations into its neuropeptide systems. Furthermore, knowledge of the interaction of bioactive ligands with their cognate receptors is thought to be very helpful for drug research using the GPCRs as a target and aiming for the development of selective bio-rational insecticides [24–26].

Historically, the *A. aegypti* peptides were first predicted from genomic work [27], and the AKH and ACP precursors were then cloned, although the ACP was named Aedae-AKH-II at the time [28]. The presence of mature Aedae-AKH-I and corazonin was shown by direct mass profiling, but evidence of the ACP peptide was not found in brain or CC tissue, possibly on account of a low concentration [29]. One Crz receptor (CrzR) and variants of the AKHR and ACP receptor (ACPR) were cloned from *A. aegypti* [28,30,31]. Each receptor was shown to be very selective, accepting only the cognate peptide, thus signifying that there are three separate and independent endocrine systems active in this mosquito species.

Structure-activity relationship (SAR) studies supply information about how a ligand interacts with its cognate receptor, especially which amino acid residue of the ligand is important for this interaction. Thus, by replacing each residue successively with simple amino acids, such as Gly or Ala, or by using bio-analogues (naturally occurring peptides with one or two known differences from the endogenous ligand), the importance of each amino acid's side chain can be probed with respect to functional or receptor binding outputs. Such SAR studies were conducted on the AKH system in a few insects and a crustacean either by measuring physiological actions in vivo [32,33] or in a mammalian cellular expression system [34,35]. For *A. aegypti* very informative data sets exist on the AKH and the ACP signalling system [36]: for the first time ever, SAR studies were performed with an ACP ligand/receptor system, and it was clear that the chain length of the ligand is important for receptor activation (no activity with 8 but with 10 amino acids), as well as C-terminal amidation, and aromatic amino acids (Phe and Trp at positions 4 and 8, respectively). A 400- to 500-fold loss of activity was measured when the N-terminal pyroglutamate (pGlu) or Thr at position 3 was replaced individually by Ala. Replacements at positions 2, 5, 6, and 7 were well tolerated, so it seems that they are not as intricately involved in receptor activation. For the *A. aegypti* AKHR, it was shown that, in general, the C-terminal portion of the AKH octapeptide, excluding the Trp at position 8, is not as critical for activation as are N-terminal positions 2, 3, and 4; and a longer chain length from ten amino acids appears permissible [36]. Hence, there is some information available on ligand-receptor requirements for two of the three GnRH superfamily signalling systems of *A. aegypti*.

In conjunction with nuclear magnetic resonance (NMR) data on the secondary structure of AKHs [37,38] and knowledge of the receptor sequence, molecular dynamics (MD) methods can derive models of how the ligand interacts with its receptor [39–41]. Such data are missing for the yellow fever mosquito and the ACP signalling system of any insect. The current study, hence, investigates the properties of the ligands Aedae-ACP (pEVTFSRDWNA-NH_2) and Aedae-AKH (pELTFTPSW-NH_2) by NMR spectroscopy in SDS (sodium dodecyl-d_{25} sulfate) micelle solution to determine their secondary structures, models the interaction of the ligands with the respective receptor and evaluates the predicted models by using the published structure-activity data. Note that Aedae-ACP is the same peptide sequence as in *A. gambiae* [1], and in many insect species [5]. Aedae-AKH is not only endogenous in *A. aegypti* and in the alderfly, *Sialis lutaria* [42], but is also encoded in the genome of *L. migratoria* [43] and *Schistocerca gregaria* [44]. In the context of examining the AKH signalling system of the desert locust, the solution structure of Aedae-AKH was previously determined along with the other two endogenous AKHs of *S. gregaria* [45]. This supplies us with valuable comparative information.

2. Materials and Methods

2.1. NMR Spectroscopy

NMR samples were prepared by dissolving the dry peptides in 150 mM sodium dodecyl-d_{25} sulfate (SDS), 20 mM phosphate buffer pH 4.5, 0.05 mM TSP (trimethylsilyl-propanoic acid), and 10% v/v D_2O, to reach a final peptide concentration of 2 mM. All NMR spectra were obtained at 310 K on an 800 MHz Bruker Advance II equipped with a 5 mm TCI cryoprobe. ^1H homonuclear TOtal Correlation SpectroscopY (TOCSY) (mixing time τ_{mix} = 80 ms) and Nuclear Overhauser Effect SpectroscopY (NOESY) (τ_{mix} = 150 and 300 ms) were acquired with 512 points and 1 k points in F1 dimension, respectively, and 4 k points in F2 dimension, between 16 and 32 transients were accumulated with 1.5 s recycle delay and multiplied with squared sine bell functions shifted by 90°. The ^1H spectral window was set to 9600 Hz. ^{13}C-1H, Heteronuclear Single Quantum Coherence (HSQC) experiments were performed with 256 points in F1 dimension and 4 k points in F2 dimension, and 64 transients were accumulated with 2 s recycle delay. The ^{13}C spectral window was set to 33,200 Hz. Non-uniform sampling ^{15}N-^1H HSQC experiments were performed with 25% of 128 points in F1 dimension and 4 k points in F2 dimension, 1024 transients were accumulated with 1.5 s recycle delay. The ^{15}N spectral window was set to 3240 Hz.

All data dimensions were zero-filled to twice the respective Free Induction Decay (FID) size. ^1H chemical shifts were referenced to TSP at 0 ppm, and ^{13}C and ^{15}N were indirectly referenced to the ^1H reference frequency. Data were processed in TopSpin

(Bruker) and analysed using the CCPNmr analysis program [46]. Backbone and side chains were assigned using all experiments.

2.2. Structure Calculations

The NOESY cross-peak assignments were used to generate distance restraints for the structure determination. These distance restraints were supplemented with dihedral angle restraints predicted with DANGLE [47] from Hα chemical shifts. A standard CNS 1.1-based protocol was employed using the ARIA 2.2 interface [48]. The 10 lowest energy structures were refined in a water shell and evaluated with MolProbity [49].

2.3. Molecular Dynamics of Ligand

The output from the NMR structural calculations was used as input to GROMACS version 2018.6 [50] for extended MD simulation in water and dodecyl phosphocholine (DPC) micelle. For the water simulations, a box containing the peptide, chloride to neutralise any charge and 7000 water molecules was constructed. The single-point charge water model was used. For the membrane simulations, the lowest energy structure from the simulations in water was placed in the centre of a 7 nm cubic box filled with approximately 10,000 water molecules and a micelle of 50 DPC molecules [51]. The micelle was translated so that, using periodic boundary conditions, half the micelle was at the bottom of the box and the other half was at the top. Energy minimisation was carried out using the steepest descent method for 10,000 steps to a tolerance of 10 kJ mol^{-1}. A series of constant pressure, temperature, and number of particles (NPT) equilibration steps were performed to solvate the peptide before the final MD simulation for 50 ns under constant temperature, volume and number of particles (NVT) conditions at 300 K.

The OPLS-AA/L force field [52] was used to describe the molecule bond energies. All bonds were constrained using the LINCS algorithm [53]. A cut-off of 1.0 nm was used for van der Waals and electrostatic interactions. Following equilibration, MD was performed for 50 ns at 300 K under NVT conditions. For each simulation, 100 snapshots were collected over the course of the simulation. Cluster analysis of the resulting structures was performed using the linkage algorithm of GROMACS with a cut-off of 0.1 nm on the backbone atoms.

2.4. Construction of Receptor Models, Ligand Docking and Molecular Dynamics

The primary sequence of the adipokinetic hormone/corazonin-related peptide receptor, *Aedes aegypti* ACPR-I (Genbank MF461644; protein: AVA08868.1), was used to construct the 3D structure of the receptor at the atomic level. The primary sequence of the *Aedes aegypti* AKH receptor was taken from Genbank MF988326 (protein AV109459.1). Swiss-Model [54] was used to search for target templates. For both receptors, the NMR structure of active β_2 androgenic receptor, 6kr8.1.A, was selected. For the inactive or 'open' model of Aedae-ACPR the 5D5A X-ray crystal structure of the β_2 androgenic receptor at 100 K was chosen. For Aedae-AKHR the Xray structure 6tpk was selected as a template of the inactive conformation. The same website was then used to construct 3D models of the receptors, based on these two templates. The resulting structures were imported into Maestro 13.1 [55] for visualisation, ligand docking, and MD calculations. The proteins were first prepared using the Maestro Protein Preparation Wizard, and the quality of the models was checked with Ramachandran plots. The Maestro Glide module was used with SP-Peptide precision to find the best poses of the ligand in the receptor binding pocket. The pose with the best glide score was used for MD simulation. For this the receptor/ligand construct was imbedded in a (1-palmitoyl-2-eleoyl-3-phosphocholin) (POPC) membrane, neutralised with Cl^- and solvated with SPC water, using the membrane setup of Desmond [56]. Molecular dynamics was performed using Desmond and the free energy of binding was calculated using MM/GBSA (Prime version 2019, Schrödinger, LLC, New York, NY, USA, 2019).

3. Results and Discussion

3.1. Aedae-ACP NMR Results

For small and partially folded peptides with affinity for lipid membranes, NMR is a very well-suited structural technique compared to cryo-EM or X-ray techniques which rely on ordered or large homogenous copies of folded molecules. The NMR assignments and chemical shift of Aedae-ACP in SDS micelle solution are given in Table 1. Some ideas of the secondary structure and flexibility of the peptide can be obtained by comparing these chemical shifts to those of the same residue in a random coil environment [57,58]. These chemical shift indices are plotted in Figure 1a. Both the H_α and H^N protons are consistently shifted up-field suggesting some type of turn structure [59]. This is consistent with the review of Tyndall et al. [60] of over 100 mammalian GPCR ligands, which all had a turn structure. The chemical shift indices are also consistent with our results for members of the AKH family, such as Melme-CC [61], Declu-CC [61], Dappu-RPCH [40], Schgr-AKH-II [40], Anoga-HrTH [39] and including Aedae-AKH [39].

Table 1. NMR assignments for Aedae-ACP in SDS micelles [a].

Residue	N	H	HA	HB	HG	CA	CB	CG	Others
1 Glu	-	-	4.42	2.53, 1.96	2.36 *	59.7	28.4	32.3	
2 Val	120.0	7.96	4.11	1.97	0.88, 0.78	62.6	33.0	21.7, 21.2	
3 Thr	117.7	7.93	4.36	4.10	1.08	61.4	70.6	21.5	
4 Phe	122.3	8.02	4.70	3.19, 3.01		57.9	40.0		HD 7.24, HE 7.20, HZ 7.10, CD 131.8, CE 131.2, CZ 129.4
5 Ser	116.9	8.01	4.40	3.83, 3.75		58.5	64.3		
6 Arg	121.1	7.74	4.10	1.41, 1.52	1.33 *	55.9	30.7	27.3	NE 124.4, HD1 2.89, HD2 2.93, HE 6.87, CD 43.5
7 Asp	119.2	8.05	4.58	2.62, 2.50		-	39.2	-	
8 Trp	122.0	7.71	4.52	3.21, 3.26		57.9	29.7		NE 128.7, HD1 7.22, HE1 9.82, HE3 7.00, HZ2 7.37, HZ3 7.55, HH2 7.04, CD1 127.5, CE3 121.6, CZ2 114.5, CZ3 121.1, CH2 124.3
9 Asn	120.3	8.02	4.61	2.65, 2.48					ND2 112.4, HD2a 6.67, HD2b 7.32
10 Ala	124.0	7.71	4.13	1.31		52.8	19.6		

[a] 2 mM peptide in 150 mM SDS micelles. Experiments were run at 310 K and referenced to TSP. * Identical chemical shift for both protons. - Not observed.

The NMR chemical shifts can also be used to estimate the flexibility of the peptide [57]. The results (Figure 1b) show that the peptide is quite flexible with an order parameter (S^2) ranging from 0 to only 0.36. A perfectly ordered (rigid) structure has an S^2 of 1. The Aedae-ACP order parameter results are the same as those found for Aedae-AKH (S^2 = 0.1–0.3) [45], Schgr-AKH-II (S^2 = 0.1–0.4) [45] which are similar to that of the crustacean member of the AKH family, Dappu-RPCH (S^2 = 0.1–0.25) [40]. However, the order parameter contrasts with the rigid conformations of a number of insect AKHs; Melme-CC (S^2 = 0.85) [61], Declu-CC (S^2 = 0.7–0.9) [61], Locmi-AKH-I (S^2 = 0.9) [45] and Anoga-HrTH (S^2 = 0.7–0.8) [39]. As expected, Aedae-ACP is more ordered in the middle of the peptide than at the termini. The NMR-derived root mean square fluctuation (RMSF) of the Aedae-ACP backbone (Figure 1c) also shows that the peptide is flexible, with RMSF values ranging from 3.5 to 8.7 Å. The RMSF values of the more rigid Melme-CC [61], Declu-CC [61] and Anoga-HrTH [39] range from 0.3 to 1.7 Å. In contrast, Dappu-RPCH has RMSF values ranging from 5 to 8 Å [40].

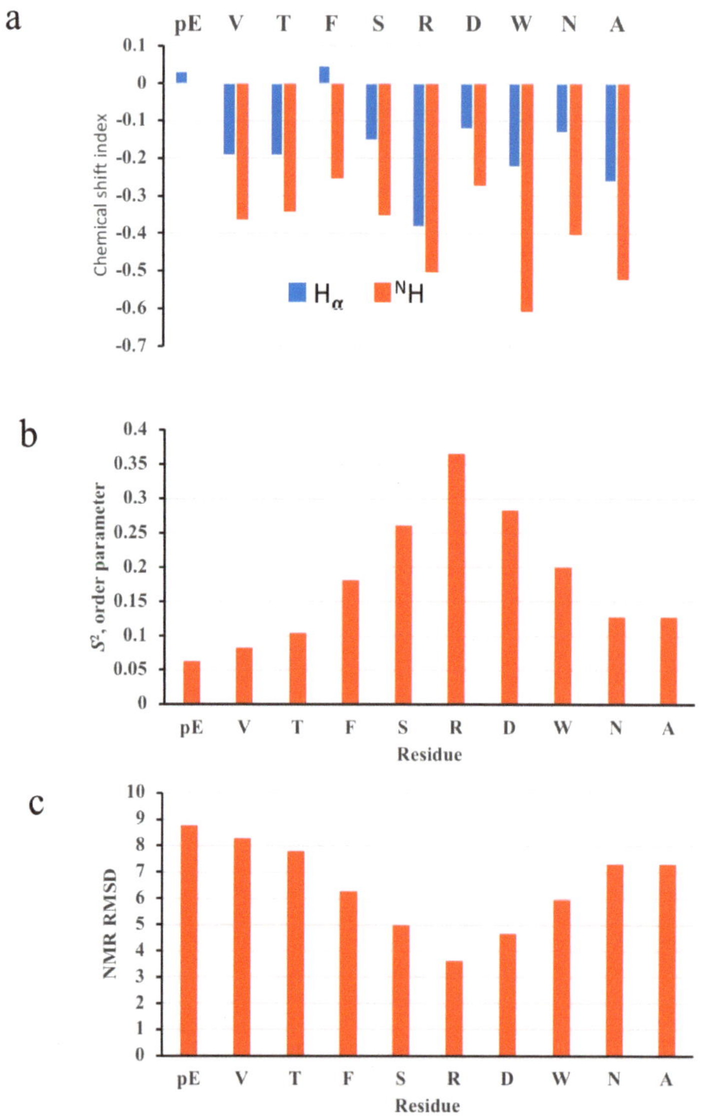

Figure 1. NMR results for Aedae-ACP in SDS micelle solution. (**a**) H_{α} and ^{N}H random coil NMR chemical shift deviations; (**b**) S^2 order parameter; and (**c**) NMR root mean square fluctuations.

The NMR restraints were used to search the conformational space of Aedae-ACP. The resulting structures were grouped according to the similarity of their backbone conformation. The root conformer of the largest cluster was placed in a solution with a DPC micelle and MD was performed for 50 ns. Figure 2a shows an overlay of the largest cluster. This cluster is extended at the C-terminus but has a β-turn around threonine at position 3 from the N-terminus. This conformation had no restraint violations and agreed with the NMR chemical shift results.

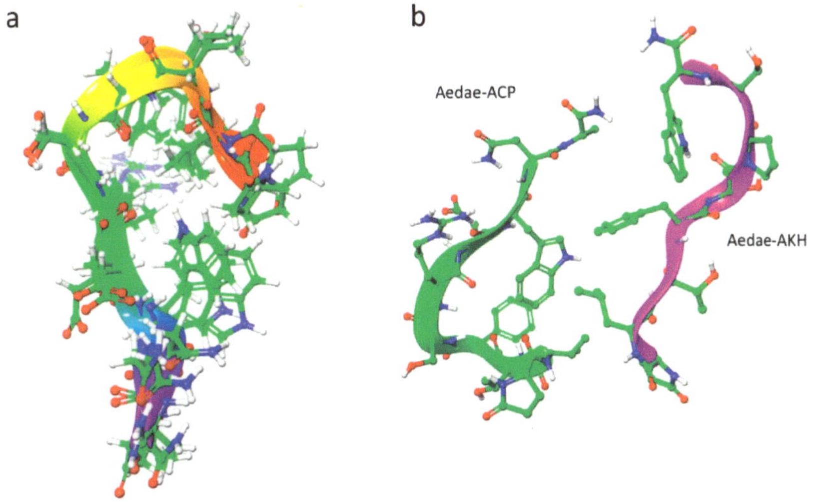

Figure 2. (**a**) Overlay of the largest cluster (49 members) from a 50 ns MD simulation of Aedae-ACP in DPC micelle solution. For clarity, every 10th snapshot is shown; (**b**) Comparison of Aedae-ACP and Aedae-AKH.

3.2. Structural Comparison of Aedae-ACP and Aedae-AKH

Previously, we had determined the solution structure of Aedae-AKH as one of the locust AKHs, using NMR-restrained molecular dynamics [45]. Here we compare the predominant solution conformations of Aedae-ACP and Aedae-AKH (Figure 2b). Aedae-AKH has a more linear structure than Aedae-ACP, which has a pronounced β-turn at Thr^3. This β-turn brings Phe^4 and Trp^8 onto the same side of the peptide. In contrast, Aedae-AKH has a proline at position 6, which introduces a turn, and again, brings Trp^8 to the same side as Phe^4. Hence, these two peptides have the same orientation of Phe^4 and Trp^8, albeit from different mechanisms. It is well known that these two aromatic residues are the most conserved AKH/ACP ones in AKH and ACP peptides, and are reportedly essential for receptor activation [8,44]. It is noted, however, that these two peptides are very flexible. The S^2 order parameter of both Aedae-ACP and Aedae-AKH is only 0.36.

3.3. Aedae-Receptor Homology Modelling

Homology modelling was used to construct two 3D models of each of the Aedae-ACP and Aedae-AKH receptors. Two templates were used for each receptor, one with the receptor in an active state (X-ray structure 6kr8.1.A) and one with the receptor in an inactive state (X-ray structure 5D5A for Aedae-ACPR and 6tpk for Aedae-AKHR). The quality of all 4 models was tested using Ramachandran plots. Each had torsion angles in the disallowed region of conformational space, but these outliers disappeared upon MD optimisation of the models. Both Aedae-ACPR and Aedae-AKHR have the conserved residues, typical of the rhodopsin superfamily of GPCRs, namely (using the Ballesteros and Weinstein numbering system [62]): $N^{1.50}$; $D^{2.50}$, $P^{2.59}$; $C^{3.25}$, the $DR^{3.50}x$ motif (DRY for the AKHR and DRC for ACPR), $W^{4.50}$; $P^{5.50}$; $F^{6.44}$, the CWxPY motif ($CWxP^{6.50}Y$), and the $NPxxY^{7.53}$ motif. These conserved residues are essential for maintaining the structure of the receptors and for their activation. Figure 3 shows the optimised structures of the two receptor models [63].

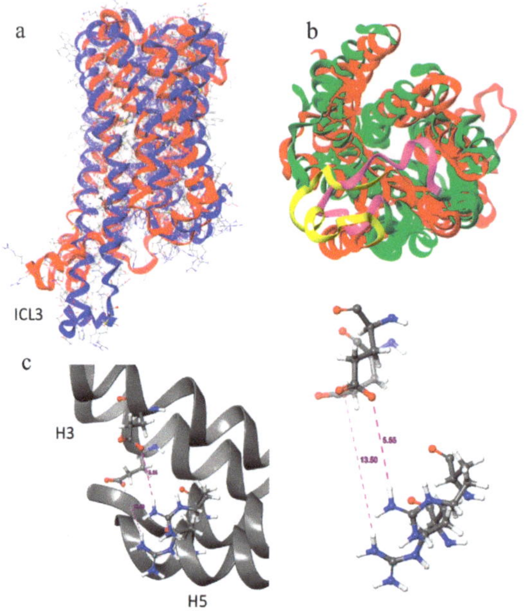

Figure 3. Overlay of two structures of Aedae-ACPR: (**a**) Side view, red = active state (6kr8); blue = inactive state (5D5A); (**b**) Top view highlighting the different positions of ECL2, yellow = inactive state; purple = active state; and (**c**) Ionic lock, distance between Glu^{299} and Arg^{205}. Inactive (5D5A) 5.56 Å, active (6kr8) 13.5 A. Note how H3 and H5 have moved away from each other upon activation.

Blind docking was performed on each of the ligands and receptor models of Aedae-ACPR. In each case the same binding pocket was found, which corresponded to the binding region found for the Dappu-RPCH [40], Melme-CC [61], Declu-CC [61], Schgr-AKH-II [45] and Anoga-HrTH [39] receptors. Glide scores ranged from −6.6–−16.9. The docked structures with the highest glide scores were placed in a POPC membrane and MD performed for 200–2200 ns.

3.4. Aedae-ACPR Models

The two homology models of Aedae-ACPR are given in Figure 3a,b. Essentially, their backbone structures are the same except for small, but essential, relative movement of the helices. Also, the orientation of ECL2 and ICL3 are different. In the active state, ECL2 lies over the binding pocket, preventing the egress of the ligand. At the same time, ICL3 moves away from the G-protein binding site. In the inactive state, ECL2 moves to the side allowing the ligand access to the binding site, and ICL3 projects further from the membrane.

A more noticeable difference in the two models is shown by the ionic lock between Arg^{205} and Glu^{299} (Figure 3c). In the inactive model, the lock is closed with an inter-residue distance of 5.56 Å, while in the active model, the lock is open with an inter-residue distance of 13.5 Å. Aedae-ACPR also has a number of other switches found in class A GPCRs. These include the DRC switch, the tyrosine toggle switch, and the hydrophobic connector shown in Figure 4.

Water is integrally involved in the action of GPCRs. The crystal structures of B2AR all have internal water molecules, and it has been postulated that these waters are necessary for ligand and G-protein binding [64]. A plot of water density (above bulk) in the active model of Aedae-ACPR is shown in Figure 4d. In the figure, water is clustered, internally, at both ends of the receptor where the ligand and G-protein bind.

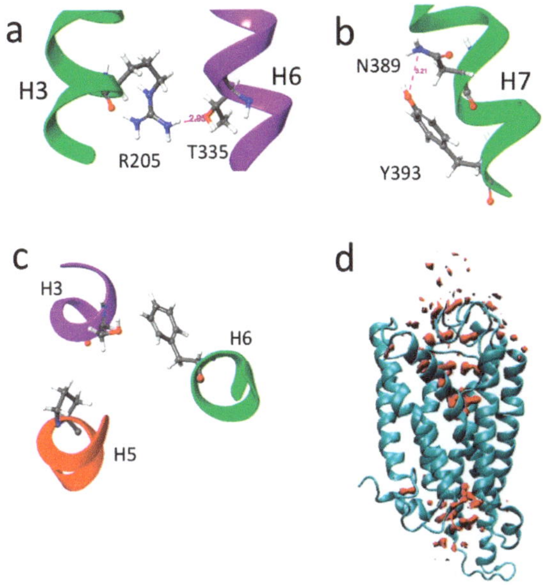

Figure 4. Aedae-ACP 6kr8 model: (**a**) DRC switch; (**b**) Tyrosine toggle switch; (**c**) hydrophobic connector switch; (**d**) Water density (above bulk) map of ACPR.

3.4.1. Aedae-ACP Docked to Aedae-ACPR

With the generated Aedae-ACPR models, ligand docking was performed to study specific interactions, for the first time, between an ACPR and its peptide ligand, Aedae-ACP. Figure 5a shows the protein root mean square deviation (RMSD) of the 6kr8 (active) model of Aedae-ACPR with Aedae-ACP docked. The blue curve is the displacement of the receptor C_α atoms relative to the starting structure and the red curve is the ligand heavy atom displacement relative to the receptor. The ligand-heavy atoms move ~3 Å from their original position to their final position. This happens in the first 0.5 ns of the simulation. The C_α atoms of the receptor, being larger, take ~40 ns to adopt their final position. Note the two curves run essentially parallel to each other, indicating that the ligand does not move relative to the receptor. The model is well equilibrated as the RMSD does not change over time.

The RMSF of the C_α atoms of the active receptor model is shown in Figure 6a. Apart from ICL3, which fluctuates 4.8 Å, there is very little change in the conformation of the receptors. The conformation of the trans-membrane helices remains fairly rigid. Protein residues that interact with the ligand are shown as vertical green lines. Aedae-ACP interacts with ECL1 and the adjacent residues of H2 and H3. Another two regions of ligand/protein contact are ECL2, H5, H6, and ECL3. The RMSF profile of Aedae-ACPR is similar to those found for several AKH insect receptor models [40].

The RMSD profile of the 5D5A (inactive model) model (Figure 5b) is very different. Here, the ligand and the receptor continue to move throughout the 2.2 μs simulation. Essentially the inactive conformer is slowly changing into the active conformer. This is shown by the change in RMSD between the inactive and active models over time. Note, however, that the protein continues to move but the ligand settles down, indicating that it is in the correct binding orientation at the start of the simulation.

The RMSF of the C_α atoms of the 5D5A receptor model (Figure 6b) shows a similar pattern to the 6kr8 model, albeit with larger fluctuations of ICL3. The ligand interacts with the same region of the protein as the 6kr8 model.

The RMSF of the ligand (Figure S1) shows how the ligand atoms interact with the protein and their entropic role in the binding event. Here the protein-ligand complex (Aedae-ACPR–Aedae-ACP) was first aligned onto the protein backbone and then the RMSF of the ligand atoms was calculated, so that the RMSF indicates the movement of the ligand within the receptor binding pocket. The RMSF of both models is very similar. There is very little fluctuation (~1 Å) of the ligand backbone and sidechains, except for Phe^4 and Arg^6. The ACP N-terminus of the active model fluctuates more than that of the inactive model. This is because the ACP C-terminus projects into the core of the receptor, while the N-terminus is towards the extra-cellular region of the receptor. The C-terminus of both models has ~2.5 Å fluctuations. Of interest is the lack of motion of Trp^8, which indicates that it is tightly bound in the active site. These results indicate that the ligand does not move substantially in the binding pocket.

Figure S2 gives more detail about which ACP receptor residues interact with Aedae-ACP. Here protein contacts with the ligand are normalised over the trajectory such that a value of 1.0 means that the contact is maintained for 100% of the simulation. Since a particular residue may have more than one contact, values above 1 are possible. The interactions are also categorised by type: H-bond, hydrophobic, ionic, and water bridges. In the inactive state, Aedae-ACP has multiple, short-term, interactions with its receptor. However, only a few are persistent: Asn^{274} has a persistent H-bond and water bridge with the ligand; and Arg^{187} forms a H-bond for 30% of the simulation, a hydrophobic interaction for 50% of the simulation, and a water bridge for the entire simulation. Also, there are H-bonds and water bridges with the receptor: Pro^{266} and Pro^{267} H-bond to the ligand for the entire simulation; Val^{246} has a water bridge to the ligand.

a

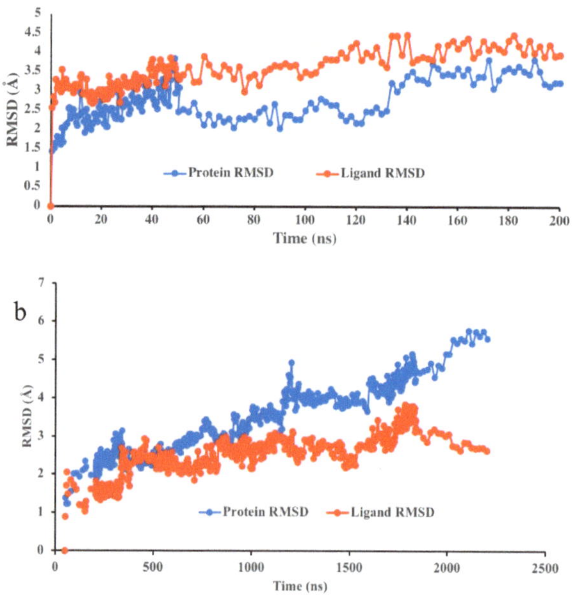

Figure 5. Protein RMSD during MD simulation of Aedae-ACP bound to Aedae-ACPR: (**a**) 6kr8 model; and (**b**) 5D5A model.

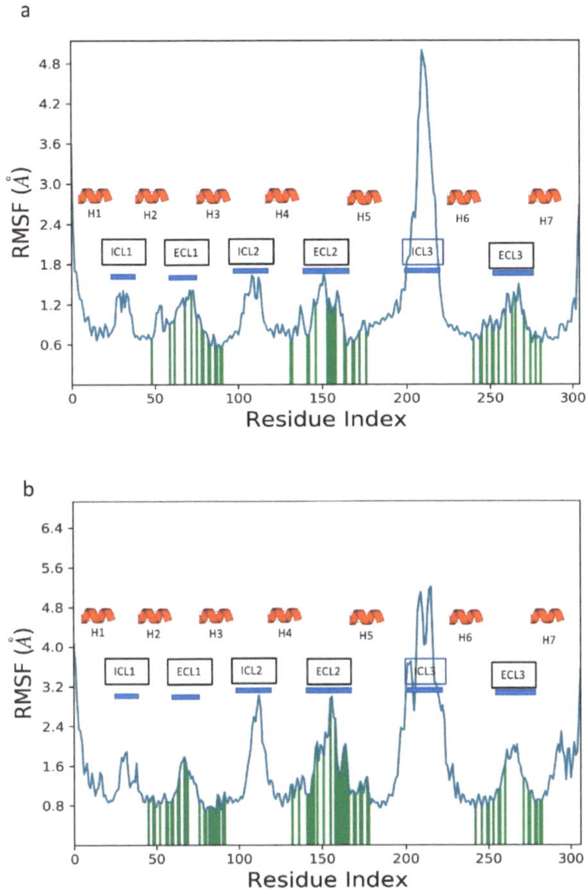

Figure 6. Protein RMSF of Aedae-ACPR + Aedae-ACP: (**a**) 6kr8 model; and (**b**) 5D5A model.

In the active state, Aedae-ACP has 14 persistent contacts with the receptor (Figure S2a). Asn^{274}, Arg^{187}, and Val^{246} contacts are still present, but there are now persistent contacts with Asp^{153}; Ala^{188}, Leu^{192} and Ser^{195} on H3; Asn^{236}; Gln^{247}, Phe^{261}, Met^{269}, and Cys^{277} on ECL2; and Trp^{350}, Tyr^{357}, Thr^{357} and Tyr^{360} on H6. Since this is the first modelling and in silico docking of ACPR and ACP as ligands, we have no other comparisons for discussion. However, a study on a GPCR from the stick insect *Carausius morosus* (touted as an AKHR but without empirical evidence) also noted that residue $Arg^{187(3.32)}$ is critical for AKH binding to the putative AKH receptor [65]. In the ligand docking of desert locust AKHs to the cognate AKHR model, Arg of Schgr-AKHR was also found to be instrumental/involved in the binding of Schgr-AKH-II [45].

The simulation interaction diagram (SID) gives details of which ligand atoms interact with the receptor. In Figure 7 the interactions between Aedae-ACP and Aedae-ACPR are colour-coded such that H-bonding is depicted in purple, while π-cation interactions are shown in red. For the duration of the simulation, contacts between the ligand and receptor are formed and broken. This is recorded as a % of the simulation time. Only interactions that persist for more than 30% of the simulation are shown. The surface of the receptor is shown as a solid line, again colour coded, polar, hydrophobic, etc., according to the nature of the receptor residues. The active model (Figure 7a) has many interactions with the central residues of the ligand. The serine OH, H-bonds to Gln^{247}, Met^{269}, and Val^{246}

for the entire simulation. The SID of the active model has a number of water molecules in the binding site, which Yuan et al. [64] have postulated are essential for receptor activation. These water molecules bridge between the ligand and the receptor. Interestingly, Trp[8] of Aedae-ACP, which is postulated to be essential for binding, interacts with Arg[187] in both ACP receptor models. The inactive model (Figure 7b) does not have as many interactions between the ligand and receptor but does have several internal H-bonds, which help to maintain the conformation of the ligand.

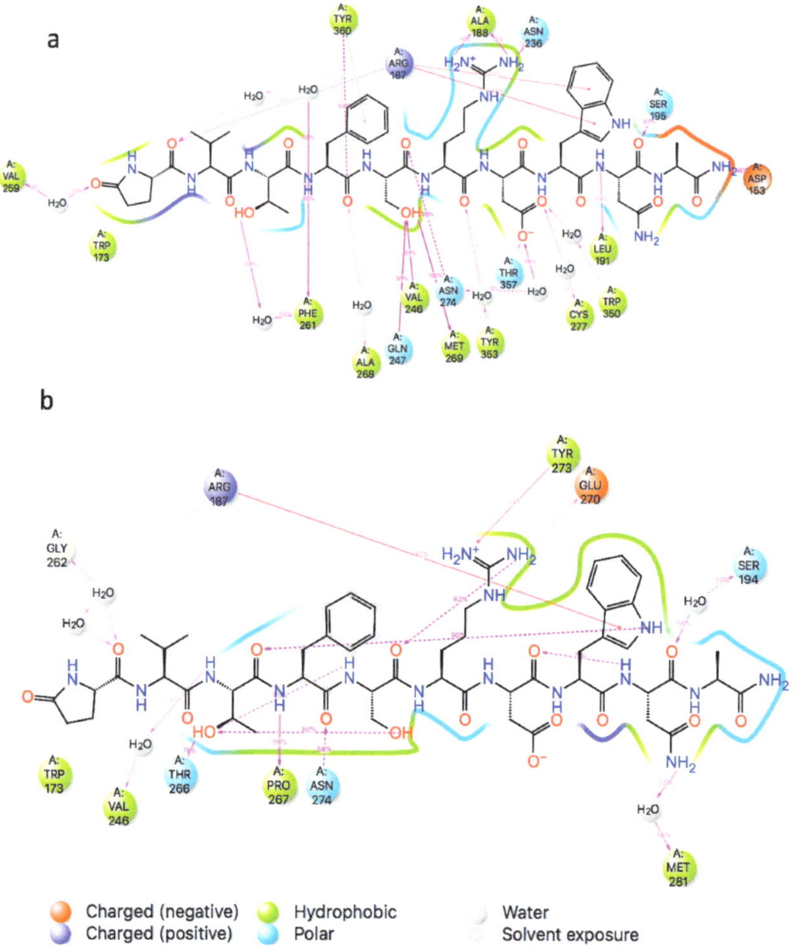

Figure 7. Simulation interaction diagram Aedae-ACPR + EVTFSRDWNAamide: (**a**) 6kr8 model; and (**b**) 5D5A model. A schematic of detailed ligand atom interactions with the protein residue interactions that occur more than 30.0% of the simulation time.

The strength of the ligand-receptor binding is best measured by the free energy of binding (ΔG_{bind}) averaged over the course of the trajectory. The free energy of binding of Aedae-ACP bound to the active model of Aedae-ACPR is -137 ± 10 kcal mol^{-1}, but only -88 ± 9 kcal mol^{-1} for the inactive model of Aedae-ACPR. It is the closing of the receptor around the ligand that is responsible for the increased binding energy.

3.4.2. Residue Scanning of Aedae-ACPR

The best way to validate a computational receptor model with simulated ligand docking is to follow up with experiments involving the physical GPCR, its cognate ligand, and a variety of other ligands that may be more- or less-suited for interacting with and activating the GPCR according to the modelled data. In the case of Aedae-ACPR and Aedae-ACP, receptor functional activation studies were completed 5 years ago in vivo in a mammalian cell line and the EC_{50} (the concentration of the ligand that produces 50% of the maximum response) was recorded in a typical SAR study via the well-known bioluminescence reporter assay [36]. In the current study, hence, we tried to replicate those experimental results computationally by using our generated Aedae-ACPR models and simulating ligand docking with the same series of ACP analogues used by Wahedi et al. [36] in their heterologous expression of Aedae-ACPR. Computationally, the ligand-receptor binding strength was measured by the free energy of binding (ΔG_{bind}) and so an inverse relationship between ΔG_{bind} and EC_{50} was expected between these two parameters.

Figure 8 shows the computational results of sequentially replacing the residues of Aedae-ACP with an alanine: substitution of Val^2, Thr^3, Phe^4, Ser^5, Arg^6, and Asn^9 all decreased the affinity slightly relative to the native peptide. On the other hand, mutation of Asp^7 increased the binding affinity, while mutation of Trp^8 decreased the binding affinity by 19 kcal mol^{-1}. Also shown in Figure 8 are the EC_{50} values taken from Washedi et al. [36] as a comparison to our computationally derived results—note that EC_{50} values could not be calculated in the case of ACP analogues with Ala^4 and Ala^8 substituted for Phe^4 and Trp^8, respectively, for those substitutions resulted in very little to no detectable activation of Aedae-ACPR even at a peptide dose of 10 μM. An inverse relationship between ΔG_{bind} and EC_{50} is evident for the Ala-substituted ACP analogues, except for the Ala^4 and Ala^7 mutations (Figure 8). This indicates that the proposed model may be virtually correct with a few possible complications. Further modelled results show a good correlation: Aedae-ACP (native ligand) and the Ala^9 substituted ACP has the lowest EC_{50} values and the highest binding affinities, while the replacement of Trp^8 with Ala, had the lowest binding affinity thus, fitting with the receptor assay data of an inactive peptide even at a very high dose. This begged the question as to why the modelled/calculated binding affinity failed to predict the experimental loss of activity upon replacement of Phe^4 by alanine. In fact, this is not the first occurrence, for the same mismatch was previously established in the simulated residue scanning of the octapeptide Dappu-RPCH with Ala^4 substitution for Phe^4 and activation of Dappu-RPCHR [40]. In the same vein, the Ala^7 mutation of Aedae-ACP had the highest binding affinity in the current study (Figure 8), whereas this analogue had only the same level of receptor activation in receptor assays as the Ala^2, Ala^5, and Ala^6 mutants [36] (Wahedi et al. 2019). Evidently, ligand binding is only one of the steps that may lead to receptor activation or not. This notion of a ligand binding without activating the receptor and the subsequent signal transduction cascade is borne out by pharmacological studies with inhibitors (antagonists) and when simply considering the idea of drug "efficacy", loosely defined as the size or strength of a response produced by a particular agonist in a particular tissue [66]. Thus, just because a ligand has affinity it does not necessarily mean that it will have efficacy; for example, a simple antagonist will have affinity but an efficacy of zero. When it comes to drug studies, the ability to bind to a receptor may determine the ability to produce a response and to some extent the size of that response; however, the two are seldom linked in a linear fashion [66]. We, therefore, conclude that certain changes to the peptide ligand may result in binding with the ACPR but not in activating the receptor and that our proposed in silico models are not fully able to distinguish between receptor binding and ligand efficacy. It is advisable, therefore, to use complementary methodologies to rigorously test model predictions. A point in the case can be found in Jackson et al. [67] where a computationally predicted antagonist of a locust AKHR was, indeed, proven to be a competitive inhibitor of AKH through the use of in vivo biological assays.

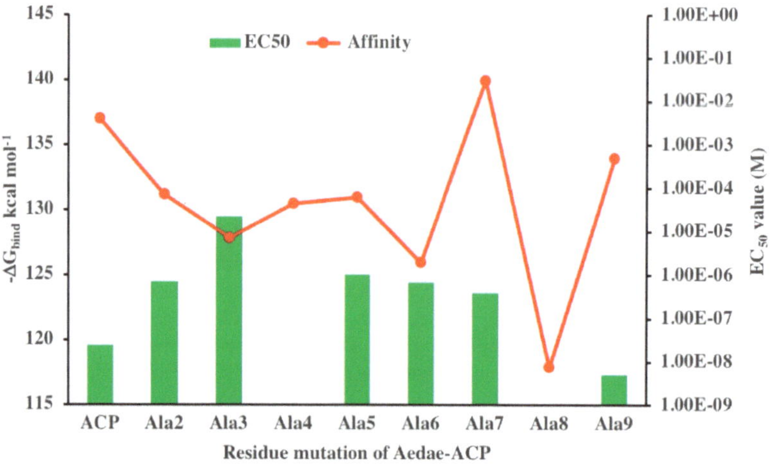

Figure 8. Free energy of binding and EC_{50} values for a series of alanine mutations of Aedae-ACP binding to Aedae-ACPR.

Analysis of the current data shows that, although Trp^8 is 79% buried within the receptor, mutation to Ala^8 leads to an increase in solvent-accessible surface area (Δ_{SASA} = 90 Å^2). It is also interesting to note that Trp^8 has a surface complementarity of 0.88 where a complementarity of 1 means the two surfaces match perfectly and 0 means the two surfaces have no complementarity.

Wahedi et al. [36] further tested the receptor activation ability of a number of other synthetic and natural analogues of ACP, and those same analogues were modelled and docked to the Aedae-ACPR models in the current study. C-terminal amidation was found to be critical for receptor activation. MD of the non-amidated peptide with the inactive receptor model had free energy of binding some 50 kcal mol^{-1} greater than the amidated peptide. This is mainly due to the very strong H-bonding between the free acid and Asp^{153}. On the other hand, binding to the active model was ~20 kcal mol^{-1} less stable than native ACP. This is the same binding as the Trp^8 mutation. In the bioassay, both Trp^8 and C-terminal amidation were essential for receptor activation.

MD of pETFSRDWNA-NH_2, an internally truncated ACP by deletion of valine in the second position, had free energy of binding ~30 kcal mol^{-1} less than native ACP and, so by analogy with [Ala^8]ACP and ACP[COOH], is predicted to be inactive. These results of the current study, indeed, corroborate the receptor assay findings of [36].

3.5. *Aedae-AKHR Models*

The AKHR of *A. aegypti* has never before been modelled. Here, we attempted to remedy this and to use the information to determine whether there could be cross-activity between AKHs and ACPs. The overlay of the two models (active and inactive) of Aedae-AKHR is shown in Figure 9. The two structures are very similar but the transmembrane helices of the 6kr8 (active) model are twisted relative to the 6tpk (inactive) model. This opens the intracellular side of the active receptor model and closes the extra-cellular side. At the same time the extra-cellular loops move, as shown in Figure 9b. ECL1 does not move. In the inactive model, ECL2 and ECL3 are positioned away from the central axis of the receptor, allowing free access of the ligand to the binding site. In the active model, ECL2 and ECL3 have moved over the top of the receptor preventing the ligand from leaving. This is particularly so for ECL2. At the same time, the orientation of the helices and loops on the intracellular side of the receptor are different (Figure 9c). In the inactive model the helices and loops close the binding site of the G-protein, while in the active model, ICL1 and ICL3 have opened up allowing the G-protein free access. This movement of the helices and loops is typical of GPCR activation [63].

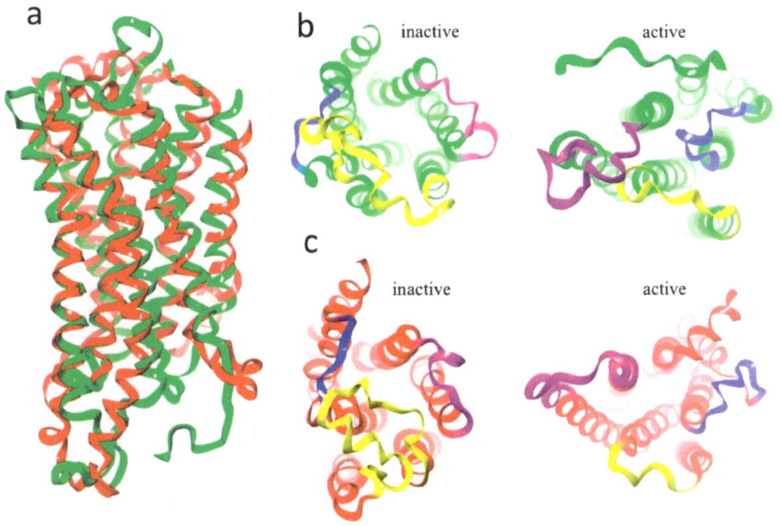

Figure 9. Aedae-AKHR: (**a**) Overlay of two models, inactive-green, active-red; (**b**) Top view showing extracellular loops blue = ECL1, yellow = ECL2, and purple = ECL3; and (**c**) Bottom view showing intracellular loops. Blue = ICL1, yellow = ICL2, plum = ICL3. For clarity, the clipping plan has been set so that only to top or bottom half of the receptor is shown.

Like Aedae-ACPR, Aedae-AKHR has a number of switches. There is the conserved DRY motif on TM3 but there is no conserved $Glu^{6.30}$ on TM6. Instead, there is a lysine which can H-bond to $Arg^{3.50}$.

Figure S3a shows the protein RMSD of the 6kr8 (active) model of Aedae-AKHR with Aedae-AKH docked. The blue curve is the displacement of the receptor C_α atoms relative to the starting structure and the red curve is the ligand heavy atom displacement relative to the receptor. The ligand-heavy atoms move ~2 Å from their original position to their final position. This happens in the first 0.5 ns of the simulation. The receptor C_α atoms have not settled down even after 300 ns.

The RMSF of the C_α atoms of the active receptor model is shown in Figure S4a. The conformation of the trans-membrane helices remains fairly rigid. The loop regions fluctuate ~2 Å, except for ICL3, which fluctuates ~5.2 Å. Protein residues that interact with the ligand are shown as vertical green lines. The ligand interacts with ECL1 and the adjacent residues of H2 and H3. The ligand also contacts receptor residues in ECL2, H5 and H6, and ECL3. The RMSF profile of Aedae-AKHR is like that of Aedae-ACPR and all other AKH receptors we have studied [37,38,45,61].

The RMSD profile of the 6tpk (inactive model) model (Figure S3b) is different. Here, both the ligand and the receptor settle down very rapidly and then do not change position for the rest of the simulation. This is different from the Aedae-ACPR simulation, where the inactive model continued to change conformation for 2.2 μs. The receptor and ligand curves run essentially parallel to each other, indicating that the ligand is not moving relative to the receptor. The model is well equilibrated as the RMSD does not change over time.

The only notable difference between the C_α atom RMSF profile of the 6tpk (inactive) and 6kr8 (active) receptor models of Aedae-AKHR, (Figure S4) is the large fluctuations of ICL2. This is the loop that moves to trap the ligand in the receptor binding site. The ligand interacts with the same region of the protein as the 6kr8 model. In both models, ICL3 moves substantially to allow the G-protein access to the receptor.

Aedae-AKH does not move substantially in the binding pocket of Aedae-AKHR, as shown by the ligand RMSF (Figure S5). In the 6kr8 model of Aedae-AKHR, the backbone atoms of docked Aedae-AKH, do not fluctuate significantly. There are ~2 Å fluctuations of all the side chain atoms, except for Trp^{8} and possibly Phe^{4}. The lack of motion of Trp^{8} indicates that it is tightly bound in the active site. The ligand atom fluctuations in the 6tpk model are greater than in the 6kr8 model. The largest variation was seen in the Phe^{4} side chain atoms. There is also substantial variation in the N-terminal atoms.

Figure S6 shows which receptor residues interact with the ligand, while Figure S7 shows which ligand residues interact with the receptor. Combining these two diagrams, the details of the receptor-ligand interactions become apparent. In the two models of the Aedae-AKH receptor, the ligand, Aedae-AKH, binds to the same region of the receptor, but the details of the interaction are different. In the active model, Trp^{133} on helix 2 H-bonds to Pro^{6}(CO) for the entire simulation. In the inactive model, Trp^{133} still H-bonds but now to Trp^{8}, with which it also has a π-π interaction. In both models, Asn^{238} on H5 interacts with Val^{2} of the ligand. These are the only two common receptor residues, in the two models, that bind to the ligand. All the other receptor-binding site residues are displaced slightly in the two models. Thus, in the active model, Asn^{226} on ECL2, H-bonds to Thr^{5}(CO), while in the inactive model, Thr^{224} on ECL2, H-bonds to Thr^{3}(CO). Ser^{313} on H6 of the active model has a water bridge with pE(CO) of the ligand, while in the inactive model, Trp^{317} H-bonds to Val^{2}(CO) and has a π-π interaction with Phe^{4} and Tyr^{316}, and H-bonds to Phe^{4}(NH) and Ser^{5}(CO). In addition, in the active model, Tyr^{233} on ECL2 has multiple interactions with ligand Phe^{4}; Lys^{332} on H7, H-bonds to Thr^{5}(OH) and has a water bridge with Phe^{4}(CO); and Arg^{153} on H3 H-bonds to Thr^{3}(OH). The similarity of binding of the active and inactive Aedae-AKHR models is reflected in their free energy of binding. For the active model, ΔG_{bind} is -137 ± 10 kcal/mol^{-1}, while for the inactive model, it is -121 ± 8 kcal/mol^{-1}.

In the Ballesteros and Weinstein numbering system, Arg^{153} is denoted 3.32 and corresponds to Arg^{269} of the stick insect (*Carausius morosus*) AKH receptor and Arg^{107} of Schgr-AKHR. In the stick insect, Arg^{269} was found to be critical for ligand binding [65], and in Schgr-AKHR, Arg^{107}, H-bonds to Schgr-AKH-II [45]. In addition, Iyison et al. [65] found very stable interactions between the ligand and $Gln^{7.35}$, and $Tyr^{6.51}$ and π-π stacking to $Phe^{3.36}$ and $Trp^{6.59}$ of the stick insect putative AKHR. We do not find the interaction between residue 3.36 and the ligand but there is a hydrophobic interaction between residue 6.59 (Trp^{317}) on Aedae-AKHR and Phe^{4} of Aedae-AKH and residue 7.35 (Gln^{331}) and Thr^{3}(OH). There is also H-bonding and a water bridge between residue $Lys^{332(7.36)}$ and Thr^{5}(OH) of Aedae-AKH. In the inactive model of Aedae-AKHR, $Glu^{130(2.61)}$ binds to Thr^{5}(CO). In the stick insect residue, 2.61 corresponds to Glu^{246}, which binds to Carmo-HrTH-I.

3.5.1. Comparison of Aedae-AKH Bound to Aedae-AKHR and Schgr-AKHR

In addition to being found in the yellow fever mosquito, *Aedes aegypti*, Aedae-AKH is also found in the desert locust, *Schistocerca gregaria*. The conformation of Aedae-AKH is similar when bound to the two receptors Aedae-AKHR and Schgr-AKHR (Figure 10a,b). The binding pocket of Schgr-AKHR consists of a cleft running across the top of the extracellular domain of the receptor between helices 2, 6, and 7 and extracellular loops 2 and 4. Aedae-AKH fits into this cleft with the central portion of the peptide fitting into the binding pocket and the two termini pointing outwards (Figure 10d). The ΔG_{bind} of Aedae-AKH to Schgr-AKHR is -88 kcal/mol^{-1}. This contrasts with Aedae-AKH binding to Aedae-AKHR, where the N-terminus of the ligand extends into the receptor with Trp^{8} at the surface of the receptor (Figure 10c). This different orientation of the ligand in the binding pocket of Schgr-AKHR and Aedae-AKHR is the reason for the much higher free energy of binding of Aedae-AKH to Aedae-AKHR. It may also account for the promiscuity of Schgr-AKHR [45].

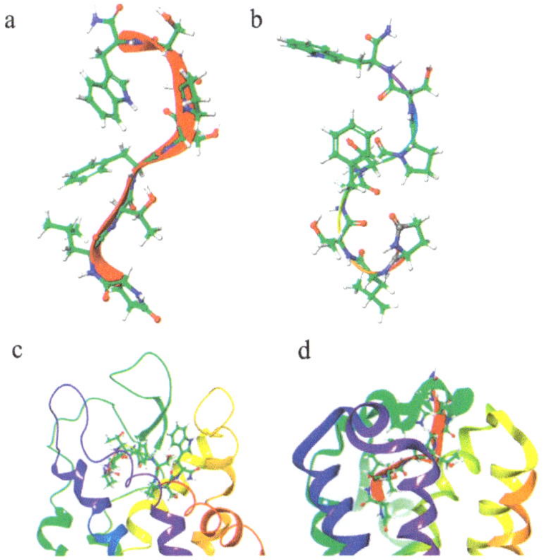

Figure 10. Conformation of Aedae-AKH bound to (**a**) Aedae-AKHR, and (**b**) Schgr-AKHR. The binding pocket of (**c**) Aedae-AKHR and (**d**) Schgr-AKHR shows the different orientations of the Aedae-AKH in the two receptors.

3.5.2. Binding of Natural Arthropod AKH Analogues to Aedae-AKHR

To test and validate our Aedae-AKHR receptor models, we modelled the docking of various AKH analogues to the receptor, including the native octapeptide Aedae-AKH (pELTFTPSWamide). Once again, we modelled insect bioanalogues (i.e., naturally occurring AKH ligands), as well as specifically modified ligands, that were previously tested in an in vitro functional Aedae-AKH receptor activation assay by Wahedi et al. [36]. In this way (as for our ACPR models above), we could directly compare and assess the accuracy of the computationally generated ligand-receptor (Aedae-AKHR-1A) models. Several authors have found an aromatic residue at position 8 to be essential for AKH receptor activation and the biological activity of AKH peptides. We have simulated this by replacing Trp^8 with alanine. The results show a much-reduced binding of the mutated analogue, with a $\Delta_{binding}$ of -89 kcal mol^{-1}, compared to -120 kcal mol^{-1} for the native peptide. The main reason for this difference in binding energy is the lipophilic interaction of Trp^8. In the native Aedae-AKH peptide, Trp^8 sits in a lipophilic pocket of the Aedae-AKHR created by Trp^{139}, Trp^{133}, Phe^{208}, and Leu^{129}. The Δ_{lipo} for this is -30 kcal mol^{-1}. For the Ala^8 mutation, Δ_{lipo} is -23 kcal mol^{-1} and the ligand has a completely different orientation in the binding pocket (Figure S8). There is no interaction with Arg^{153}. Thus [Ala^8]AKH does not interact with the receptor residues necessary for activation. This mutation was not tested by Wahedi et al. [36], but a designed, synthetic analogue of Lacol-AKH, Lacol-AKH-7mer (pELTFTSS-NH_2), was tested in the receptor bioassay and found to be only 7% active at the highest concentration of 10 µM tested. Thus, this peptide did not activate Aedae-AKHR. Since Lacol-AKH-7mer differs from [Ala^8]Aedae-AKH in being C-terminally truncated (no Trp^8) and having Pro^6 replaced by Ser^6, we also simulated the binding of this 7-mer peptide to Aedae-AKHR. Here a $\Delta_{binding}$ of only -78 kcal mol^{-1} was obtained, a difference of some 43 kcal mol^{-1} less compared to native Aedae-AKH. Interestingly, the 7-mer form of Lacol-AKH had a better solvation energy (16 kcal mol^{-1}) than Aedae-AKH but a poorer Coulombic (-27 kcal mol^{-1}) and van der Waals (-24 kcal mol^{-1}) interaction. Lacol-AKH also had a weak interaction with Arg^{153}.

To better understand the importance of N-terminal residues, Wahedi et al. [36] measured the activity of Erysi-AKH, a peptide that occurs naturally in the dragonfly *Erythemis simplicicollis*. This peptide differs from Aedae-AKH at position 3 (threonine to asparagine exchange). This substitution resulted in a 310-fold reduction in the receptor activity study. The Δ_{binding} of Erysi-AKH was calculated in the current study to be 38 kcal mol^{-1} less than Aedae-AKH. Further substitution at position 2 (leucine to valine) as the peptide code-named Libau-AKH, a natural peptide isolated from the dragonfly *Libellula auripennis*, resulted in an activity of 1.7-fold less than Erysi-AKH. Docking of Libau-AKH to Aedae-AKHR had free energy of binding 1.7 kcal mol^{-1} less than Erysi-AKH. An AKH from the firebug, *Pyrrhocoris apterus* (Pyrap-AKH), also has two amino acid substitutions relative to Aedae-AKH (N^3 and N^7 vs. T^3 and S^7) and relative to Libau-AKH (L^2 and N^7 vs. V^2 and S^7). In the Aedae-AKHR activation bioassay, Pyrap-AKH was found to be more active than Libau-AKH but less active than Aedae-AKH and Erysi-AKH. Our simulation results are at odds with this observation. The Δ_{binding} of Pyrap-AKH was −153 kcal mol^{-1}, which is even more stable than Aedae-AKH. In all, Pyrap-AKH has 9, 11, and 12 kcal mol^{-1} more favourable Coulombic, lipophilic, and van der Waals energies with the Aedae-AKH receptor than Aedae-AKH. Hence, based on the free energy of binding alone, Pyrap-AKH should be more active than Aedae-AKH. Looking at the details of Pyrap-AKH binding, however, it is oriented differently in the binding pocket to Aedae-AKH. It does not interact with the same receptor residues identified previously as essential for receptor activation, which is why it is not active in the receptor assay. On the other hand, there is a very stable interaction between the mutated asparagine in position 7 and the receptor residues Arg^{153}, Tyr^{309}, Tyr^{310}, Gln^{204}, and Tyr^{237}. It is this strong H-bonding between Asn^7 on the ligand and the five receptor residues that accounts for the large free energy of binding. This dichotomy again illustrates the disconnect between binding affinity and activity as discussed above.

The importance of proline in position 6 was tested using Hipes-AKH-I from the sphingid moth, *Hippotion eson*. This peptide has the same sequence as Aedae-AKH, except that the proline in position 6 is changed to serine. In the receptor bioassay, Hipes-AKH-I had a very similar activity to Aedae-AKH and hence Wahedi et al. [36] concluded that position 6 is not very important for receptor activation. In our simulation, Hipes-AKH had free energy of binding of −85 kcal mol^{-1}, which is better than Lacol-AKH and Erysi-AKH but is less than Aedae-AKH; this result concurs with that of Wahedi et al. [36]. Hipes-AKH does bind to Arg^{153}, previously identified as essential for activity.

Finally, Wahedi et al. [36], used the AKH analogue, Tabat-AKH, from the black horse-fly, *Tabanus atratus*, where glycine is substituted for serine at position seven, to test the importance of this position. Here they found that Tabat-AKH was 30% more active than Aedae-AKH. Our simulation results, however, show that, while Tabat-AKH has very similar interactions with the receptor as Aedae-AKH, its free energy of binding to the receptor is only 0.5 kcal mol^{-1} better. Given the standard deviation in the free energies of binding, this result is in accord with the bioassay results. Also, Tabat-AKH does interact with Arg^{153}.

3.6. Docking of Aedae-AKH and Aedae-ACP to the Non-Cognate Receptor

Aedes aegypti has two well-characterised signalling systems with the ligands AKH and ACP. The ACP system appears to be more prescriptive than the AKH system in that it does not tolerate shorter peptides, whereas the AKH system is activated by a decapeptide [36].

The selectivity of Aedae-ACPR and Aedae-AKHR for their cognate peptides was checked by cross-binding of Aedae-ACP to Aedae-AKHR and Aedae-AKH to Aedae-ACPR. Docking of Aedae-AKH to Aedae-ACPR resulted in multiple poses with glide scores ranging from −8.7 to −2.3. Contrary to all other studies on AKH peptides, here the peptide did not have a β-turn but only a kink at proline. The ligand was not found in the receptor binding site but across the opening with the Trp^8 residue projecting into the binding site (Figure S9a). MD of the docked ligand had a free energy of binding of -129 ± 6 kcal mol^{-1}, which is a rather high free energy of binding. The simulation interaction diagram shows that AKH binds strongly to residues Arg^{187}, Glu^{164}, Tyr^{192}, Asn^{274}, Arg^{245}, Tyr^{353}, and Thr^{357}. These are all Aedae-ACP receptor residues outside the binding pocket we had established with Aedae-ACP (see above). The N-terminal pyroglutamic acid of Aedae-AKH had water bridges to a number of Aedae-ACP receptor residues (364, 367, and 368) and the tryptophan side chain sits in a positively charged pocket. All these interactions make for strong ligand/receptor binding but in the wrong place for receptor activation.

Aedae-ACP docks to Aedae-AKHR with glide scores ranging from −10 to −4. The best pose had a $\Delta G_{binding}$ of −80 kcal mol^{-1}, which is low. The ligand is oriented with the C-terminus projected inside the receptor and the N-terminus pointing out of the binding pocket (Figure S9b). The ligand interacts with receptor residues Ser^{313}, Tyr^{316}, Asn^{325}, Asn^{327}, Gln^{328} and Gln^{331}. None of these residues are essential for receptor activation. Hence the simulation results predict that Aedae-ACP should not activate Aedae-AKHR.

Both docking attempts are pointing clearly to two independent signalling systems with no overlap.

4. Conclusions

In this study, homology modelling was used to construct 3D models of the AKH and ACP receptors from the yellow fever mosquito, *Aedes aegypti*. At the same time, NMR-constrained MD was used to determine the preferred conformation of Aedae-ACP in a lipid micelle environment. The structure of Aedae-ACP, together with our previously determined structure of Aedae-AKH, were then used to identify the ligand binding pockets of their respective receptors.

Aedae-ACP was found to have a pronounced β-turn at Thr^3, which brought Phe^4 and Trp^8 onto the same side of the peptide. This conformation was stabilised by intramolecular hydrogen bonds. Aedae-AKH had a more linear structure, but a proline kink at position 6 also moved Trp^8 to the same side as Phe^4. Phe^4 and Trp^8 are reportedly essential for receptor activation, so it is interesting that these two residues had the same orientation, albeit arising from different mechanisms, in both ligands.

The structure of both receptors was typical of class A, GPCRs, with 7 transmembrane helices and an eighth helix lying in the plane of the membrane's inner surface. Each had a disulfide bridge between helix 3 and ECL2 and the conserved residues typical of this class of receptor. The requisite switches and locks were found except that Aedae-ACPR had a $DR^{3.50}C$ motif instead of the normal DRY motif.

The binding pocket of Aedae-ACPR comprised residues from all the helices, except helix one, and ECL2. $Ser^{194(3.39)}$ defined the bottom of the binding pocket with ECL2 closing the top. In the inactive model, ECL2 lay to the side allowing the ligand access to the binding pocket, and then moved over the ligand upon receptor activation, preventing egress of the ligand.

Ligand residue substitution studies show that strong ligand-receptor binding is a necessary but not sufficient condition for receptor activation. It appears that binding to Arg^{153} is also essential for receptor activation of both Aedae-ACPR and Aedae-AKHR. This is the same residue that was postulated to be essential for the activation of the stick insect (*C. morosus*) and the desert locust (*S. gregaria*) AKHRs. Docking studies also showed why cross-activation of Aedae-ACPR and Aedae-AKHR by Aedae-ACP and Aedae-AKH is not possible.

The results of this NMR-MD study are the first of its kind to give more insight into the adipokinetic hormone/corazonin-related peptide signalling systems of the yellow fever mosquito, *Aedes aegypti*, and is novel in providing a plausible comparison between the two similar receptors (ACPR and AKHR) and the reason why they bind and are activated by their respective cognate ligand and are not activated by the non-cognate ligand. Having validated the receptor models it should now be possible to search for or design, species-specific, molecules that may act as insecticides. Furthermore, the current results put into question those studies that indicate that the ACPR may be activated by AKHs or that the AKHR is activated by ACP.

Supplementary Materials: The following supporting information can be downloaded at: https://www.mdpi.com/article/10.3390/biom14030313/s1, Figure S1: RMSF of Aedae-ACP aligned onto the two Aedae-ACPR protein models. Figure S2: Protein interaction fraction Aedae-ACPR + Aedae-ACP: (a) active model, and (b) inactive model. Figure S3: Protein RMSD: (a) Aedae-AKH docked to Aedae-AKHR_6kr8 (active), and (b) Aedae-AKH docked to Aedae-AKHR_6tpk (inactive). Figure S4: Protein RMSF: (a) Aedae-AKH docked to Aedae-AKHR_6kr8, and (b) Aedae-AKH docked to Aedae-AKHR_6tpk. Figure S5: Ligand RMSF: (a) Aedae-AKH docked to Aedae-AKHR_6kr8, and (b) Aedae-AKH docked to Aedae-AKHR_6tpk. Figure S6: Protein-ligand contacts: (a) Aedae-AKH docked to Aedae-AKHR_6kr8, and (b) Aedae-AKH docked to Aedae-AKHR_6tpk. Figure S7: Ligand-Receptor contacts: (a) Aedae-AKH docked to Aedae-AKHR_6kr8, and (b) Aedae-AKH docked to Aedae-AKHR_6tpk. Figure S8: Binding pocket of active Aedae-AKHR model bound ligand: (a) Aedae-AKH, and (b) [Ala8]Aedae-AKH. Figure S9: (a) Aedae-ACPR showing binding of Aedae-AKH (red). For comparison, the orientation of the active peptide Aedae-ACP (orange) is shown. For clarity H6 is not displayed. W8 is displayed as ball and stick, and (b) Aedae-AKHR with Aedae-ACP docked. For clarity, the helices in front of the ligand are not shown.

Author Contributions: Conceptualization, G.G. and G.E.J.; methodology, G.E.J., M.-A.S. and F.S.; formal analysis, G.E.J., G.G., H.G.M. and M.-A.S.; investigation, G.E.J. and M.-A.S.; resources, G.E.J., G.G., H.G.M., M.-A.S. and F.S.; data curation, G.E.J.; writing—original draft preparation, G.E.J. and M.-A.S.; writing—review and editing, G.E.J., G.G., H.G.M., M.-A.S. and F.S.; funding acquisition, G.E.J., G.G., H.G.M., M.-A.S. and F.S. All authors have read and agreed to the published version of the manuscript.

Funding: This research was funded by the National Research Foundation of South Africa (grant Nos 93450 and 85466 to Graham E. Jackson; grant numbers 85768 [IFR13020116790] to GG and 150678 to HGM, and the University of Cape Town Research Committee. The Centre for High-Performance Computing (CHPC), South Africa, provided computational resources for this research project.

Institutional Review Board Statement: Not applicable.

Informed Consent Statement: Not applicable.

Data Availability Statement: Data are contained within the article and Supplementary Materials.

Acknowledgments: M.-A.S. and F.S. acknowledge access to the Bio21 NMR Facility.

Conflicts of Interest: The authors declare no conflict of interest.

References

1. Hansen, K.K.; Stafflinger, E.; Schneider, M.; Hauser, F.; Cazzamali, G.; Williamson, M.; Kollmann, M.; Schachtner, J.; Grimmelikhuijzen, C.J.P. Discovery of a Novel Insect Neuropeptide Signaling System Closely Related to the Insect Adipokinetic Hormone and Corazonin Hormonal Systems. *J. Biol. Chem.* **2010**, *285*, 10736–10747. [CrossRef]
2. Roch, G.J.; Busby, E.R.; Sherwood, N.M. Evolution of GnRH: Diving deeper. *Gen. Comp. Endocrinol.* **2011**, *171*, 1–16. [CrossRef]
3. Gäde, G.; Šimek, P.; Marco, H.G. An invertebrate [hydroxyproline]-modified neuropeptide: Further evidence for a close evolutionary relationship between insect adipokinetic hormone and mammalian gonadotropin hormone family. *Biochem. Biophys. Res. Commun.* **2011**, *414*, 592–597. [CrossRef]
4. Li, S.; Hauser, F.; Skadborg, S.K.; Nielsen, S.V.; Kirketerp-Møller, N.; Grimmelikhuijzen, C.J.P. Adipokinetic hormones and their G protein-coupled receptors emerged in Lophotrochozoa. *Sci. Rep.* **2016**, *6*, 32789. [CrossRef] [PubMed]
5. Marco, H.G.; Glendinning, S.; Ventura, T.; Gäde, G. The Gonadotropin-releasing hormone (GnRH) superfamily across Pancrustacea/Tetraconata. *Mol. Cell. Endocrinol.* 2024, *under review*.
6. Gäde, G.; Auerswald, L. Mode of action of neuropeptides from the adipokinetic hormone family. *Gen. Comp. Endocrinol.* **2003**, *132*, 10–20. [CrossRef] [PubMed]
7. Gäde, G. Regulation of intermediary metabolism and water balance of insects by neuropeptides. *Annu. Rev. Entomol.* **2004**, *49*, 93–113. [CrossRef] [PubMed]
8. Marco, H.G.; Gäde, G. Adipokinetic Hormone: A Hormone for all Seasons? In *Arthropoda. Advances in Invertebrate (Neuro)Endocrinology*; Saleuddin, S., Lange, A., Orchard, I., Eds.; Apple Academic Press: Palm Bay, FL, USA, 2020; Volume 2, pp. 129–176.
9. Kodrík, D. Adipokinetic hormone functions that are not associated with insect flight. *Physiol. Entomol.* **2008**, *33*, 9. [CrossRef]
10. Kodrík, D.; Bednárová, A.; Zemanová, M.; Krishnan, N. Hormonal regulation of response to oxidative stress in insects—An update. *Int. J. Mol. Sci.* **2015**, *16*, 25788–25816. [CrossRef] [PubMed]

11. Predel, R.; Neupert, S.; Russell, W.K.; Scheibner, O.; Nachman, R.J. Corazonin in insects. *Peptides* **2007**, *28*, 3–10. [CrossRef] [PubMed]
12. Veenstra, J.A. Isolation and structure of corazonin, a cardioactive peptide from the American cockroach. *FEBS Lett.* **1989**, *250*, 231–234. [CrossRef]
13. Tawfik, A.I.; Tanaka, S.; De Loof, A.; Schoofs, L.; Baggerman, G.; Waelkens, E.; Derua, R.; Milner, Y.; Yerushalmi, Y.; Pener, M.P. Identification of the gregarization-associated dark-pigmentotropin in locusts through an albino mutant. *Proc. Natl. Acad. Sci. USA* **1999**, *96*, 7083–7087. [CrossRef] [PubMed]
14. Tanaka, Y.; Hua, Y.; Roller, L.; Tanaka, S. Corazonin reduces the spinning rate in the silkworm, *Bombyx mori*. *J. Insect. Physiol.* **2002**, *48*, 707–714. [CrossRef] [PubMed]
15. Kim, Y.J.; Spalovská-Valachová, I.; Cho, K.H.; Zitnanova, I.; Park, Y.; Adams, M.E.; Zitnan, D. Corazonin receptor signaling in ecdysis initiation. *Proc. Natl. Acad. Sci. USA* **2004**, *101*, 6704–6709. [CrossRef] [PubMed]
16. Gospocic, J.; Shields, E.J.; Glastad, K.M.; Lin, Y.; Penick, C.A.; Yan, H.; Mikheyev, A.S.; Linksvayer, T.A.; Garcia, B.A.; Berger, S.L.; et al. The Neuropeptide Corazonin Controls Social Behavior and Caste Identity in Ants. *Cell* **2017**, *170*, 748–759.e12. [CrossRef] [PubMed]
17. Kaufmann, C.; Brown, M.R. Regulation of carbohydrate metabolism and flight performance by a hypertrehalosaemic hormone in the mosquito *Anopheles gambiae*. *J. Insect Physiol.* **2008**, *54*, 367–377. [CrossRef] [PubMed]
18. Patel, H.; Orchard, I.; Veenstra, J.A.; Lange, A.B. The distribution and physiological effects of three evolutionarily and sequence-related neuropeptides in *Rhodnius prolixus*: Adipokinetic hormone, corazonin and adipokinetic hormone/corazonin-related peptide. *Gen. Comp. Endocrinol.* **2014**, *195*, 1–8. [CrossRef]
19. Zhou, Y.J.; Fukumura, K.; Nagata, S. Effects of adipokinetic hormone and its related peptide on maintaining hemolymph carbohydrate and lipid levels in the two-spotted cricket, *Gryllus bimaculatus*. *Biosci. Biotechnol. Biochem.* **2018**, *82*, 274–284. [CrossRef]
20. Hou, L.; Guo, S.; Wang, Y.; Nie, X.; Yang, P.; Ding, D.; Li, B.; Kang, L.; Wang, X. Neuropeptide ACP facilitates lipid oxidation and utilization during long-term flight in locusts. *eLife* **2021**, *10*, e65279. [CrossRef]
21. Afifi, S.; Wahedi, A.; Paluzzi, J.P. Functional insight and cell-specific expression of the adipokinetic hormone/corazonin-related peptide in the human disease vector mosquito, *Aedes aegypti*. *Gen. Comp. Endocrinol.* **2023**, *330*, 114145. [CrossRef]
22. Centers for Disease Control. 2018. Available online: https://archive.cdc.gov/#/details?url=https://www.cdc.gov/globalhealth/newsroom/topics/yellowfever/index.html (accessed on 3 March 2024).
23. World Health Organization. Launch of the WHO Global Arbovirus Initiative, Meeting Report. 2022. Available online: https://cdn.who.int/media/docs/default-source/world-health-data-platform/technical-advisory-groups/arbovirus/glai-launch-meeting-summary_webinar_31-march-2022.pdf (accessed on 3 March 2024).
24. Verlinden, H.; Vleugels, R.; Zels, S.; Dillen, S.; Lenaerts, C.; Crabbé, K.; Spit, J.; Vanden Broeck, J. Receptors for neuronal or endocrine signalling molecules as potential targets for the control of insect pests. *Adv. Insect Physiol.* **2014**, *46*, 167–303.
25. Audsley, N.; Down, R.E. G protein coupled receptors as targets for next generation pesticides. *Insect Biochem. Mol. Biol.* **2015**, *67*, 27–37. [CrossRef] [PubMed]
26. Hill, C.A.; Sharan, S.; Watts, V.J. Genomics, GPCRs and new targets for the control of insect pests and vectors. *Curr. Opin. Insect Sci.* **2018**, *30*, 99–106. [CrossRef] [PubMed]
27. Nene, V.; Wortman, J.R.; Lawson, D.; Haas, D.; Kodira, C.; Tu, Z.J. Genome sequence of *Aedes aegypti*, a major arbovirus vector. *Science* **2007**, *316*, 1718–1723. [CrossRef] [PubMed]
28. Kaufmann, C.; Merzendorfer, H.; Gäde, G. The adipokinetic hormone system in Culicinae (Diptera: Culicidae): Molecular identification and characterization of two adipokinetic hormone (AKH) precursors from *Aedes aegypti* and *Culex pipiens* and two putative AKH receptor variants from *A. aegypti*. *Insect Biochem. Mol. Biol.* **2009**, *39*, 770–781. [CrossRef]
29. Predel, R.; Neupert, S.; Garczynski, S.F.; Crim, J.W.; Brown, M.R.; Russell, W.K.; Kahnt, J.; Russell, D.H.; Nachman, R.J. Neuropeptidomics of the mosquito *Aedes aegypti*. *J. Proteome Res.* **2010**, *9*, 2006–2015. [CrossRef]
30. Wahedi, A.; Paluzzi, J.P. Molecular identification, transcript expression, and functional deorphanization of the adipokinetic hormone/corazonin-related peptide receptor in the disease vector, *Aedes aegypti*. *Sci. Rep.* **2018**, *8*, 2146. [CrossRef] [PubMed]
31. Oryan, A.; Wahedi, A.; Paluzzi, J.-P.-V. Functional characterization and quantitative expression analysis of two GnRH-related peptide receptors in the mosquito, *Aedes aegypti*. *Biochem. Biophys. Res. Commun.* **2018**, *497*, 550–557. [CrossRef] [PubMed]
32. Gäde, G.; Hayes, T.K. Structure-activity relationships for *Periplaneta americana* hypertrehalosemic hormone I: The importance of side chains and termini. *Peptides* **1995**, *16*, 1173–1180. [CrossRef] [PubMed]
33. Ziegler, R.; Cushing, A.; Walpole, P.; Jasensky, R.; Morimoto, H. Analogs of *Manduca* adipokinetic hormone tested in a bioassay and in a receptor-binding assay. *Peptides* **1998**, *19*, 481–486. [CrossRef]
34. Caers, J.; Peeters, L.; Janssen, T.; De Haes, W.; Gäde, G.; Schoofs, L. Structure-activity studies of *Drosophila* adipokinetic hormone (AKH) by a cellular expression system of dipteran AKH receptors. *Gen. Comp. Endocrinol.* **2012**, *177*, 332–337. [CrossRef] [PubMed]
35. Marco, H.G.; Verlinden, H.; Broeck, J.V.; Gäde, G. Characterisation and pharmacological analysis of a crustacean G protein-coupled receptor: The red pigment-concentrating hormone receptor of *Daphnia pulex*. *Sci. Rep.* **2017**, *7*, 6851. [CrossRef]
36. Wahedi, A.; Gäde, G.; Paluzzi, J.-P. Insight into mosquito GnRH-related neuropeptide receptor specificity revealed through analysis of naturally occurring and synthetic analogs of this neuropeptide family. *Front. Endocrinol.* **2019**, *10*, 742. [CrossRef]

37. Zubrzycki, I.Z.; Gäde, G. Conformational Study on an Insect Neuropeptide of the AKH/RPCH-Family by Combined 1H-NMR Spectroscopy and Molecular Mechanics. *Biochem. Biophys. Res. Commun.* **1994**, *198*, 228–235. [CrossRef] [PubMed]
38. Nair, M.M.; Jackson, G.E.; Gäde, G. Conformational study of insect adipokinetic hormones using NMR constrained molecular dynamics. *J. Comput.-Aided Mol. Des.* **2001**, *15*, 259–270. [CrossRef] [PubMed]
39. Mugumbate, G.; Jackson, G.E.; van der Spoel, D.; Koever, K.E.; Szilagyi, L. *Anopheles gambiae*, Anoga-HrTH hormone, free and bound structure—A nuclear magnetic resonance experiment. *Peptides* **2013**, *41*, 94–100. [CrossRef]
40. Jackson, G.E.; Pavadai, E.; Gäde, G.; Timol, Z.; Andersen, N.H. Interaction of the red pigment-concentrating hormone of the crustacean *Daphnia pulex*, with its cognate receptor, Dappu-RPCHR: A nuclear magnetic resonance and modeling study. *Int. J. Biol. Macromol.* **2018**, *106*, 969–978. [CrossRef]
41. Abdulganiyyu, I.A.; Sani, M.-A.; Separovic, F.; Marco, H.; Jackson, G.E. Phote-HrTH (*Phormia terraenovae* hypertrehalosaemic hormone), the metabolic hormone of the fruit fly: Solution structure and receptor binding model. *Aust. J. Chem.* **2020**, *73*, 202–211. [CrossRef]
42. Gäde, G.; Šimek, P.; Marco, H.G. The first identified neuropeptide in the insect order Megaloptera: A novel member of the adipokinetic hormone family in the alderfly *Sialis lutaria*. *Peptides* **2009**, *30*, 477–482. [CrossRef] [PubMed]
43. Veenstra, J.A. The contribution of the genomes of a termite and a locust to our understanding of insect neuropeptides and neurohormones. *Front. Physiol.* **2014**, *5*, 454. [CrossRef] [PubMed]
44. Marchal, E.; Schellens, S.; Monjon, E.; Bruyninckx, E.; Marco, H.; Gäde, G.; Vanden Broeck, J.; Verlinden, H. Analysis of Peptide Ligand Specificity of Different Insect Adipokinetic Hormone Receptors. *Int. J. Mol. Sci.* **2018**, *19*, 542. [CrossRef]
45. Jackson, G.E.; Pavadai, E.; Gäde, G.; Andersen, N. The adipokinetic hormones and their cognate receptor from the desert locust, *Schistocerca gregaria*: Solution structure of endogenous peptides and models of their binding to the receptor. *PeerJ* **2019**, *7*, e7514. [CrossRef] [PubMed]
46. Vranken, W.F.; Boucher, W.; Stevens, T.J.; Fogh, R.H.; Pajon, A.; Llinas, M.; Ulrich, E.L.; Markley, J.L.; Ionides, J.; Laue, E.D. The CCPN data model for NMR spectroscopy: Development of a software pipeline. *Proteins Struct. Funct. Bioinform.* **2005**, *59*, 687–696. [CrossRef]
47. Cheung, M.-S.; Maguire, M.L.; Stevens, T.J.; Broadhurst, R.W. DANGLE: A Bayesian inferential method for predicting protein backbone dihedral angles and secondary structure. *J. Magn. Reson.* **2010**, *202*, 223–233. [CrossRef]
48. Rieping, W.; Habeck, M.; Bardiaux, B.; Bernard, A.; Malliavin, T.E.; Nilges, M. ARIA2: Automated NOE assignment and data integration in NMR structure calculation. *Bioinformatics* **2007**, *23*, 381–382. [CrossRef]
49. Chen, V.B.; Arendall, W.B.; Headd, J.J.; Keedy, D.A.; Immormino, R.M.; Kapral, G.J.; Murray, L.W.; Richardson, J.S.; Richardson, D.C. MolProbity: All-atom structure validation for macromolecular crystallography. *Acta Crystallogr. Sect. D Biol. Crystallogr.* **2010**, *66*, 12–21. [CrossRef] [PubMed]
50. Abraham, M.J.; Murtola, T.; Schulz, R.; Páll, S.; Smith, J.C.; Hess, B.; Lindahl, E. GROMACS: High performance molecular simulations through multi-level parallelism from laptops to supercomputers. *SoftwareX* **2015**, *1–2*, 19–25. [CrossRef]
51. Tieleman, D.P.; Van Der Spoel, D.; Berendsen, H.J.C. Molecular dynamics simulations of dodecylphosphocholine micelles at three different aggregate sizes: Micellar structure and chain relaxation. *J. Phys. Chem. B* **2000**, *104*, 6380–6388. [CrossRef]
52. Robertson, M.J.; Tirado-Rives, J.; Jorgensen, W.L. Improved peptide and protein torsional energetics with the OPLS-AA force field. *J. Chem. Theory Comput.* **2015**, *11*, 3499–3509. [CrossRef]
53. Hess, B.; Bekker, H.; Berendsen, H.J.; Fraaije, J.G. LINCS: A linear constraint solver for molecular simulations. *J. Comput. Chem.* **1997**, *18*, 1463–1472. [CrossRef]
54. Kiefer, F.; Arnold, K.; Künzli, M.; Bordoli, L.; Schwede, T. The SWISS-MODEL Repository and associated resources. *Nucleic Acids Res.* **2009**, *37* (Suppl. S1), D387–D392. [CrossRef] [PubMed]
55. *Schrödinger Release 2021-1: Maestro*; Schrödinger, LLC.: New York, NY, USA, 2021.
56. *Desmond Molecular Dynamics System*; D.E. Shaw Research: New York, NY, USA, 2021.
57. Berjanskii, M.; Wishart, D.S. NMR: Prediction of protein flexibility. *Nat. Protoc.* **2006**, *1*, 683–688. [CrossRef] [PubMed]
58. Tremblay, M.-L. The predictive accuracy of secondary chemical shifts is more affected by protein secondary structure than solvent environment. *J. Biomol. NMR* **2010**, *46*, 257. [CrossRef] [PubMed]
59. Szilágyi, L. Chemical shifts in proteins come of age. *Prog. Nucl. Magn. Reson. Spectrosc.* **1995**, *27*, 325–442. [CrossRef]
60. Tyndall, J.D.A.; Pfeiffer, B.; Abbenante, G.; Fairlie, D.P. Over one hundred peptide-activated G protein-coupled receptors recognize ligands with turn structure. *Chem. Rev.* **2005**, *105*, 793–826. [CrossRef] [PubMed]
61. Jackson, G.E.; Gamieldien, R.; Mugumbate, G.; Gäde, G. Structural studies of adipokinetic hormones in water and DPC micelle solution using NMR distance restrained molecular dynamics. *Peptides* **2014**, *53*, 270–277. [CrossRef]
62. Ballesteros, J.A.; Weinstein, H. Integrated methods for the construction of three-dimensional models and computational probing of structure-function relations in G protein-coupled receptors. In *Methods in Neurosciences*; Elsevier: Amsterdam, The Netherlands, 1995; Volume 25, pp. 366–428.
63. Schöneberg, T.; Schultz, G.; Gudermann, T. Structural basis of G protein-coupled receptor function. *Mol. Cell. Endocrinol.* **1999**, *151*, 181–193. [CrossRef]
64. Yuan, S.; Filipek, S.; Palczewski, K.; Vogel, H. Activation of G-protein-coupled receptors correlates with the formation of a continuous internal water pathway. *Nat. Commun.* **2014**, *5*, 4733. [CrossRef]

65. Iyison, N.B.; Sinmaz, M.G.; Sahbaz, B.D.; Shahraki, A.; Aksoydan, B.; Durdagi, S. In silico characterization of adipokinetic hormone receptor and screening for pesticide candidates against stick insect, *Carausius morosus*. *J. Mol. Graph. Model.* **2020**, *101*, 107720. [CrossRef] [PubMed]
66. Lambert, D. Drugs and receptors. *Contin. Educ. Anaesth. Crit. Care Pain* **2004**, *4*, 181–184. [CrossRef]
67. Jackson, G.E.; Gäde, G.; Marco, H.G. In Silico Screening for pesticide Candidates against the Desert Locust *Schistocerca gregaria*. *Life* **2022**, *12*, 387. [CrossRef] [PubMed]

biomolecules

MDPI

Article

Revisiting Concurrent Radiation Therapy, Temozolomide, and the Histone Deacetylase Inhibitor Valproic Acid for Patients with Glioblastoma— Proteomic Alteration and Comparison Analysis with the Standard-of-Care Chemoirradiation

Andra V. Krauze [1,*], Yingdong Zhao [2], Ming-Chung Li [2], Joanna Shih [2], Will Jiang [1], Erdal Tasci [1], Theresa Cooley Zgela [1], Mary Sproull [1], Megan Mackey [1], Uma Shankavaram [1], Philip Tofilon [1] and Kevin Camphausen [1]

1 Radiation Oncology Branch, Center for Cancer Research, National Cancer Institute, National Institutes of Health (NIH), 9000 Rockville Pike, Building 10, CRC, Bethesda, MD 20892, USA; erdal.tasci@nih.gov (E.T.); theresa.cooleyzgela@nih.gov (T.C.Z.); uma@mail.nih.gov (U.S.); philip.tofilon@nih.gov (P.T.)

2 Computational and Systems Biology Branch, Biometric Research Program, Division of Cancer Treatment and Diagnosis, National Cancer Institute, National Institutes of Health, Rockville, Maryland 20850, USA; limingc@mail.nih.gov (M.-C.L.); jshih@mail.nih.gov (J.S.)

* Correspondence: andra.krauze@nih.gov

Citation: Krauze, A.V.; Zhao, Y.; Li, M.-C.; Shih, J.; Jiang, W.; Tasci, E.; Cooley Zgela, T.; Sproull, M.; Mackey, M.; Shankavaram, U.; et al. Revisiting Concurrent Radiation Therapy, Temozolomide, and the Histone Deacetylase Inhibitor Valproic Acid for Patients with Glioblastoma—Proteomic Alteration and Comparison Analysis with the Standard-of-Care Chemoirradiation. *Biomolecules* **2023**, *13*, 1499. https://doi.org/10.3390/biom13101499

Academic Editors: Hyung-Sik Won and Ji-Hun Kim

Received: 24 August 2023
Revised: 19 September 2023
Accepted: 20 September 2023
Published: 10 October 2023

Abstract: Background: Glioblastoma (GBM) is the most common brain tumor with an overall survival (OS) of less than 30% at two years. Valproic acid (VPA) demonstrated survival benefits documented in retrospective and prospective trials, when used in combination with chemo-radiotherapy (CRT). Purpose: The primary goal of this study was to examine if the differential alteration in proteomic expression pre vs. post-completion of concurrent chemoirradiation (CRT) is present with the addition of VPA as compared to standard-of-care CRT. The second goal was to explore the associations between the proteomic alterations in response to VPA/RT/TMZ correlated to patient outcomes. The third goal was to use the proteomic profile to determine the mechanism of action of VPA in this setting. Materials and Methods: Serum obtained pre- and post-CRT was analyzed using an aptamer-based SOMAScan® proteomic assay. Twenty-nine patients received CRT plus VPA, and 53 patients received CRT alone. Clinical data were obtained via a database and chart review. Tests for differences in protein expression changes between radiation therapy (RT) with or without VPA were conducted for individual proteins using two-sided *t*-tests, considering *p*-values of <0.05 as significant. Adjustment for age, sex, and other clinical covariates and hierarchical clustering of significant differentially expressed proteins was carried out, and Gene Set Enrichment analyses were performed using the Hallmark gene sets. Univariate Cox proportional hazards models were used to test the individual protein expression changes for an association with survival. The lasso Cox regression method and 10-fold cross-validation were employed to test the combinations of expression changes of proteins that could predict survival. Predictiveness curves were plotted for significant proteins for VPA response (*p*-value < 0.005) to show the survival probability vs. the protein expression percentiles. Results: A total of 124 proteins were identified pre- vs. post-CRT that were differentially expressed between the cohorts who received CRT plus VPA and those who received CRT alone. Clinical factors did not confound the results, and distinct proteomic clustering in the VPA-treated population was identified. Time-dependent ROC curves for OS and PFS for landmark times of 20 months and 6 months, respectively, revealed AUC of 0.531, 0.756, 0.774 for OS and 0.535, 0.723, 0.806 for PFS for protein expression, clinical factors, and the combination of protein expression and clinical factors, respectively, indicating that the proteome can provide additional survival risk discrimination to that already provided by the standard clinical factors with a greater impact on PFS. Several proteins of interest were identified. Alterations in GALNT14 (increased) and CCL17 (decreased) ($p = 0.003$ and 0.003, respectively, FDR 0.198 for both) were associated with an improvement in both OS and PFS. The pre-CRT protein expression revealed 480 proteins predictive for OS and 212 for PFS ($p < 0.05$), of which 112 overlapped between OS and PFS. However, FDR-adjusted *p* values were high, with OS (the smallest p value of 0.586) and PFS (the smallest *p* value of 0.998). The protein PLCD3 had the lowest p-value (p = 0.002 and 0.0004 for OS and PFS, respectively), and its elevation prior to CRT predicted superior OS and PFS with VPA administration. Cancer hallmark genesets associated with proteomic alteration observed with the administration of VPA aligned with known signal transduction pathways of this agent in malignancy and non-malignancy settings, and GBM signaling, and included epithelial–mesenchymal transition, hedgehog signaling, Il6/JAK/STAT3, coagulation, NOTCH, apical junction, xenobiotic metabolism, and complement signaling. Conclusions: Differential alteration in proteomic expression pre- vs. post-completion of concurrent chemoirradiation (CRT) is present with the addition of VPA. Using pre- vs. post-data, prognostic proteins emerged in the analysis. Using pre-CRT data, potentially predictive proteins were identified. The protein signals and hallmark gene sets associated with the alteration in the proteome identified between patients who received VPA and those who did not, align with known biological mechanisms of action of VPA and may allow for the identification of novel biomarkers associated with outcomes that can help advance the study of VPA in future prospective trials.

Keywords: glioma; radiation; proteomic; valproic acid; HDAC inhibitor

1. Introduction

Glioblastoma (GBM) is the most common and the most aggressive brain tumor [1]. The current standard of care involves maximal surgical resection followed by concurrent radiation therapy (RT) and temozolomide (TMZ), followed by adjuvant TMZ [2]. The prognosis in GBM remains poor, with an overall survival (OS) of less than 30% at two years. Several therapies [3] have been studied to improve outcomes beyond the chemoirradiation (CRT) Stupp regimen, which was the first to result in improvement in OS by adding TMZ to RT [2]; however, while some benefits were described in some, none of these attempts have made an appreciable impact on OS. Valproic acid (VPA) has been one of the agents studied in this context, given its use as an antiepileptic agent in glioma patients who often present with seizures. Its activity as an HDAC inhibitor [4–6], its use as an antiepileptic agent [7–9], its association with improvement in survival [7,8,10–13], as well as its value given the cost of care [14], have made VPA an attractive agent of study [15–18] and the subject of several reviews [19–21]. Several studies have revealed potential anti-tumor effects via several cancer hallmark pathways, including angiogenesis, DNA repair, stemness, cellular reprogramming, apoptosis, and the epithelial-to-mesenchymal transition [22–25], including synergism in conjunction with TMZ [26,27]. The precise mechanisms of action that may underlie possible improvements in outcomes have, however, remained ill-defined even as a relationship between VPA dose [9,22,28,29] and duration [30] emerged that may well explain discordant outcome results in meta-analyses [11,31] given the use of seizure dose VPA as compared to high-dose VPA [17] and treatment duration as well as evolving seizure management over time transitioning from VPA to increase use of Levetiracetam [9,31–33]. The addition of VPA to concurrent RT/TMZ in patients with newly diagnosed GBM in our previous phase II trial was well tolerated, resulted in a favorable toxicity profile, had no late effects (neurological, pain, and blood/ bone marrow toxicity and mostly grade 1/2 and only two grade 3/4 toxicities), and improved outcomes (median OS 29.6 months (range: 21–63.8 months) [15–17]. The analysis of the proteomic alteration signatures post chemoirradiation in conjunction with OS was previously described [34]. In this study, we aimed to determine whether differential alteration in proteomic expression pre- vs. post-completion of concurrent chemoirradiation (CRT) is present with the addition of VPA to CRT, and if present, link proteomic alteration to both OS and PFS, and the biological mechanisms of action of VPA via prognostic and predictive protein signals.

2. Materials and Methods

2.1. Patients

Twenty-nine patients who received concurrent valproic acid (VPA) were compared to 53 patients who received CRT alone. All patients had pathology-proven GBM (diagnosed 2005–2013) and were enrolled on NCI NIH IRB-approved protocols. The patients who received concurrent high-dose VPA were treated on the open-label, NCI NIH phase 2 study (NCT00302159). To be included in this analysis in the VPA class, the patients needed to have received $\geq$1 week of VPA as per the original analysis [17] and have biospecimen obtained amenable to proteomic analysis. Patients who received CRT alone needed to have documented tissue diagnosis of glioblastoma and have received standard of care concurrent chemoirradiation defined as 59.4–60 Gy in 30–33 fractions with concurrent TMZ on natural history protocols (NCT00027326, NCT00083512). Blood biospecimens obtained before and after CRT completion were included in the study. In the patients who received VPA, this was initiated one week before the first day of RT at 10 to 15 mg/kg/day and subsequently increased up to 25 mg/kg/day over the week before RT. Analysis of their initial outcomes and late toxicity was previously published [15–17]. Serum samples were screened using the multiplexed, aptamer-based approach (SOMAScan® assay) to measure the relative concentrations of 7596 protein targets (7289 human) for changes in expression using approximately 150 ul of serum [35,36]. Clinical data (age, gender), tumor characteristics (location, MGMT methylation status), management-related factors (extent of resection), radiation therapy volumes (GTV T1, GTV T2), recursive partitioning analysis score (RPA) [37], and outcomes (PFS, OS) were obtained or derived (RPA) from the protocol database and electronic health record with GTV T1, GTV T2, generated per ICRU report 83 [38] obtained from the radiation therapy treatment planning (contoured on the T1 gadolinium sequence of the MRI scan employed for RT planning per standard guidelines).

2.2. SomaLogic SOMAScan® Assays

Serum samples were obtained before initiation of CRT (average seven days, range (0 to 23)) and following completion of CRT (average seven days, range (−1 to 30)) with the time between pre- and post-sample acquisition averaging 49 days (range 27–83 days). Following the acquisition, samples were frozen at −80 for an average of 3442 days (range 800–5788 days) and then defrosted and screened using the aptamer-based SOMAScan® proteomic assay technology for changes in the expression of 7000+ protein analytes [35,36]. SOMAScan® data were filtered to remove non-human and non-protein targets, resulting in 7289 aptamers targeting 6386 unique gene symbols. RFU values reported by SOMAScan® were log2-transformed.

2.3. Data Process

There were 7596 proteins on the chip. We selected 7289 human proteins for the subsequent analyses. There were 82 patients with data before CRT (PRE) and post-completion of CRT (COT (Completion of Treatment)). Log base 2 (COT/PRE) represented the protein expression change between after-treatment and pre-treatment conditions.

2.4. Class Comparisons

Tests for differences in clinical characteristics and protein expression changes between CRT with or without VPA were conducted using two-sided *t*-tests, considering *p*-values of <0.05 as significant. Adjustment for age, sex, and other clinical covariates was performed separately when appropriate. The Benjamini and Hochberg method was used to estimate the false discovery rate [39]. Hierarchical clustering of significant differentially expressed proteins was carried out using BRB-ArrayTools Dynamic Heatmap [40].

2.5. Gene Set Enrichment Analysis

Fifty Cancer Hallmark gene sets were downloaded from MSigDB. Gene Set Enrichment analyses were performed in BRB-ArrayTools [40]. The Kolmogorov–Smirnov (KS) tests are applied separately to each of the 50 gene sets. A gene set is considered significant if its corresponding KS re-sampling *p*-value is below the specified threshold (*p*-values < 0.05). GSEA with adjustments for age and sex were performed.

2.6. Survival Analysis

In the previous iteration of proteomic sample analysis in this cohort, univariate and multivariate Cox analysis was carried out for OS [34]. This iteration aimed to examine potential differential protein alteration pre- vs. post-CRT, seeking to define protein expression between patients who received VPA and those who did not. Univariate Cox proportional hazards models were fit to test individual protein expression change levels for association with both OS and PFS. Regression coefficients from these models were tested using a two-sided Wald test, considering *p*-values < 0.05 as significant. First, we examined the association between the expression of individual proteins and survival in unadjusted and adjusted analyses. Using protein expression changes above and below 0 Kaplan–Meier survival curves were plotted using the R statistical package [41].

Two models were employed to examine whether alteration in the protein expression with the administration of VPA can provide additional survival risk discrimination to that already provided by the standard covariates and, if so, to evaluate how much risk discrimination power the protein expression can add to the clinical covariates. To test the combinations of expression changes of proteins that could predict survival, we used the Lasso Cox regression method [42,43] implemented in BRB-ArrayTools [40]. To avoid overfitting due to the initial supervised selection of proteins to define the prognostic index, we used 10-fold cross-validation. A log-rank statistic is computed to assess whether the association of expression data to survival data is statistically significant. The significance of the log-rank statistics is determined by the permutation test. In the combined model, permutation test is performed by shuffling expression profiles while preserving survival data and covariates. Cross-validated Kaplan-Meier curves and log-rank statistics are generated, yielding a *p*-value that assesses whether expression data significantly enhances risk prediction compared to covariates. Cross-validated time-dependent ROC curves were employed for the model containing standard covariates and including both standard covariates and protein expression to evaluate whether the expression data provide more accurate predictions than those provided by standard clinical covariates in the case without separate test data [44].

Based on the pre-CRT protein measurement, predictiveness curves were plotted for each significant protein that is predictive for VPA response (*p*-value < 0.005) to show the survival probability vs. the protein expression percentiles [45]. Based on the cross point of the predictiveness curves, any new samples/patients would thus be evaluated for the superior response given the addition of VPA treatment. Furthermore, Kaplan–Meier curves were generated for both VPA groups using the stratified data in the low-/high-score cohorts in OS and PFS, respectively.

In summary, this study primarily focused on analyzing protein expression changes induced by treatment, with the exception of predictive protein identification using the pre-CRT measurement. The data analysis workflow is visually represented in Figure 1B and the models with mathematical formulas are available as supplementary materials in Supplementary File S1.

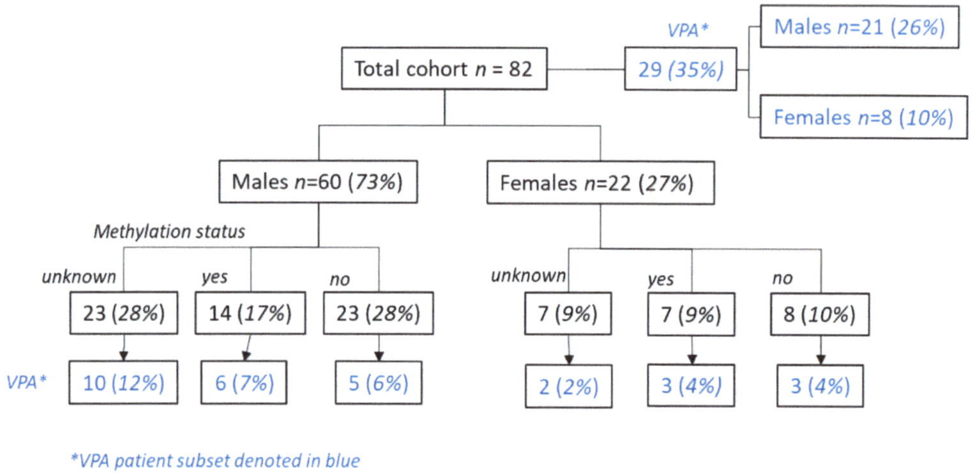

(A)

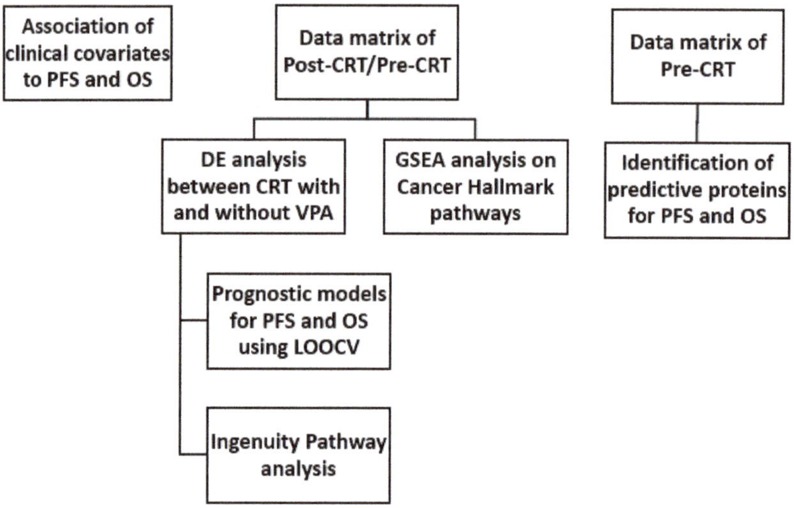

(B)

Figure 1. (**A**) Patient cohort breakdown by gender, methylation status and valproic acid (VPA) administration. (**B**) Data analysis workflow.

3. Results

3.1. Clinical Features Comparison between VPA and Non-VPA Cohort

Twenty-nine patients received VPA, and 53 received CRT alone (Figure 1A). MGMT methylation status was 9/29 (31%) vs. 12/53 (23%) methylated, 8/29(28%) vs. 23/53(43%) unmethylated, and 12/29(41%) vs. 18/53(34%) unknown, for VPA vs. non-VPA cohorts, respectively (Figure 1A) and MGMT methylation status was not statistically significant between the two cohorts (Table 1). VPA patients were statistically different from non-VPA patients with respect to age, extent of resection KPS, RPA, and RT technique (Table 1), with VPA patients being younger (mean age 52 vs. 58, but similar range 31–71), enriched in GTR resection status and fewer biopsies and superior KPS and RPA.

Table 1. Clinical covariate comparison of patients who received concurrent CRT vs. patients who received CRT plus VPA.

VPA Administration	No	Yes	*p*-Value
Total cohort n = 82 (%)	53 (*64.6*)	29 (*35.4*)	
Age (mean (SD))	58.06 (10.54)	52.34 (9.60)	*0.018*
Age Range	*31–70*	*31–71*	
Gender = Male (%)	39 (*73.6*)	21 (*72.4*)	*1*
Location			
Periventricular or Cortical = Periventricular (%)	22 (*41.5*)	6 (*20.7*)	*0.097*
Hemisphere			*0.614*
Left	23 (*43.4*)	15 (*51.7*)	
Right	29 (*54.7*)	14 (*48.3*)	
Both	1 (*1.9*)	0 (*0.0*)	
Extent of Resection			*0.04*
GTR	15 (*28.3*)	16 (*55.2*)	
STR	31 (*58.5*)	12 (*41.4*)	
Biopsy	7 (*13.2*)	1 (*3.4*)	
MGMT status			*0.361*
methylated	12 (*22.6*)	9 (*31.0*)	
unmethylated	23 (*43.4*)	8 (*27.6*)	
unknown	18 (*34.0*)	12 (*41.4*)	
KPS			*0.014*
60–80	14 (*26.4*)	3 (*10.3*)	
90	24 (*45.3*)	12 (*41.4*)	
100	10 (*18.9*)	14 (*48.3*)	
Unknown	5 (*9.4*)	0 (*0.0*)	
RPA			*0.019*
3	5 (*9.4*)	9 (*31.0*)	
4	29 (*54.7*)	17 (*58.6*)	
5	16 (*30.2*)	3 (*10.3*)	
Unknown	3 (*5.7*)	0 (*0.0*)	
RT volumes			
GTV T1 (cc)			*0.437*
<20 cc	13 (*24.5*)	11 (*37.9*)	
20–40 cc	19 (*35.8*)	9 (*31.0*)	
>40 cc	21 (*39.6*)	9 (*31.0*)	
GTV T2 (cc)			*0.152*
<10 cc	8 (*15.1*)	0 (*0.0*)	
10–50 cc	13 (*24.5*)	8 (*27.6*)	
50–100 cc	15 (*28.3*)	8 (*27.6*)	
>100 cc	17 (*32.1*)	13 (*44.8*)	
RT Technique			*<0.001*
3D	15 (*28.3*)	9 (*31.0*)	
IMRT	18 (*34.0*)	20 (*69.0*)	
Arc	20 (*37.7*)	0 (*0.0*)	

3.2. Clinical Factors Survival and Progression-Free Survival Analysis

In the VPA cohort, MGMT methylation status and RPA were statistically significant for OS. On univariate analysis, MGMT unmethylated status and RPA class 4 were associated with adverse outcomes (HR 3.2 and 2.86, respectively) (Supplementary Table S1). RPA was the only clinical feature statistically significant for PFS.

When combining VPA and non-VPA cohorts on Cox regression analysis (Supplementary Table S2, Figure S1) age, RPA, MGMT status, GTV T1, cortical vs. periventricular location, either hemisphere vs. bilateral disease, tumor location, and the administration of VPA were statistically significant for OS. The administration of VPA resulted in superior OS ($p = 0.011$) in Kaplan–Meier analysis (Supplementary Figure S2A). Age, BMI, RPA, MGMT status, cortical vs. periventricular location, tumor location, and the administration of VPA were statistically significant for PFS. The administration of VPA resulted in superior PFS ($p = 0.015$) in Kaplan–Meier analysis (Supplementary Figure S2B).

3.3. *Differentially Expressed Proteins VPA vs. No VPA*

The protein signal was not affected by the time in the freezer from collection to analysis (Supplementary Figure S3 showing a signal for proteins GALNT14 and SKP1). Differentially expressed proteins were examined between two classes: patients who received CRT alone (class 0) and patients who received CRT plus VPA (class 1) (Figure 2, Table 2). One hundred twenty-three proteins were identified that were altered pre- vs. post-CRT between the two classes. T-test results for the number of significant proteins between classes were adjusted for the impact of clinical covariates (Table 2). Similar numbers of significantly differentially expressed proteins were identified when adjusting for clinical variables compared to the unadjusted model (row #1) except for tumor location, wherein multiple categories were present with few samples in each category. Overall, this indicates that the results are globally not confounded by clinical covariates, including MGMT status (the last two rows), which are very similar (57 vs. 59) (Table 2). Hierarchical clustering of the 124 differentially expressed proteins revealed distinct proteomic clustering in the VPA-treated population (Figure 3, Supplementary Figure S4A,B display the gene names for the top (Figure S4A) and bottom cluster (Figure S4B), respectively) with significance level unadjusted $p < 0.001$ and FDR-adjusted p-value below 0.058 for all identified proteins (Supplementary File S2). Of the proteins statiscally significant for OS (GALNT14, CCL17, CTSV, ACP6, BMP6, SLITRK6, MSTN, NPTX1, ICAM4, SLITRK5), the top 10 displayed in Table 3 sorted in ascending order by OS FDR (all proteins displayed in Supplementary File S2), GALNT14 and CCL17 were the only two proteins with an FDR of 0.198 (Table 3). For PFS, GALNT14, ACP6, FBLN7, ALB, SLITRK5, TLNRD1, GNS, FCGRT, STAP1 and PRTG were stastically significant; the FDR, however, was 0.232 or higher for all proteins (Table 3, Supplementary File S2).

Table 2. The number of significant proteins in different class comparisons adjusted by clinical covariates.

Class Comparison	Class 0	Class 1	Adjusted by	# of Significant Proteins ($p < 0.001$)
VPA	VPA = 0 (53)	VPA = 1 (29)		124
VPA	VPA = 0 (53)	VPA = 1 (29)	age (>65)	109
VPA	VPA = 0 (53)	VPA = 1 (29)	sex	128
VPA	VPA = 0 (53)	VPA = 1 (29)	GTV-T1 (median)	127
VPA	VPA = 0 (53)	VPA = 1 (29)	Resection type	134
VPA	VPA = 0 (53)	VPA = 1 (29)	KPS	110
VPA	VPA = 0 (53)	VPA = 1 (29)	RPA	108
VPA	VPA = 0 (53)	VPA = 1 (29)	Radiation Technique	89
VPA	VPA = 0 (53)	VPA = 1 (29)	GTV-V2 (median)	125
VPA	VPA = 0 (53)	VPA = 1 (29)	Infiltration	104
VPA	VPA = 0 (52)	VPA = 1 (29)	Hemisphere	120
VPA	VPA = 0 (51)	VPA = 1 (28)	BMI (median)	114
VPA	VPA = 0 (53)	VPA = 1 (29)	Location	83
VPA with known MGMT	VPA = 0 (35)	VPA = 1 (17)		57
VPA with known MGMT	VPA = 0 (35)	VPA = 1 (17)	MGMT	59

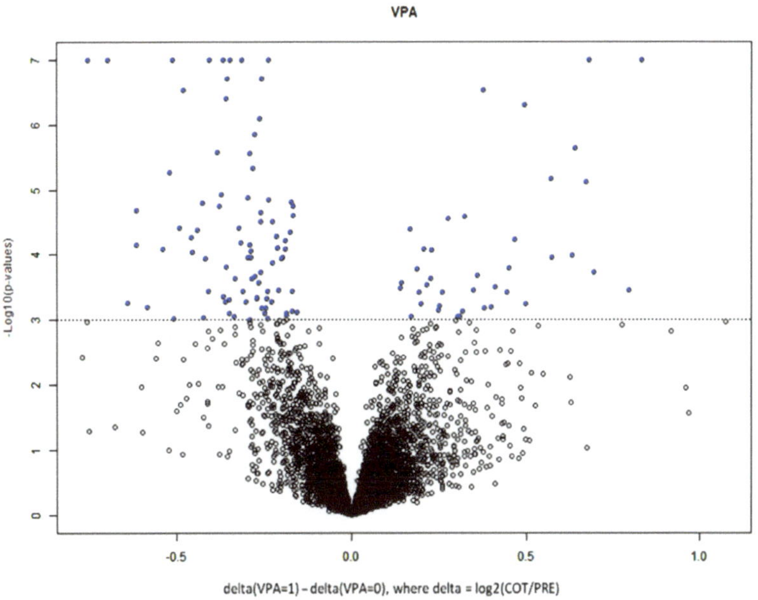

Figure 2. Volcano plot of class comparison of patients who received chemoirradiation (53 samples, class 0) and patients who received chemoirradiation plus VPA (29 sample, class 1) for the 7289 measured proteins using log2(cot-pre) data. Blue dots indicate the 124 differentially expressed proteins in the VPA-treated population with significance level unadjusted $p < 0.001$ and FDR-adjusted p-value below 0.058.

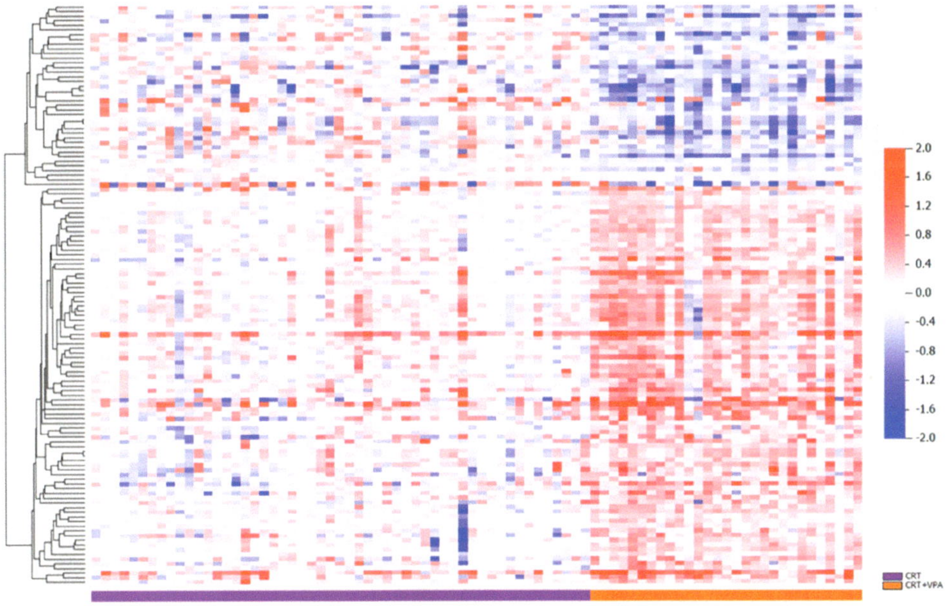

Figure 3. Hierarchical clustering of 124 significantly differentially expressed proteins between patients treated with CRT and concurrent VPA vs. CRT. Supplementary Figure S4A,B display the protein names for top (Figure S4A) and bottom cluster (Figure S4B), respectively.

Table 3. Top 10 protein signals significant for overall survival (OS) and progression-free survival (PFS) by *p*-value based on the results from 124 significantly differentially expressed proteins from the comparison of patients treated with CRT plus VPA vs. CRT alone.

Symbol	Name	EntrezID	Fold-Change	Mean log2(COT/PRE)	OS *p*-Value	OS FDR	OS HR	PFS *p*-Value	PFS FDR	PFS HR
CCL17	*C-C motif chemokine ligand 17*	6361	1.620	−0.004	0.003	0.198	1.513	0.024	0.232	1.363
GALNT14	*polypeptide N-acetylgalactosaminy-ltransferase 14*	79623	0.780	0.186	0.003	0.198	0.407	0.004	0.232	0.388
CTSV	*chathepsin V*	1515	1.160	−0.088	0.009	0.285	3.647	0.024	0.232	3.031
ACP6	*acid phosphatase 6, lysophosphatidic*	51205	0.810	0.184	0.011	0.285	0.408	0.007	0.232	0.378
BMP6	*bone morphogenetic protein 6*	654	0.850	0.134	0.012	0.285	0.344	0.027	0.240	0.369
MSTN	*myostatin*	2660	0.850	0.089	0.019	0.304	0.277	0.093	0.339	0.424
SLITRK6	*SLIT and NTRK like family protein 6*	84189	0.770	0.116	0.021	0.304	0.494	0.194	0.496	0.729
ICAM4	*intercellular adhesion molecule 4 (Landsteiner-Wiener blood group)*	3386	1.240	−0.267	0.027	0.304	2.002	0.039	0.246	1.806
NPTX1	*neuronal pentraxin 1*	4884	0.870	0.050	0.029	0.304	0.286	0.280	0.504	0.615
SLITRK5	*SLIT and NTRK like family protein 5*	26050	0.720	0.229	0.031	0.304	0.542	0.013	0.232	0.475

3.4. Survival Models for OS and PFS

To evaluate whether clinical covariates can predict survival, three statistically significant clinical variables identified in the univariate analysis, i.e., age, GTV-T1, and VPA, were included in a multivariate Cox model for overall OS and PFS, respectively (Supplementary Table S2 and Figure S1). The other covariates not retained were RPA ("unknown" status was significant), MGMT status (unknown in 34% and 41% of the non-VPA and VPA cohorts, respectively), hemisphere vs. bilateral disease, and location (too few samples in each category). To examine whether protein expression provides additional survival risk discrimination to that already provided by the three clinical covariates, protein signals identified as significantly differentially expressed between VPA and non-VPA (Supplementary File S2) were included in survival models for OS and PFS and Lasso regression was used to build the survival risk prediction models. Landmark times were selected based on the clinically observed and published literature median survival and progression times for GBM [46–48]. Cross-validated time-dependent ROC curves for OS and PFS for landmark times of 20 months and 6 months, respectively, were generated revealing AUC of 0.0.531, 0.756, 0.774 for OS and 0.535, 0.723, 0.806 for PFS for protein expression, clinical covariates and the combination thereof, respectively, indicating improved risk discrimination power with the addition of protein expression to the clinical covariates. A more significant impact on PFS as compared to OS was observed (Figure 4). As shown in Supplementary Figure S5, the cross-validated Kaplan–Meier curves and log-rank tests indicated that protein-only models were not statistically significant for OS or PFS, clinical covariates were significant for both OS and PFS, and combined models versus covariates only model were not significant for PFS or OS (Supplemental Figure S5). GALNT14, ACP, SLITRK5 and CCL17 were associated with both OS and PFS (Table 3). Among the above four proteins, GALNT14 was retained in univariate Cox proportional hazard models with an increased pre- vs. post-CRT value associated with improved OS and PFS (Table 3, Figure 5). We experimented with a survival model employing GALNT14 without other protein signals; however, this did not improve AUC (Supplementary Figure S6).

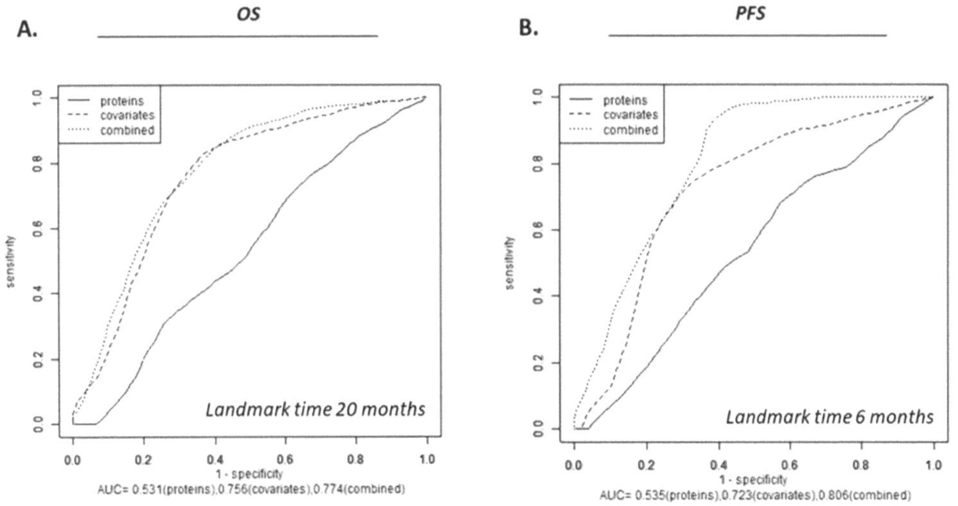

Figure 4. Time-dependent ROC curve for overall survival (OS) (**A**) and progression-free survival (PFS) (**B**) prediction model. (**A**) OS by proteins, covariates and combination of proteins and covariates. (**B**) PFS by proteins, covariates and combination of proteins and covariates.

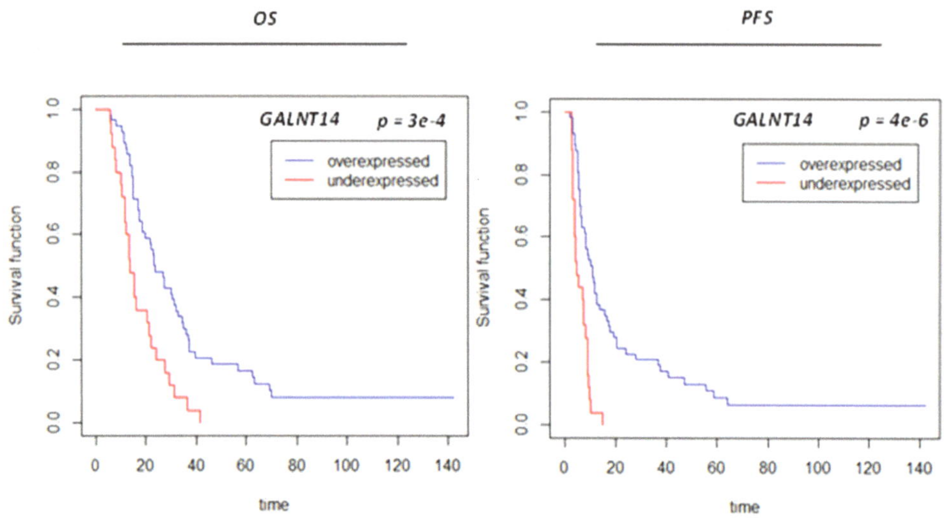

Figure 5. Kaplan–Meier curves for overall survival (OS) (**A**) and progression-free survival (PFS) (**B**) by difference in GALNT14 expression pre- vs. post-completion of chemoirradiation.

3.5. Protein Signals Predictive of VPA Response

The pre-CRT protein expression was analyzed for predictive proteins and, with $p < 0.05$, revealed 480 proteins associated with OS and 212 associated with PFS, of which 112 overlapped between OS and PFS (Supplementary File S3). PLCD3, VARS1, CYREN and KIR2DL4 emerged as predictive protein signals with $p < 0.005$ for both OS and PFS. For PLCD3, a higher score predicting superior OS and PFS with VPA administration ($p < 0.0005$) and a robust differential survival probability vs. the protein expression percentiles (Figure 6).

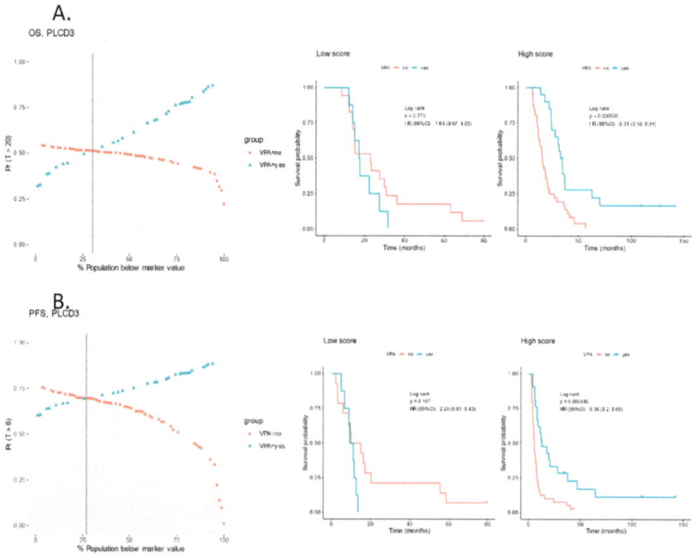

Figure 6. Predictiveness curves for the PLCD3 protein for (**A**) OS and (**B**) PFS and KM survival curves for high- and low-score groups. Vertical grey line indicates crossing point/threshold percentile of 30% and 27% for OS and PFS respectively.

3.6. Pathway Analysis

Cancer hallmark genesets associated with VPA administration were analyzed. They identified several pathways related to the signal transduction pathways of VPA in malignancy and non-malignancy settings as well as tumor proliferation and migration, including the epithelial–mesenchymal transition (EMT), hedgehog signaling, Il6/JAK/STAT3, coagulation, NOTCH, apical junction, xenobiotic metabolism, and complement signaling (Supplementary Table S3). EMT had the most significant number of matched proteins (150).

4. Discussion

The ability to evaluate proteomic changes in a cohort of patients, such as the one in this study, represents a unique opportunity to analyze the impact of an additive component to the standard-of-care CRT by, in this case, examining the effect of VPA administered as part of a prospective protocol. We have previously shown that the patient population treated with concurrent VPA in this trial [17] had superior outcomes as compared to those described in the literature [15] and in modern-day trials [46–48], with an acceptable toxicity profile [16]. We have previously reported on the global proteomic alteration identified pre- vs. post-CRT in GBM [34]. The current analysis aims to define the effect of VPA administration on the proteome pre- vs. post-CRT in GBM compared to patients who received standard-of-care CRT alone.

In this study, we identified differential proteomic expression between patients who received CRT and those who received CRT plus VPA with 124 proteins differentially expressed, indicating that the effects of VPA provide a sufficiently enriched proteomic signal. We note that the sample size employed in this study [49,50] compares favorably with previous studies of similar scope [51], aligning with the design of similar studies that employ large-scale data [52] (Supplementary Table S4). We also note that serum sample acquisition before and after CRT is feasible despite the time range from collection to analysis (2003–2015), with time spent in storage ranging from 2 to 15 years. The proteomic signal remains robust, unaffected by storage, and significantly altered to capture intervention with VPA and CRT. The analysis of the proteomic signal revealed that protein expression was distinctly clustered in the patients who received VPA. This is interesting given that although this is a large-scale proteomic data set, it still represents only a tiny subset of the proteome overall, and it is presumably impacted by innumerable competing factors: clinical factors, medications, and other factors that have yet to be proteomically defined.

We found that in the OS and PFS models, the proteomic signal conferred additive risk discrimination power as compared to the proteome or the clinical data in isolation, and this was more pronounced for PFS in the context of VPA treatment. This is logical given that the signal alteration resulted from pre- vs. post-CRT proteome, which would more likely impact PFS since it represents a "closer" outcome endpoint to sample acquisition compared to OS, which occurs later. OS is also subject to multiple other factors, including further resection, additional systemic management, patient performance status, and comorbidities. It should also be noted that the ability to capture and interpret progression as an endpoint is limited and, thus, PFS remains flawed with clinical information limited by inconsistencies (clinical, radiographic, or both); hence, presumably, PFS remains relatively insensitive. Based on this analysis, employing proteomic alteration with validation in larger cohorts may be possible to identify more robust signals and better predict progression.

The GALNT14 protein was identified in both protein and protein-plus-covariate models, and was significant for both OS and PFS, with an increase following CRT and VPA treatment, measured as an improvement in OS and PFS and thus prognostic for both. GALNT14 is a member of the polypeptide N-acetylgalactosaminyltransferase (GALNT) family comprised of enzymes that catalyze mucin-type O-glycosylation of proteins. Alterations in components of this family have been associated with several hallmarks of cancer, including migration, proliferation, and treatment resistance [53,54]. GALNT14 has been expressed in multiple cancers altering several biological functions, and was recently described as an emerging marker capable of predicting outcomes [53]. Previous data have shown that GALNT14 correlates with Apo2L/TRAIL sensitivity in pancreas cancer, non-small-cell lung cancer, and melanoma cell lines, with overexpression increasing response to treatment by leveraging O-glycosylation to mediate apoptosis-initiating protease caspase-8 [55], decreasing resistance to apoptosis. The impact of altered O-glycosylation by members of the GALNT family is wide-ranging, as recently described in genome-wide analyses, and under- and over-expressed genes likely exhibit different effects on different cancers [54]. The role of GALNT14 in glioma has not been described, nor has its role as part of the human proteome and, thus, requires more research and validation. However, alternation in this protein in our study appears to correlate to the administration of VPA and survival. VPA, as noted, impacts multiple signaling pathways [21], and its mechanism as a radiation modifier has yet to be fully understood. Our study is the first to connect GALNT14, an emerging oncologic marker, to VPA administration, GBM biology, and the human proteome. Additional markers were identified (Supplemental material File 4). CTSV (Cathepsin V), ACP6 (Acid phosphatase 6, lysophosphatidic), BMP6 (Bone morphogenetic protein 6), MSTN (Myostatin), SLITRK6 (SLIT and NTRK like family member 6), ICAM4 (Intercellular adhesion molecule 4 (Landsteiner-Wiener blood group), NPTX1 (Neuronal pentraxin 1) and SLITRK5 (SLIT and NTRK like family member 5). All these proteins have relevance to cancer (Supplemental material File 4), while BMP6, MSTN, SLITRK5 and 6 and ICAM4 and NPTX1 have specific relevance to GBM with, in the case of SLTGK5 and 6 and NPTX1 having been linked to neural tissue and neurodegeneration respectively.

PLCD3 emerged as one of the most statistically significant predictive proteins by p-value for both OS and PFS, in addition to VARS1, CYREN, KIR2DL4 all with $p < 0.005$ for both OS and PFS. PLCD3 had a higher value before CRT associated with the improved outcomes with the administration of VPA, and this bears further investigation, as do the additional predictive proteins identified in this study. Several predictive proteins identified have connections to known pathways in cancer, including PLCD3 (phospholipase C delta3), VARS1 (Valyl-tRNA synthetase 1), CYREN (Cell cycle regulator of NHEJ), KIR2DL4 (Killer cell immunoglobulin-like receptor 2DL4) and SKP1(S-phase kinase-associated protein 1), and have a direct link to GBM [56,57] (Supplemental File 4). PLCD3 connects to PI3K (Phosphatidylinositol-4,5-bisphosphate 3-kinase) and EGFR, which are both critical in GBM, with PI3K signaling exhibiting heterogeneous signaling that is the subject of ongoing investigation [58,59]. Notably VARS1 may relate to seizure presentation and management in the context of GBM, while CYREN likely relates to radiation and chemotherapy managements given its association with non homologous end joing DNA repair pathways. KIR2DL4 has been implicated in cancer in relationship to the immune microenviroment and is subject to evolving mangement avenues for targeted cancer immunotherapy (Supplemental File 4). SKP1 is the most significant predictive protein for OS and a transcription regulator with significant connections to molecular pathways in cancer and GBM specifically [60,61]. In its interaction with β-transducin repeat-containing E3 ubiquitin-protein ligase (β-TrCP), itself a substrate recognition subunit for the Skp1-Cullin1-F-box protein E3 ubiquitin ligase, it has been implicated in tumorigenesis and regulation of pathways with β-TrCP suppressing progression and cell migration in glioma. It has also been reported to induce chromosome instability via cyclin E1 in other cancers [62]. Additional proteins, including AGR3, APPL1, CCL17, CLU, and FBLN7, are all supported by data in GBM, with their role an ongoing research interest [63–67].

The statistically significant proteins identified in this study and hallmark gene sets associated with the alteration in the proteome observed between patients who received CRT plus VPA and those who received CRT alone align with known biological mechanisms of action of VPA as an HDACi [21], including effects on apoptosis [28,68], DNA repair and damage response [23], signaling via Notch and TGF [30], BMP [69,70], NF-κB and STAT3 [6] (Figure 7, Supplementary Figure S7) [71]. Understanding the effect of VPA by exploiting observed proteomic alteration may allow for understanding the benefit observed with its administration in glioma patients and identifying novel biomarkers that can help advance the study of VPA in future prospective trials to improve outcomes.

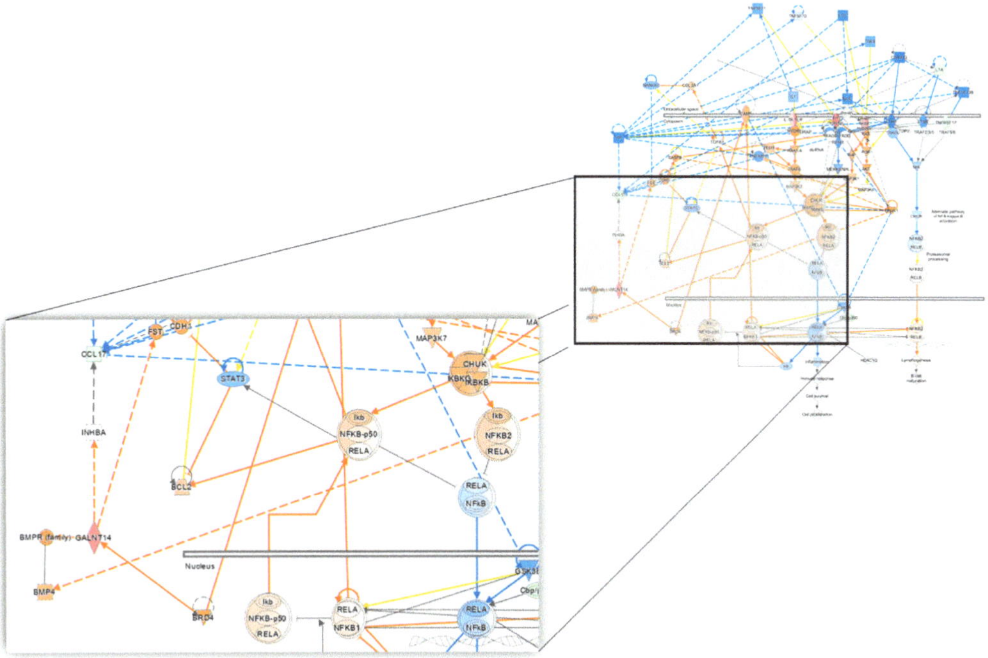

Figure 7. Ingenuity Pathway Analysis (IPA) overlaying the alteration of 124 differentially expressed proteins onto the NF-κB and STAT3 pathways showcasing the effect of GALNT14 and CCL17. (QIAGEN Inc., https://www.qiagenbioinformatics.com/products/ingenuitypathway-analysis, accessed on 24 July 2023 [71]).

This study's limitations include the small cohort and retrospective nature of the study, given the comparison with patients who did not receive VPA and were not treated on trial. The outcomes were superior to real-world data and thus may not be representative. The data set was missing MGMT in 37% of patients, and IDH status was unavailable. The data can not be validated with additional cohorts since no such cohorts are treated with high-dose VPA and available proteome, and large-scale proteomic data are lacking. Moreover, while adjusting for clinical covariates in the prognostic models, the potential interactions among these covariates were not incorporated. This omission could introduce bias if significant interactions exist and are associated with survival outcomes. Future directions include building prediction models wherein we will explore several techniques to mitigate class imbalance [72]. There are also additional impacts of other factors on the proteome, including steroids, thrombosis, and medications that are not captured in the clinical classification, and these can impact the analysis and interpretation. We also do not know if the changes in the proteome stem from the tumor or from normal tissues, or if the changes observed are representative of cause or effect.

5. Conclusions

Differentially expressed proteins were identified in a large-scale proteomic panel carried out before and post-completion of CRT with the addition of high-dose VPA. GALNT14 and CCL17 were identified as potential prognostic markers based on their expression changes between pre- and post-treatment proteomic profiles. Additionally, PLCD3, SKP1, VARS1, CYREN, and KIR2DL4 were found to be potentially predictive biomarkers solely from the expression levels in the pre-treatment proteomic profile. Those findings were supported by existing data in cancer with several proteins specifically reported on in GBM with growing associations to treatment resistance or response. The predictive and prognostic ability following measurement in serum in GBM patients with the addition of VPA to the standard-of-care CRT is novel, as is the identification of several proteins that, collectively or individually, may be explored as biomarkers. Predictive markers may point to biological risk groups that may benefit from administering VPA to result in superior outcomes. Given these findings, VPA benefits from additional studies in prospective trials.

Supplementary Materials: The following supporting information can be downloaded at https://www.mdpi.com/article/10.3390/biom13101499/s1. File S1: Survival models with mathematical formulas; File S2: The 124 differentially expressed proteins in the VPA-treated population; File S3: Pre-CRT protein expression analyzed for predictive proteins showing the 112 proteins overlapped between OS and PFS; File S4: Additional identified proteins in the reanalysis post data correction; Figure S1: Forest plot for covariates for overall survival (OS) and progression free survival (PFS); Figure S2: KM curves for OS (A) and PFS (B) for the administration of VPA; Figure S3: Protein signal vs. time in freezer from collection to analysis in days for. (A) GALNT14, statistically significant for OS and PFS in Cox analysis and survival. (B) SKP1, predictive for response to VPA in prediction model; Figure S4: Figure 3 displayed as the two separate zoom-in figures with gene names to represent the top (A) and bottom (B) clusters of proteins in the original heatmap; Figure S5: Kaplan Meier curves for survival (OS) (A-C) and progression free survival (PFS) (D–F) with patient population risk stratified (high(red), low (blue)) by protein expression (A,D), covariates (B,E) and combination of protein expression and covariates (C,F) Protein data is based on the results from 124 significantly differentially expressed proteins from class comparison between patients treated with CRT and concurrent VPA vs CRT. Figure S6: Time-dependent ROC curve for overall survival (OS) (A) and progression free survival (PFS) (B) prediction model based on GALNT14; Figure S7: GALNT14 and CCL17, the two proteins associated with OS with FDR 0.104 with potential function between two major signaling pathways driven by TGF and NF-κB. (QIAGEN Inc., https://www.qiagenbioinformatics.com/products/ingenuitypathway-analysis) accessed on 24 July 2023 [71]; Table S1: Patient characteristics table and cox regression analysis of clinical covariates in the VPA cohort; Table S2: Cox analysis for overall survival (OS) and progression free survival (PFS) with hazard ratio and p-value for VPA and no VPA patients.; Table S3: Cancer Hallmark GeneSets associated with Valproic acid (VPA) administration; Table S4: Results of online sample size calculation tool to calculate the minimum sample size for PFS and OS. References [73–92] were cited in Supplementary Materials.

Author Contributions: Conceptualization, A.V.K., P.T. and K.C.; Data curation, A.V.K., W.J., T.C.Z., M.S., M.M. and U.S.; Formal analysis, A.V.K., Y.Z., M.-C.L. and J.S.; Funding acquisition, A.V.K. and K.C.; Investigation, A.V.K., Y.Z., M.-C.L., E.T. and M.S.; Methodology, A.V.K., Y.Z., M.-C.L., J.S. and K.C.; Project administration, A.V.K. and K.C.; Resources, A.V.K., Y.Z. and K.C.; Software, Y.Z., M.-C.L. and W.J.; Supervision, A.V.K., Y.Z. and K.C.; Validation, Y.Z. and M.-C.L.; Visualization, A.V.K., Y.Z. and M.-C.L.; Writing—original draft, A.V.K. and Y.Z.; Writing—review and editing, A.V.K., Y.Z., M.-C.L., J.S., E.T., T.C.Z., M.S., M.M., U.S., P.T. and K.C. All authors have read and agreed to the published version of the manuscript.

Funding: Funding is provided in part by NCI NIH intramural program (ZID BC 010990).

Institutional Review Board Statement: All patients were treated on NCI NIH IRB (IRB00011862)-approved protocols 02C0064, 04C0200 and 06C0112.

Informed Consent Statement: Patient consent was obtained per the above-listed protocols.

Data Availability Statement: The data pertaining to this study has been made available as supplementary material to this manuscript.

Acknowledgments: The results shown here are in whole or part based upon data generated by the aptamer-based proteomics technology SOMAScan® Assay by SomaLogic. Palantir Foundry was used in the integration, harmonization, and analysis of clinical and proteomic data inside the secure NIH Integrated Data Analysis Platform (NIDAP).

Conflicts of Interest: The authors declare that they have no conflicts of interest.

Abbreviations

CRT	Concurrent Chemoirradiation
EMT	Epithelial–Mesenchymal Transition
GBM	Glioblastoma
GTV T1	Gross Tumor Volume on T1 Gadolinium-Enhanced MRI Sequence
GTV T2	Gross Tumor Volume on T2 FLAIR Signal Sequence
MGMT	O6-Methylguanine-DNA Methyltransferase
OS	Overall survival
PFS	Progression-Free Survival
RPA	Recursive Partitioning Analysis
RT	Radiation Therapy
TMZ	Temozolomide
VPA	Valproic Acid
WHO	World Health Organisation

References

1. Ostrom, Q.T.; Patil, N.; Cioffi, G.; Waite, K.; Kruchko, C.; Barnholtz-Sloan, J.S. CBTRUS Statistical Report: Primary Brain and Other Central Nervous System Tumors Diagnosed in the United States in 2013–2017. *Neuro-Oncol.* **2020**, *22*, iv1–iv96. [CrossRef]
2. Stupp, R.; Mason, W.P.; van den Bent, M.J.; Weller, M.; Fisher, B.; Taphoorn, M.J.; Belanger, K.; Brandes, A.A.; Marosi, C.; Bogdahn, U.; et al. Radiotherapy plus concomitant and adjuvant temozolomide for glioblastoma. *N. Engl. J. Med.* **2005**, *352*, 987–996. [CrossRef]
3. Mathen, P.; Rowe, L.; Mackey, M.; Smart, D.; Tofilon, P.; Camphausen, K. Radiosensitizers in the temozolomide era for newly diagnosed glioblastoma. *Neuro-Oncol. Pract.* **2020**, *7*, 268–276. [CrossRef]
4. Cornago, M.; Garcia-Alberich, C.; Blasco-Angulo, N.; Vall-Llaura, N.; Nager, M.; Herreros, J.; Comella, J.X.; Sanchis, D.; Llovera, M. Histone deacetylase inhibitors promote glioma cell death by G2 checkpoint abrogation leading to mitotic catastrophe. *Cell Death Dis.* **2014**, *5*, e1435. [CrossRef] [PubMed]
5. Zhou, Y.; Xu, Y.; Wang, H.; Niu, J.; Hou, H.; Jiang, Y. Histone deacetylase inhibitor, valproic acid, radiosensitizes the C6 glioma cell line in vitro. *Oncol. Lett.* **2014**, *7*, 203–208. [CrossRef] [PubMed]
6. Berendsen, S.; Frijlink, E.; Kroonen, J.; Spliet, W.G.M.; van Hecke, W.; Seute, T.; Snijders, T.J.; Robe, P.A. Effects of valproic acid on histone deacetylase inhibition in vitro and in glioblastoma patient samples. *Neuro-Oncol. Adv.* **2019**, *1*, vdz025. [CrossRef]
7. Kerkhof, M.; Dielemans, J.C.; van Breemen, M.S.; Zwinkels, H.; Walchenbach, R.; Taphoorn, M.J.; Vecht, C.J. Effect of valproic acid on seizure control and on survival in patients with glioblastoma multiforme. *Neuro-Oncol.* **2013**, *15*, 961–967. [CrossRef]
8. Guthrie, G.D.; Eljamel, S. Impact of particular antiepileptic drugs on the survival of patients with glioblastoma multiforme. *J. Neurosurg.* **2013**, *118*, 859–865. [CrossRef]
9. Redjal, N.; Reinshagen, C.; Le, A.; Walcott, B.P.; McDonnell, E.; Dietrich, J.; Nahed, B.V. Valproic acid, compared to other antiepileptic drugs, is associated with improved overall and progression-free survival in glioblastoma but worse outcome in grade II/III gliomas treated with temozolomide. *J. Neuro-Oncol.* **2016**, *127*, 505–514. [CrossRef]
10. Weller, M.; Gorlia, T.; Cairncross, J.G.; van den Bent, M.J.; Mason, W.; Belanger, K.; Brandes, A.A.; Bogdahn, U.; Macdonald, D.R.; Forsyth, P.; et al. Prolonged survival with valproic acid use in the EORTC/NCIC temozolomide trial for glioblastoma. *Neurology* **2011**, *77*, 1156–1164. [CrossRef] [PubMed]
11. Lu, V.M.; Texakalidis, P.; McDonald, K.L.; Mekary, R.A.; Smith, T.R. The survival effect of valproic acid in glioblastoma and its current trend: A systematic review and meta-analysis. *Clin. Neurol. Neurosurg.* **2018**, *174*, 149–155. [CrossRef] [PubMed]
12. Kuo, Y.J.; Yang, Y.H.; Lee, I.Y.; Chen, P.C.; Yang, J.T.; Wang, T.C.; Lin, M.H.; Yang, W.H.; Cheng, C.Y.; Chen, K.T.; et al. Effect of valproic acid on overall survival in patients with high-grade gliomas undergoing temozolomide: A nationwide population-based cohort study in Taiwan. *Medicine* **2020**, *99*, e21147. [CrossRef] [PubMed]
13. Wang, G.; Guan, S.; Yang, X.; Sun, S.; Huang, B.; Li, X. Administration of Valproic Acid Improves the Survival of Patients with Glioma Treated with Postoperative Radiotherapy. *Oncol. Res. Treat.* **2022**, *45*, 650–659. [CrossRef]
14. Fisher, C.; Broderick, W. Sodium valproate or valproate semisodium: Is there a difference in the treatment of bipolar disorder? *Psychiatr. Bull.* **2003**, *27*, 446–448. [CrossRef]
15. Krauze, A.V.; Megan, M.; Theresa, C.Z.; Peter, M.; Shih, J.H.; Tofilon, P.J.; Rowe, L.; Gilbert, M.; Camphausen, K. The addition of Valproic acid to concurrent radiation therapy and temozolomide improves patient outcome: A Correlative analysis of RTOG 0525, SEER and a Phase II NCI trial. *Cancer Stud. Ther.* **2020**, *5*. [CrossRef]
16. Krauze, A.V.; Mackey, M.; Rowe, L.; Chang, M.G.; Holdford, D.J.; Cooley, T.; Shih, J.; Tofilon, P.J.; Camphausen, K. Late toxicity in long-term survivors from a phase 2 study of concurrent radiation therapy, temozolomide and valproic acid for newly diagnosed glioblastoma. *Neuro-Oncol. Pract.* **2018**, *5*, 246–250. [CrossRef]
17. Krauze, A.V.; Myrehaug, S.D.; Chang, M.G.; Holdford, D.J.; Smith, S.; Shih, J.; Tofilon, P.J.; Fine, H.A.; Camphausen, K. A Phase 2 Study of Concurrent Radiation Therapy, Temozolomide, and the Histone Deacetylase Inhibitor Valproic Acid for Patients With Glioblastoma. *Int. J. Radiat. Oncol. Biol. Phys.* **2015**, *92*, 986–992. [CrossRef]

18. Su, J.M.; Murray, J.C.; McNall-Knapp, R.Y.; Bowers, D.C.; Shah, S.; Adesina, A.M.; Paulino, A.C.; Jo, E.; Mo, Q.; Baxter, P.A.; et al. A phase 2 study of valproic acid and radiation, followed by maintenance valproic acid and bevacizumab in children with newly diagnosed diffuse intrinsic pontine glioma or high-grade glioma. *Pediatr. Blood Cancer* **2020**, *67*, e28283. [CrossRef]
19. Yuan, Y.; Xiang, W.; Qing, M.; Yanhui, L.; Jiewen, L.; Yunhe, M. Survival analysis for valproic acid use in adult glioblastoma multiforme: A meta-analysis of individual patient data and a systematic review. *Seizure* **2014**, *23*, 830–835. [CrossRef]
20. Ochiai, S.; Nomoto, Y.; Yamashita, Y.; Watanabe, Y.; Toyomasu, Y.; Kawamura, T.; Takada, A.; Ii, N.; Kobayashi, S.; Sakuma, H. Roles of Valproic Acid in Improving Radiation Therapy for Glioblastoma: A Review of Literature Focusing on Clinical Evidence. *Asian Pac. J. Cancer Prev.* **2016**, *17*, 463–466. [CrossRef]
21. Han, W.; Guan, W. Valproic Acid: A Promising Therapeutic Agent in Glioma Treatment. *Front. Oncol.* **2021**, *11*, 687362. [CrossRef]
22. Osuka, S.; Takano, S.; Watanabe, S.; Ishikawa, E.; Yamamoto, T.; Matsumura, A. Valproic acid inhibits angiogenesis in vitro and glioma angiogenesis in vivo in the brain. *Neurol. Med.-Chir.* **2012**, *52*, 186–193. [CrossRef]
23. Hoja, S.; Schulze, M.; Rehli, M.; Proescholdt, M.; Herold-Mende, C.; Hau, P.; Riemenschneider, M.J. Molecular dissection of the valproic acid effects on glioma cells. *Oncotarget* **2016**, *7*, 62989–63002. [CrossRef]
24. Han, W.; Yu, F.; Cao, J.; Dong, B.; Guan, W.; Shi, J. Valproic Acid Enhanced Apoptosis by Promoting Autophagy Via Akt/mTOR Signaling in Glioma. *Cell Transpl.* **2020**, *29*, 963689720981878. [CrossRef]
25. Yang, Z.Y.; Wang, X.H. Valproic Acid Inhibits Glioma and Its Mechanisms. *J. Healthc. Eng.* **2022**, *2022*, 4985781. [CrossRef] [PubMed]
26. Ryu, C.H.; Yoon, W.S.; Park, K.Y.; Kim, S.M.; Lim, J.Y.; Woo, J.S.; Jeong, C.H.; Hou, Y.; Jeun, S.S. Valproic acid downregulates the expression of MGMT and sensitizes temozolomide-resistant glioma cells. *J. Biomed. Biotechnol.* **2012**, *2012*, 987495. [CrossRef] [PubMed]
27. Tsai, H.C.; Wei, K.C.; Chen, P.Y.; Huang, C.Y.; Chen, K.T.; Lin, Y.J.; Cheng, H.W.; Chen, Y.R.; Wang, H.T. Valproic Acid Enhanced Temozolomide-Induced Anticancer Activity in Human Glioma Through the p53-PUMA Apoptosis Pathway. *Front. Oncol.* **2021**, *11*, 722754. [CrossRef]
28. Zhang, C.; Liu, S.; Yuan, X.; Hu, Z.; Li, H.; Wu, M.; Yuan, J.; Zhao, Z.; Su, J.; Wang, X.; et al. Valproic Acid Promotes Human Glioma U87 Cells Apoptosis and Inhibits Glycogen Synthase Kinase-3beta Through ERK/Akt Signaling. *Cell. Physiol. Biochem.* **2016**, *39*, 2173–2185. [CrossRef]
29. Riva, G.; Cilibrasi, C.; Bazzoni, R.; Cadamuro, M.; Negroni, C.; Butta, V.; Strazzabosco, M.; Dalpra, L.; Lavitrano, M.; Bentivegna, A. Valproic Acid Inhibits Proliferation and Reduces Invasiveness in Glioma Stem Cells Through Wnt/beta Catenin Signalling Activation. *Genes* **2018**, *9*, 522. [CrossRef]
30. Riva, G.; Butta, V.; Cilibrasi, C.; Baronchelli, S.; Redaelli, S.; Dalpra, L.; Lavitrano, M.; Bentivegna, A. Epigenetic targeting of glioma stem cells: Short-term and long-term treatments with valproic acid modulate DNA methylation and differentiation behavior, but not temozolomide sensitivity. *Oncol. Rep.* **2016**, *35*, 2811–2824. [CrossRef]
31. Happold, C.; Gorlia, T.; Chinot, O.; Gilbert, M.R.; Nabors, L.B.; Wick, W.; Pugh, S.L.; Hegi, M.; Cloughesy, T.; Roth, P.; et al. Does Valproic Acid or Levetiracetam Improve Survival in Glioblastoma? A Pooled Analysis of Prospective Clinical Trials in Newly Diagnosed Glioblastoma. *J. Clin. Oncol.* **2016**, *34*, 731–739. [CrossRef]
32. Berendsen, S.; Varkila, M.; Kroonen, J.; Seute, T.; Snijders, T.J.; Kauw, F.; Spliet, W.G.; Willems, M.; Poulet, C.; Broekman, M.L.; et al. Prognostic relevance of epilepsy at presentation in glioblastoma patients. *Neuro-Oncol.* **2016**, *18*, 700–706. [CrossRef]
33. Knudsen-Baas, K.M.; Storstein, A.M.; Zarabla, A.; Maialetti, A.; Giannarelli, D.; Beghi, E.; Maschio, M. Antiseizure medication in patients with Glioblastoma- a collaborative cohort study. *Seizure* **2021**, *87*, 107–113. [CrossRef]
34. Krauze, A.V.; Sierk, M.; Nguyen, T.; Chen, Q.; Yan, C.; Hu, Y.; Jiang, W.; Tasci, E.; Cooley Zgela, T.; Sproull, M.; et al. Glioblastoma survival is associated with distinct proteomic alteration signatures post chemoirradiation in a large-scale proteomic panel. *Front. Oncol.* **2023**, *13*, 1127645. [CrossRef]
35. Gold, L.; Walker, J.J.; Wilcox, S.K.; Williams, S. Advances in human proteomics at high scale with the SOMAscan proteomics platform. *New Biotechnol.* **2012**, *29*, 543–549. [CrossRef]
36. Tuerk, C.; Gold, L. Systematic evolution of ligands by exponential enrichment: RNA ligands to bacteriophage T4 DNA polymerase. *Science* **1990**, *249*, 505–510. [CrossRef]
37. Mirimanoff, R.O.; Gorlia, T.; Mason, W.; Van den Bent, M.J.; Kortmann, R.D.; Fisher, B.; Reni, M.; Brandes, A.A.; Curschmann, J.; Villa, S.; et al. Radiotherapy and temozolomide for newly diagnosed glioblastoma: Recursive partitioning analysis of the EORTC 26981/22981-NCIC CE3 phase III randomized trial. *J. Clin. Oncol.* **2006**, *24*, 2563–2569. [CrossRef] [PubMed]
38. Hodapp, N. The ICRU Report 83: Prescribing, recording and reporting photon-beam intensity-modulated radiation therapy (IMRT). *Strahlenther. Onkol.* **2012**, *188*, 97–99. [CrossRef] [PubMed]
39. Benjamini, Y.; Hochberg, Y. Controlling the False Discovery Rate: A Practical and Powerful Approach to Multiple Testing. *J. R. Stat.Soc. Ser. B (Methodol.)* **1995**, *57*, 289–300. [CrossRef]
40. Simon, R.; Lam, A.; Li, M.C.; Ngan, M.; Menenzes, S.; Zhao, Y. Analysis of gene expression data using BRB-ArrayTools. *Cancer Inform.* **2007**, *3*, 11–17. [CrossRef]
41. Dobbin, K.K.; Simon, R.M. Sample size planning for developing classifiers using high-dimensional DNA microarray data. *Biostatistics* **2006**, *8*, 101–117. [CrossRef] [PubMed]
42. Dobbin, K.K.; Zhao, Y.; Simon, R.M. How large a training set is needed to develop a classifier for microarray data? *Clin. Cancer Res.* **2008**, *14*, 108–114. [CrossRef] [PubMed]

43. R Core Team (2023). R: A Language and Environment for Statistical Computing. R Foundation for Statistical Computing, Vienna, Austria. Available online: https://www.R-project.org/ (accessed on 22 September 2023).
44. Tibshirani, R. The lasso method for variable selection in the Cox model. *Stat. Med.* **1997**, *16*, 385–395. [CrossRef]
45. Simon, N.; Friedman, J.; Hastie, T.; Tibshirani, R. Regularization Paths for Cox's Proportional Hazards Model via Coordinate Descent. *J. Stat. Softw.* **2011**, *39*, 1–13. [CrossRef]
46. Simon, R.M.; Subramanian, J.; Li, M.C.; Menezes, S. Using cross-validation to evaluate predictive accuracy of survival risk classifiers based on high-dimensional data. *Brief. Bioinform.* **2011**, *12*, 203–214. [CrossRef] [PubMed]
47. Janes, H.; Pepe, M.S.; Bossuyt, P.M.; Barlow, W.E. Measuring the performance of markers for guiding treatment decisions. *Ann. Intern. Med.* **2011**, *154*, 253–259. [CrossRef]
48. Stupp, R.; Taillibert, S.; Kanner, A.; Read, W.; Steinberg, D.M.; Lhermitte, B.; Toms, S.; Idbaih, A.; Ahluwalia, M.S.; Fink, K.; et al. Effect of Tumor-Treating Fields Plus Maintenance Temozolomide vs Maintenance Temozolomide Alone on Survival in Patients With Glioblastoma: A Randomized Clinical Trial. *JAMA* **2017**, *318*, 2306–2316. [CrossRef] [PubMed]
49. Stupp, R.; Hegi, M.E.; Gorlia, T.; Erridge, S.C.; Perry, J.; Hong, Y.K.; Aldape, K.D.; Lhermitte, B.; Pietsch, T.; Grujicic, D.; et al. Cilengitide combined with standard treatment for patients with newly diagnosed glioblastoma with methylated MGMT promoter (CENTRIC EORTC 26071-22072 study): A multicentre, randomised, open-label, phase 3 trial. *Lancet Oncol.* **2014**, *15*, 1100–1108. [CrossRef]
50. Weller, M.; Butowski, N.; Tran, D.D.; Recht, L.D.; Lim, M.; Hirte, H.; Ashby, L.; Mechtler, L.; Goldlust, S.A.; Iwamoto, F.; et al. Rindopepimut with temozolomide for patients with newly diagnosed, EGFRvIII-expressing glioblastoma (ACT IV): A randomised, double-blind, international phase 3 trial. *Lancet Oncol.* **2017**, *18*, 1373–1385. [CrossRef]
51. Kim, H.K.; Choi, I.J.; Kim, C.G.; Kim, H.S.; Oshima, A.; Yamada, Y.; Arao, T.; Nishio, K.; Michalowski, A.; Green, J.E. Three-gene predictor of clinical outcome for gastric cancer patients treated with chemotherapy. *Pharmacogenomics J.* **2012**, *12*, 119–127. [CrossRef]
52. Simon, R.; Radmacher, M.D.; Dobbin, K. Design of studies using DNA microarrays. *Genet. Epidemiol.* **2002**, *23*, 21–36. [CrossRef] [PubMed]
53. Lin, W.R.; Yeh, C.T. GALNT14: An Emerging Marker Capable of Predicting Therapeutic Outcomes in Multiple Cancers. *Int. J. Mol. Sci.* **2020**, *21*, 1491. [CrossRef] [PubMed]
54. Hussain, M.R.; Hoessli, D.C.; Fang, M. N-acetylgalactosaminyltransferases in cancer. *Oncotarget* **2016**, *7*, 54067–54081. [CrossRef] [PubMed]
55. Wagner, K.W.; Punnoose, E.A.; Januario, T.; Lawrence, D.A.; Pitti, R.M.; Lancaster, K.; Lee, D.; von Goetz, M.; Yee, S.F.; Totpal, K.; et al. Death-receptor O-glycosylation controls tumor-cell sensitivity to the proapoptotic ligand Apo2L/TRAIL. *Nat. Med.* **2007**, *13*, 1070–1077. [CrossRef] [PubMed]
56. Jiang, X.; Xing, H.; Kim, T.M.; Jung, Y.; Huang, W.; Yang, H.W.; Song, S.; Park, P.J.; Carroll, R.S.; Johnson, M.D. Numb regulates glioma stem cell fate and growth by altering epidermal growth factor receptor and Skp1-Cullin-F-box ubiquitin ligase activity. *Stem Cells* **2012**, *30*, 1313–1326. [CrossRef] [PubMed]
57. Wang, L.B.; Karpova, A.; Gritsenko, M.A.; Kyle, J.E.; Cao, S.; Li, Y.; Rykunov, D.; Colaprico, A.; Rothstein, J.H.; Hong, R.; et al. Proteogenomic and metabolomic characterization of human glioblastoma. *Cancer Cell* **2021**, *39*, 509–528.e520. [CrossRef] [PubMed]
58. Pridham, K.J.; Varghese, R.T.; Sheng, Z. The Role of Class IA Phosphatidylinositol-4,5-Bisphosphate 3-Kinase Catalytic Subunits in Glioblastoma. *Front. Oncol.* **2017**, *7*, 312. [CrossRef]
59. Franco, C.; Kausar, S.; Silva, M.F.B.; Guedes, R.C.; Falcao, A.O.; Brito, M.A. Multi-Targeting Approach in Glioblastoma Using Computer-Assisted Drug Discovery Tools to Overcome the Blood-Brain Barrier and Target EGFR/PI3Kp110β Signaling. *Cancers* **2022**, *14*, 3506. [CrossRef] [PubMed]
60. Liang, J.; Wang, W.F.; Xie, S.; Zhang, X.L.; Qi, W.F.; Zhou, X.P.; Hu, J.X.; Shi, Q.; Yu, R.T. β-transducin repeat-containing E3 ubiquitin protein ligase inhibits migration, invasion and proliferation of glioma cells. *Oncol. Lett.* **2017**, *14*, 3131–3135. [CrossRef]
61. Wang, H.; Pan, J.Q.; Luo, L.; Ning, X.J.; Ye, Z.P.; Yu, Z.; Li, W.S. NF-κB induces miR-148a to sustain TGF-β/Smad signaling activation in glioblastoma. *Mol. Cancer* **2015**, *14*, 2. [CrossRef]
62. Thompson, L.L.; Baergen, A.K.; Lichtensztejn, Z.; McManus, K.J. Reduced SKP1 Expression Induces Chromosome Instability through Aberrant Cyclin E1 Protein Turnover. *Cancers* **2020**, *12*, 531. [CrossRef] [PubMed]
63. Li, S.; Gao, P.; Dai, X.; Ye, L.; Wang, Z.; Cheng, H. New prognostic biomarker CMTM3 in low grade glioma and its immune infiltration. *Ann. Transl. Med.* **2022**, *10*, 206. [CrossRef] [PubMed]
64. Diggins, N.L.; Webb, D.J. APPL1 is a multifunctional endosomal signaling adaptor protein. *Biochem. Soc. Trans.* **2017**, *45*, 771–779. [CrossRef] [PubMed]
65. Korbecki, J.; Kojder, K.; Simińska, D.; Bohatyrewicz, R.; Gutowska, I.; Chlubek, D.; Baranowska-Bosiacka, I. CC Chemokines in a Tumor: A Review of Pro-Cancer and Anti-Cancer Properties of the Ligands of Receptors CCR1, CCR2, CCR3, and CCR4. *Int. J. Mol. Sci.* **2020**, *21*, 8412. [CrossRef]
66. Autelitano, F.; Loyaux, D.; Roudières, S.; Déon, C.; Guette, F.; Fabre, P.; Ping, Q.; Wang, S.; Auvergne, R.; Badarinarayana, V.; et al. Identification of novel tumor-associated cell surface sialoglycoproteins in human glioblastoma tumors using quantitative proteomics. *PLoS ONE* **2014**, *9*, e110316. [CrossRef]

67. de Vega, S.; Kondo, A.; Suzuki, M.; Arai, H.; Jiapaer, S.; Sabit, H.; Nakada, M.; Ikeuchi, T.; Ishijima, M.; Arikawa-Hirasawa, E.; et al. Fibulin-7 is overexpressed in glioblastomas and modulates glioblastoma neovascularization through interaction with angiopoietin-1. *Int. J. Cancer* **2019**, *145*, 2157–2169. [CrossRef]
68. Thotala, D.; Karvas, R.M.; Engelbach, J.A.; Garbow, J.R.; Hallahan, A.N.; DeWees, T.A.; Laszlo, A.; Hallahan, D.E. Valproic acid enhances the efficacy of radiation therapy by protecting normal hippocampal neurons and sensitizing malignant glioblastoma cells. *Oncotarget* **2015**, *6*, 35004–35022. [CrossRef]
69. Raja, E.; Komuro, A.; Tanabe, R.; Sakai, S.; Ino, Y.; Saito, N.; Todo, T.; Morikawa, M.; Aburatani, H.; Koinuma, D.; et al. Bone morphogenetic protein signaling mediated by ALK-2 and DLX2 regulates apoptosis in glioma-initiating cells. *Oncogene* **2017**, *36*, 4963–4974. [CrossRef]
70. Talwadekar, M.; Fernandes, S.; Kale, V.; Limaye, L. Valproic acid enhances the neural differentiation of human placenta derived-mesenchymal stem cells in vitro. *J. Tissue Eng. Regen. Med.* **2017**, *11*, 3111–3123. [CrossRef]
71. Krämer, A.; Green, J.; Pollard, J., Jr.; Tugendreich, S. Causal analysis approaches in Ingenuity Pathway Analysis. *Bioinformatics* **2014**, *30*, 523–530. [CrossRef]
72. Tasci, E.; Zhuge, Y.; Camphausen, K.; Krauze, A.V. Bias and Class Imbalance in Oncologic Data-Towards Inclusive and Transferrable AI in Large Scale Oncology Data Sets. *Cancers* **2022**, *14*, 2897. [CrossRef] [PubMed]
73. Xia, Y.; Ge, M.; Xia, L.; Shan, G.; Qian, J. CTSV (cathepsin V) promotes bladder cancer progression by increasing NF-κB activity. *Bioengineered* **2022**, *13*, 10180–10190. [CrossRef]
74. Mitrović, A.; Senjor, E.; Jukić, M.; Bolčina, L.; Prunk, M.; Proj, M.; Nanut, M.P.; Gobec, S.; Kosa, J. New inhibitors of cathepsin V impair tumor cell proliferation and elastin degradation and increase immune cell cytotoxicity. *Comput. Struct. Biotechnol. J.* **2022**, *20*, 4667–4687. [CrossRef]
75. Gao, L.; Xiong, D.-D.; Yang, X.; Li, J.-D.; He, R.-Q.; Huang, Z.-G.; Lai, Z.F.; Liu, L.-M.; Luo, J.-Y.; Du, X.F.; et al. The expression characteristics and clinical significance of ACP6, a potential target of nitidine chloride, in hepatocellular carcinoma. *BMC Cancer* **2022**, *22*, 1244. [CrossRef]
76. Berezovsky, A.D.; Poisson, L.M.; Cherba, D.; Webb, C.P.; Transou, A.D.; Lemke, N.W.; Hong, X.; Hasselbach, L.A.; Irtenkauf, S.M.; Mikkelsen, T.; et al. Sox2 promotes malignancy in glioblastoma by regulating plasticity and astrocytic differentiation. *Neoplasia* **2014**, *16*, 193–206. [CrossRef]
77. Ehata, S.; Miyazono, K. Bone Morphogenetic Protein Signaling in Cancer; Some Topics in the Recent 10 Years. *Front. Cell Dev. Biol.* **2022**, *10*, 883523. [CrossRef]
78. Sachdeva, R.; Wu, M.; Johnson, K.; Kim, H.; Celebre, A.; Shahzad, U.; Graham, M.S.; Kessler, J.A.; Chuang, J.H.; Karamchandani, K.; et al. BMP signaling mediates glioma stem cell quiescence and confers treatment resistance in glioblastoma. *Sci. Rep.* **2019**, *9*, 14569. [CrossRef] [PubMed]
79. Han, Y.-Q.; Ming, S.-L.; Wu, H.-T.; Zeng, L.; Ba, G.; Li, J.; Lu, W.-F.; Han, J.; Du, Q.-J.; Sun, M.-M.; et al. Myostatin knockout induces apoptosis in human cervical cancer cells via elevated reactive oxygen species generation. *Redox Biol.* **2018**, *19*, 412–428. [CrossRef] [PubMed]
80. Peng, H.; Li, Z.; Fu, J.; Zhou, R. Growth and differentiation factor 15 regulates PD-L1 expression in glioblastoma. *Cancer Manag. Res.* **2019**, *11*, 2653–2661. [CrossRef]
81. Mir, M.A.; Pandith, A.A.; Mansoor, S.; Baba, S.M.; Makhdoomi, R.; Ain, Q.-U.; Anwar, I.; Para, S.A.; Bhat, A.H.; Koul, A.M.; et al. Differential expression of SLITRK6 gene as a potential therapeutic target for urothelial carcinoma in particular upper tract cancer. *Gene* **2023**, *878*, 147583. [CrossRef]
82. Aruga, J.; Yokota, N.; Mikoshiba, K. Human SLITRK family genes: Genomic organization and expression profiling in normal brain and brain tumor tissue. *Gene* **2003**, *315*, 87–94. [CrossRef] [PubMed]
83. Kammerer, S.; Roth, R.B.; Reneland, R.; Marnellos, G.; Hoyal, C.R.; Markward, N.J.; Ebner, F.; Kiechle, M.; Schwarz-Boeger, U.; Griffiths, L.R.; et al. Large-scale association study identifies ICAM gene region as breast and prostate cancer susceptibility locus. *Cancer Res.* **2004**, *64*, 8906–8910. [CrossRef]
84. Shen, C.K.; Shen, C.-K.; Huang, B.-R.; Yeh, W.-L.; Chen, C.-W.; Liu, Y.-S.; Lai, S.-W.; Tseng, W.P.; Lu, D.-Y.; Tsai, C.-F. Regulatory effects of IL-1β in the interaction of GBM and tumor-associated monocyte through VCAM-1 and ICAM-1. *Eur. J. Pharmacol.* **2021**, *905*, 174216. [CrossRef]
85. Wang, Z.; Wang, X.; Zou, H.; Dai, Z.; Feng, S.; Zhang, M.; Xiao, G.; Liu, Z.; Cheng, Q. The Basic Characteristics of the Pentraxin Family and Their Functions in Tumor Progression. *Front. Immunol.* **2020**, *11*, 1757. [CrossRef]
86. Gómez de San José, N.; Massa, F.; Halbgebauer, S.; Oeckl, P.; Steinacker, P.; Otto, M. Neuronal pentraxins as biomarkers of synaptic activity: From physiological functions to pathological changes in neurodegeneration. *J. Neural. Transm.* **2022**, *129*, 207–230. [CrossRef] [PubMed]
87. Sun, J.; Shin, D.Y.; Eiseman, M.; Yallowitz, A.R.; Li, N.; Lalani, S.; Li, Z.; Cung, M.; Bok, S.; Debnath, S.; et al. SLITRK5 is a negative regulator of hedgehog signaling in osteoblasts. *Nat. Commun.* **2021**, *12*, 4611. [CrossRef]
88. Hiz, S.; Kiliç, S.; Bademci, G.; Karakulak, T.; Erdoğan, A.; Özden, B.; Eresen, C.; Erdal, E.; Yiş, U.; Tekin, M.; et al. VARS1 mutations associated with neurodevelopmental disorder are located on a short amino acid stretch of the anticodon-binding domain. *Turk. J. Biol.* **2022**, *46*, 458–464. [CrossRef]

89. Arnoult, N.; Correia, A.; Ma, J.; Merlo, A.; Garcia-Gomez, S.; Maric, M.; Tognetti, M.; Benner, C.W.; Boulton, S.J.; Saghatelian, A.; et al. Regulation of DNA repair pathway choice in S and G2 phases by the NHEJ inhibitor CYREN. *Nature* **2017**, *549*, 548–552. [CrossRef]
90. Ahmed, E.A.; Rosemann, M.; Scherthan, H. NHEJ Contributes to the Fast Repair of Radiation-induced DNA Double-strand Breaks at Late Prophase I Telomeres. *Health Phys.* **2018**, *115*, 102–107. [CrossRef] [PubMed]
91. Zheng, G.; Jia, L.; Yang, A.G. Roles of HLA-G/KIR2DL4 in Breast Cancer Immune Microenvironment. *Front. Immunol.* **2022**, *13*, 791975. [CrossRef]
92. Fabian, K.P.; Hodge, J.W. The emerging role of off-the-shelf engineered natural killer cells in targeted cancer immunotherapy. *Mol. Ther. Oncolytics* **2021**, *23*, 266–276. [CrossRef] [PubMed]

MDPI AG
Grosspeteranlage 5
4052 Basel
Switzerland
Tel.: +41 61 683 77 34

Biomolecules Editorial Office
E-mail: biomolecules@mdpi.com
www.mdpi.com/journal/biomolecules